Training for the
NEW
ALPINISM

Training for the
NEW
ALPINISM

A MANUAL FOR THE CLIMBER AS ATHLETE

Steve House and Scott Johnston

patagonia

Ventura, California

Training for the New Alpinism
A Manual for the Climber as Athlete

Patagonia publishes a select list of titles on wilderness, wildlife, and outdoor sports that inspire and restore a connection to the natural world.

First Edition

Disclaimer
The information provided in this book is designed to provide helpful information on the subjects covered, including endurance and strength training, nutrition, and physical and mental fitness. It is particularly designed for people who are actively participating in or would like to train for certain extreme physical activities such as rock and ice climbing.

This information is not for everyone, as many of the activities described are intense and can be dangerous. You should not undertake any of these activities unless and until you have consulted with qualified medical personnel and been cleared to participate. And, of course, if you find that you are suffering from the symptoms of any physical or medical condition, you should consult with your physician or other qualified health provider immediately. Do not avoid or disregard professional medical advice or delay in seeking it because of something you have read in this book.

All of the information contained in this book, including text, graphics, images, recipes, exercises, training regimens, diets, and references to third party materials are for informational and educational purposes only. The authors and publisher of this book shall have no liability or responsibility to any reader or any third party arising out of any injury or damage incurred as a result of the use of the information provided in this book.

Editor: John Dutton
Photo Editor: Steve House
Illustrations Editor: Scott Johnston
Design and Production: Faceout Studio

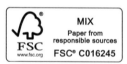

Printed in Canada on 100 percent post-consumer recycled paper

ISBN 978-1-938340-23-9
E-Book ISBN 978-1-938340-24-6

Publisher's Cataloging in Publication Data

House, Steve, 1970-

    Training for the new alpinism : a manual for the climber as athlete / by Steve House and Scott Johnston. -- 1st ed. -- Ventura, Calif. : Patagonia Books, c2014.

    p. ; cm.

    ISBN: 978-1-938340-23-9 (print) ; 978-1-938340-24-6 (ebook)
    Includes bibliographical references, glossary and index.
    Contents: The methodology and physiology of endurance training -- Planning your training -- Tools for training -- Train, practice, climb.
    Summary: Applying training practices from other endurance sports, the authors demonstrate that following a carefully designed regimen is as effective for alpinism as it is for any other endurance sport and leads to better performance. They deliver detailed instruction on how to plan and execute training tailored to your individual circumstances, translating training theory into practice to allow you to coach yourself to any mountaineering goal.-- Publisher.

    1. Mountaineering--Training. 2. Rock climbing--Training. 3. Endurance sports--Training. 4. Mountaineers--Training of. 5. Athletes--Training of. 6. Physical fitness. I. Johnston, Scott, 1953- II. Title.

GV200 .H68 2014   2013952042

Acknowledgments

Crafting this book seemed, at times, like a Sisyphean task. A task that was endurable due to the love and support of our wives, Midge Cross and Eva House. If you enjoyed this book, you have them to thank.

Issac Newton famously noted that his work stood on the shoulders of giants. In the case of athletics we have gained enormously from the works of Tudor Bompa, PhD, coach Renato Canova, coach Peter Coe, Jack Daniels, PhD, Jan Helgarud, PhD, Timothy Noakes, MD, PhD, Jan Olbrecht, PhD, Thomas Kurz, PhD, and Yuri Verkhoshansky, PhD.

Mark Twight crucially convinced us that this book "Needs to be written." back in the beginning. Stacie Wing-Gaia, PhD, reviewed the nutrition chapter, Dr. Peter Hackett (Everest 1981) and Dr. Robert Schoene reviewed and commented on the chapter on high altitude, and many persons and authors contributed to the mental chapter in innumerable ways.

A big shout of thanks goes round the world to all that contributed their voices to this book: Ueli Steck, Zoe Hart, Christophe Moulin, Krissy Moehl, Alexander Odintsov, Tony Yaniro (who wrote four essays), Caroline George, Chad Kellogg, Roger Schaeli, Kelly Cordes, Will Gadd, Peter Habeler, Gerlinde Kaltenbrunner, Marko Prezelj, Steve Swenson, Voytek Kurtyka, Stephan Siegrist, Jean Troillet, Danika Gilbert, Andreas Fransson, Scott Semple, Colin Haley, Barry Blanchard, and Ines Papert.

We'd like to extend a special thanks to the best alpine-climbing photographer in the world, Marko Prezelj, for not only the brilliant cover image but the numerous other images from his many expeditions.

As we gaze back on the three years of work that went into these pages, it is obvious that we could not have done this without Karla Olson and the entire team at Patagonia Books. Lastly a special thanks is owed to our editor, John Dutton, for his patient, thoughtful work.

Front Cover: Steve House leading during the first free ascent of the Italian Pillar route of Taulliraju, Cordillera Blanca, Peru.
Photo: Marko Prezelj

Contents

Section 3: Tools for Training

Section 4: Train, Practice, Climb

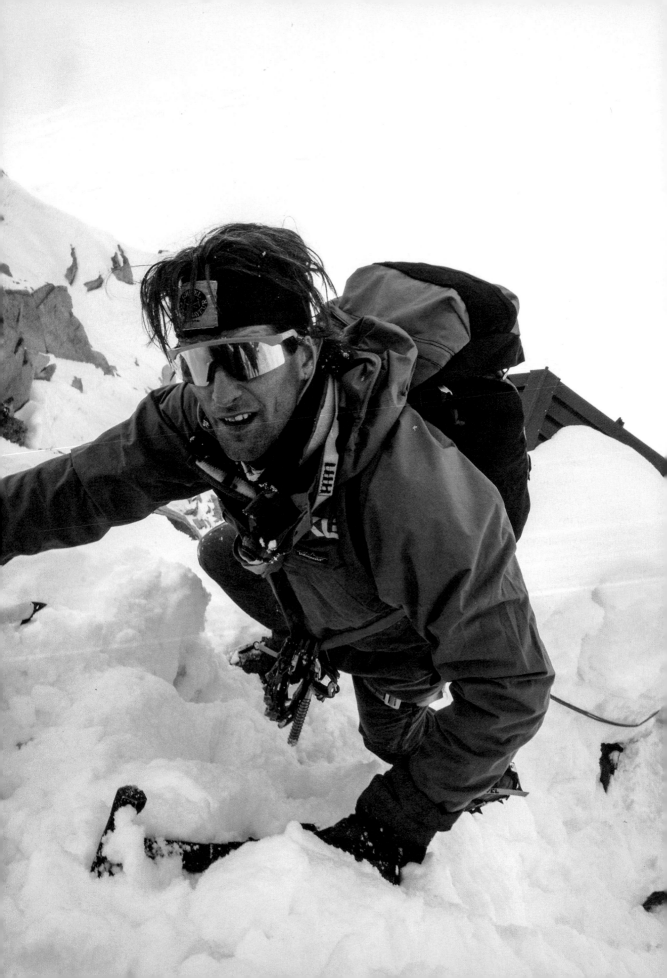

Foreword

The Edge of the Map

I consider myself a charter member of the first generation of alpine climbers who trained intentionally using artificial means.

For me, training was born of failure. When I failed—and it happened a lot—it was because ambition outstripped ability. I narrowed that lack of ability to physical issues often enough that I decided to do something about it. Chasing the first half of Brian Eno's motto, I pushed myself to "the most extreme limits" and reaped rewards, but it took years to fulfill the second half of that motto, which is "retreat to a more useful position."

My approach to training echoed how I climbed. The romance of climbing didn't interest me. I didn't seek harps and wings. I heard no opera up there. Instead, my mountains had teeth. The jagged edge we walked up there dragged itself across my throat, and the throats of my friends and peers. I took the mountains' indifference to life as aggression, and fought back. I armored myself against that indifference; with training, with thinking, with attitude. I trained with friends who shared a similar approach. Our mantra was dark, but it motivated us.

When we ran we breathed in rhythm—no matter the speed—and that beat had words: "They all died." We inhaled and exhaled the great alpine epics—like the tragedy that befell Walter Bonatti's party on the Freney Pillar—to push ourselves to a place where we would never come up short, physically.

Opposite: Mark Twight exiting the Col Fourche bivouac near Mont Maudit, France. *Photo: Ace Kvale*

The consequences of falling short made training important. I realized early that controlling the things that I could control gave me greater freedom to address the things that I could not control. And the mountains offered those in spades.

Unfortunately, I had no idea how to use the gym, and without someone to ask, I made many mistakes. I tried to mimic climbing in the weight room, but didn't comprehend how best to use this valuable tool, and wasted my time. The gym is useful as a means of overloading the organism in a way that can't (safely) be done in the real environment of alpinism.

Later, my training sessions began by pre-fatiguing my body on a Stairmaster, or treadmill, and then lifting because that's how alpinism looked to me: approach and then climb. It took years to learn that doing the opposite sent hormonal signals more appropriate to physical development for alpine climbing.

Then I read that some rock climbers used hypertrophy-style training to increase muscle mass and push limit-strength higher. So we did that until I realized that mass had to be carried whether it was being used or not. I had misused a specific training idea based on the mistaken premise that all climbing is the same. It isn't. Limit-strength was never an issue in the mountains but we wanted it to be, so that we could do that style of training.

Eventually I trained in a way that emphasized maximum recruitment of existing muscle. I had to carry my own engine so it made sense to increase my power-to-weight ratio; to extract the maximum from existing resources. Then, I reasoned, if the engine is still inadequate, I could increase its horsepower—as long as that doesn't affect fuel economy.

The engine analogy produced an accurate description of our training objectives, which allowed us to think and plan in coherent terms. We decided that the ideal "engine" for alpinism could go forever, produce explosive force on demand and keep delivering 50 to 60 percent of peak force without "overheating." Tuning such diverse characteristics into an engine requires much of the mechanic, foremost of which is an understanding of the overall objectives.

In *Extreme Alpinism: Climbing Light, Fast and High*, I described the goal of physical training for alpinism with the phrase "to make yourself as indestructible as possible." In short: resilience. For too long I thought this concept was solely contingent on physical capacities, but eventually realized that these influence mental capacities. In fact, I think we revere the physical too much when it is the mind that imagines the goal, solves the problem, and achieves it—using the body as its engine.

If physical training is a tool, it's a hammer. Often we swing it to the exclusion of all other tools because it feels like an easy fix: it features nearly immediate positive feedback as well as rapid progress, especially if you've never used one before. But increased physical capacity doesn't guarantee improvements to climbing. Often strength blinds us to the benefits of technique or efficiency. We close our eyes and pull, but alpinism rarely rewards raw strength—successful alpinists appear to be those who multiply physical force with the lever of creativity, confidence, and psychological resilience.

Undertaken correctly, physical training is a useful means of psychological manipulation: goals set, achieved, and surpassed in the gym—whether they are specifically transferable or not—stimulate psychological development we can express in the mountains. Constantly overcoming difficult training challenges and examining ourselves along the way improves self-assurance. That confidence frees imagination. It opens doors to new, more difficult projects, and expands our problem-solving repertoire.

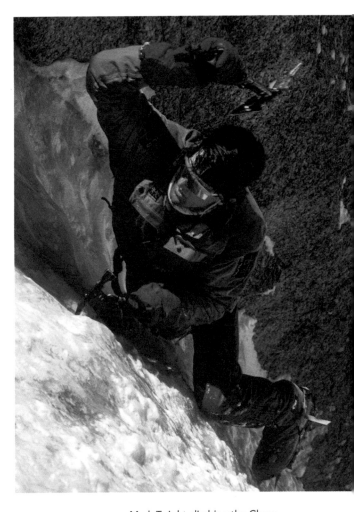

Mark Twight climbing the Chere Couloir, Mont Blanc du Tacul (13,937', 4,248m), France in 1990. *Photo: Ace Kvale*

To attempt the impossible demands a high order explosion of confidence, sustained by the diesel-fueled physical capacity to back up that hubris. Neither capacity is powerful on its own but a whole, well-trained mental-physical system is practically unstoppable. In this sense we can bring our unrealistic ambitions within reach by figuratively changing the length, and functionally increasing the strength of our arms.

The really big routes I climbed didn't happen because I trained harder. Rather they happened as result of having trained better and climbed more. Frequency and consistency and accumulation allowed me to go harder, higher, and for longer. Increasing the intensity of the "artificial" training was never critical. Intensity played a minor role: it could not shortcut experience or efficiency. Twenty years of consistent training squeezed wretched mental weakness out of me and built a vast foundation of accumulated fitness. The resulting deep physical tank and huge psychological reserve opened up terrain and timing that I

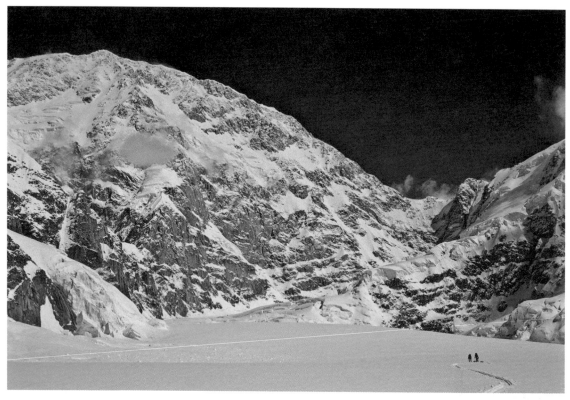

Mark Twight and Scott Backes
approaching the south face of Denali
and the Slovak Direct Route.
Photo: Steve House

could never have imagined without it. Training was one of the keys to
my success as a climber, but not in the way I believed it would be when
I hit the weight room that first time.

These days physical and mental training is my bread and butter.
Strength training directly benefits the athlete who plays a sport in
which the strongest always wins. That's not climbing. So we work indi-
rectly: When we increase an athlete's work capacity, we improve that
person's ability to recover, then climbing-specific training frequency
can be increased, which means more climbing. A greater volume of
quality sport-specific effort leads to improvement. This is training but
it is also lifestyle, and managing it wholesale.

To achieve this we need a certain quantity and quality of knowledge.
Unfortunately, much of what passes for fitness knowledge is actually
marketing, or confined to the controlled conditions of a lab with no
regard for biochemical or temperamental individuality. Steve and Scott
have collected the vast data relevant to training and preparation for
alpine climbing and are presenting it here in a practical, user-friendly
manner. They back their thesis with their own remarkable experience.
And reinforce it with unique points of view contributed by climbers
whose practice has had enormous influence on the evolution of the

sport. On its own the book is invaluable. Combined with the routes and adventures that it will surely inform, its impact on the evolution of the generations of future climbers will be great.

I often say that greater fitness leads to more opportunity. This holds true for knowledge as well. When we acquire new skills, when we develop ourselves as human beings, we uncover new potential. The map gets bigger. We increase the scope of our world and the opportunities available in it. *Training for the New Alpinism* might well take you right off the edge of the world as you know it.

MARK TWIGHT
Salt Lake City
June 2013

Mark Twight riding the cobbles in Sofia, Bulgaria, after finishing the work day training actors and stunt crew for the Warner Brothers movie: *300: Rise of an Empire. Photo: Clay Enos*

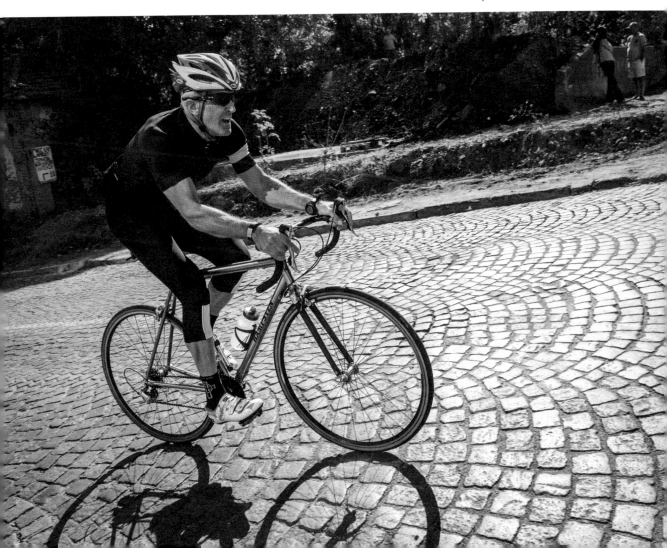

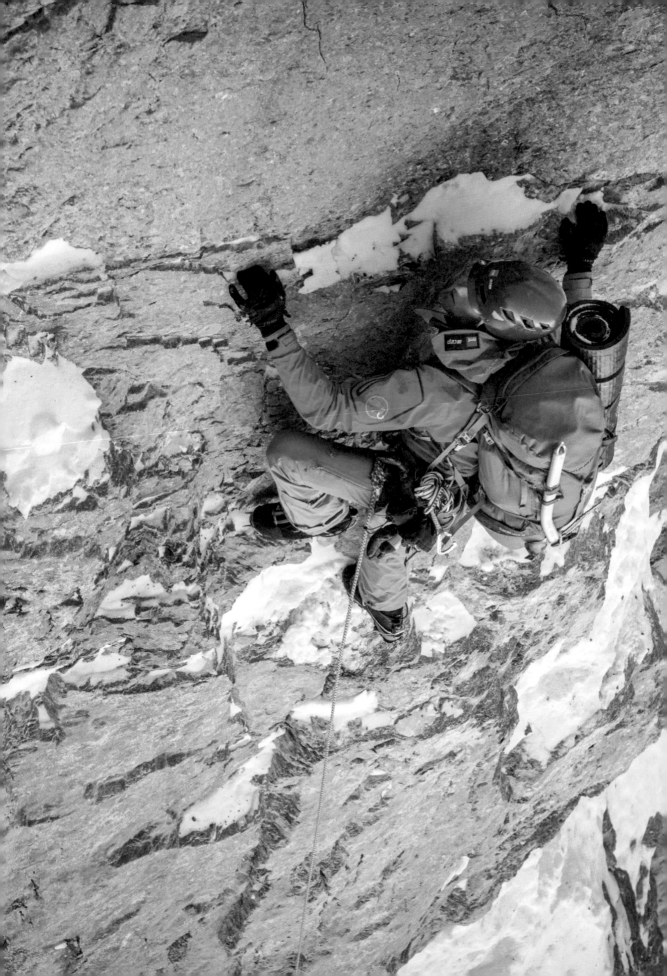

Introduction

The Old Becomes New Again

It was a close, warm, breezeless summer night,
Wan, dull, and glaring, with a dripping fog
Low-hung and thick that covered all the sky;
But, undiscouraged, we began to climb
The mountainside.

— WILLIAM WORDSWORTH, *The Prelude* (1799–1805)

Physical exploration of the world was growing rapidly during the Romantic Period, the time of Wordsworth. Early mountaineers were upper class and well educated: poets, photographers, geologists, painters, and natural historians.

In 1895 the Englishman and alpinist Albert Mummery and four men undertook the first attempt to climb one of the Himalaya's giant peaks, the 26,660-foot (8,126-meter) high Nanga Parbat. Mummery and two of his men lost their lives in an avalanche during the attempt. Thus climbing entered the twentieth century with artistic grace tainted by extreme tragedy; this began the greatest period of growth in alpinism, particularly in the Alps.

Technical standards rose rapidly. In 1906, 5.9 was first climbed in the Elbe Sandstone Mountains. Around this same time Austrian Paul Preuss trained himself to do one-armed pull-ups and climbed (and

Opposite: Swiss alpinist Stephan Siegrist climbs the Difficult Crack pitch of the 1938 Route on the north face of the Eiger (13,024', 3,970m) in Switzerland. *Photo: Thomas Senf*

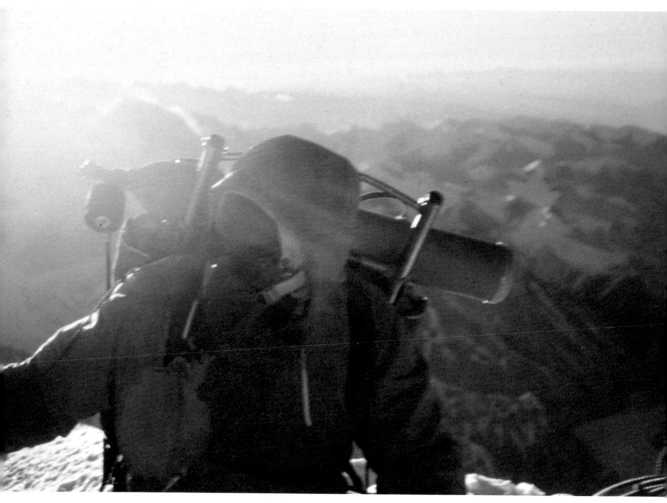

Tom Hornbein on the summit of Mount Everest (29,029', 8,848m) at 6:15 p.m., May 22, 1963, after making the first ascent of the west ridge. He and Willi Unsoeld also completed the first ever traverse of a mountain over 8,000 meters. *Photo: Willi Unsoeld*

down climbed) alpine rock routes in the Dolomites to a modern grade of 5.8, solo and in hobnailed boots. By 1922 the top grade was 5.10d. Climbers of the time climbed many beautiful, difficult routes in the mountains. To modern climbers, they seem to have been driven by an innate curiosity to ascend, explore, and observe what would unfold in the process.

The great wars twisted everything; the conquest of the world's fourteen highest peaks after World War II became surrogate battlegrounds to reinforce superiority, or symbolize rebirth, depending on whether your country had won or lost: Annapurna to the French, Everest to the British, Nanga Parbat to the Germans, K2 to the Italians. Ascent was transformed into conquest; summits became symbols of nationalistic pride. The climbing of mountains was changed forever. This ended symbolically in 1980 when Reinhold Messner was asked why he did not carry his country's flag to the top of Everest, and he replied: "I did not go up for Italy, nor for South Tyrol. I went up for myself." Though his comment angered many at the time, the line was drawn.

In the information age all must be measured. For climbing, an emphasis on difficulty and speed emerged. Hardest, highest, fastest. In the age of social media all must be shared. The resulting cocktail of cameras, danger, and testosterone are all too often tragic. Rarely graceful.

The new alpinism comes full circle as small teams of fit, trained athletes emulate Mummery, aspire to Preuss, climb like the young Messner. Because those pioneers knew that alpinism—indeed all mindful pursuits—is at its most simple level the sum of your daily choices and daily practices. Progress is entirely personal. The spirit of climbing does not lie in outcomes—lists, times, your conquests. You do keep those; you will always know which mountains you have climbed, which you have not. What you can climb is a manifestation of the current, temporary, state of your whole self. You can't fake a sub-four-minute mile just as you can't pretend to do an asana. Ascent too is an expression of many skills developed, refined, mastered.

Training is the most important vehicle for preparation. Constant practice begets examination and refinement of technique as well as fitness. It is not our natural tendency to value struggle over success, a worldview that climbing sternly enforces. Embracing struggle for its own sake is an important step on your path. Incremental vacillations in your self—your physical and mental selves—are exquisitely revealed in practicing ascent. There is no end to your progress or your process. For the two of us the pursuit of climbing mountains has been among the most powerful personal experiences we have known. Nothing else has come close to the blunt power of climbing to inform us about ourselves.

We don't presume to tell anyone what the new alpinism will actually become; no one can know this. But we do think that we have earned the perspective to point in the right general direction: Structured, progressive training will be a big component, perhaps define, the future of alpine climbing. But not because it will help you climb harder, faster— though it will. Training prepares your body and, most important, your mind for ascent through consistent, hard, disciplined practice.

Go simply, train smart, climb well.

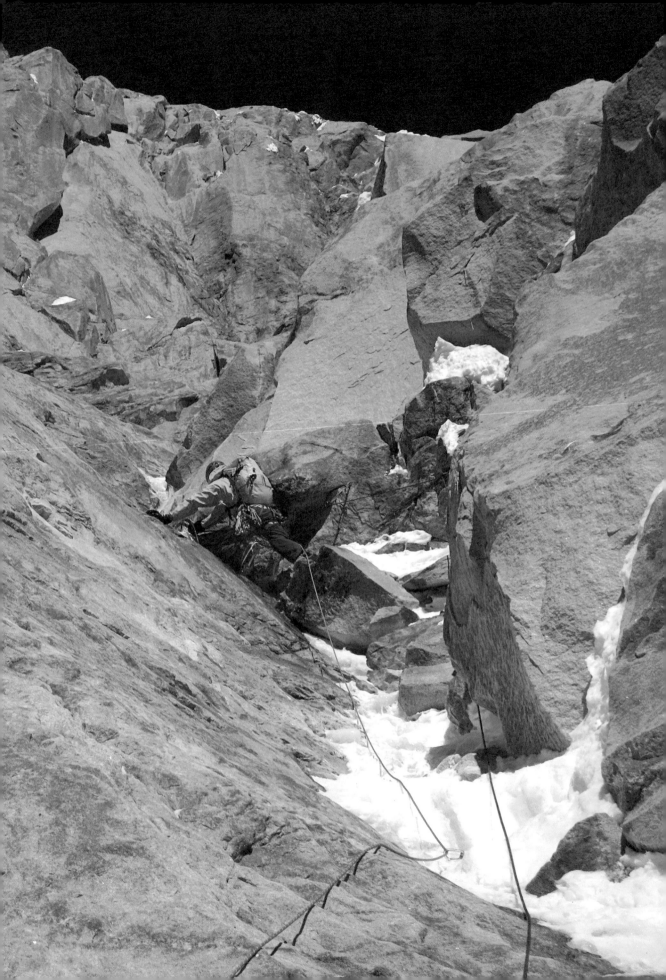

Chapter 1

Training for the New Alpinism

"What advantages do we hope to gain (from climbing mountains)? Naturally, there is the pleasure we get from the climbing process itself and from our victories, but as well as the delights of exercise in a mountain environment, there is also the process, coming every time as a surprise, of self-discovery, deepening a little further with every climb: who we are, how far we can go, what is our potential, where are the limits of our technique, our strength, our skill, our mountaineering sense: discoveries whose acceptance means that, if necessary, we may turn back and return another time, several times if need be–'Tomorrow is a new day.'"

— GASTON RÉBUFFAT, from *The Mont Blanc Massif: The Hundred Finest Routes*

Most of what climbers describe as training today happens as a substitute for climbing. You can't climb because you're far from the mountains, so you train; common examples include the lunchtime run or an after-work visit to the climbing gym. As soon as alpinists have time and access to mountains, they stop training because they can

Opposite: Hayden Kennedy leading a difficult mixed pitch high on Baintha Brakk (The Ogre, 23,901', 7,285m) during the first ascent of the south face. *Photo: Kyle Dempster*

go climbing instead. This is the wrong approach if you want to progress your climbing, and has contributed to the dead-end standards of alpine climbing.

Standards in rock climbing have skyrocketed since 1978, from 5.13 to 5.15. It's no coincidence that during this same period we've seen the emergence of climbing gyms and youth competitions. Today standards in alpinism languish. Steve attempted an unclimbed line on the west face of Makalu three times between 2008 and 2011, and was unable to match the high point established by Voytek Kurtyka and Alex MacIntyre in 1982. New routes established in alpine style on 8,000-meter peaks with sustained technical difficulties are so rare that, by our accounting, this has been accomplished only five times in history (1984 by Nil Bohigas and Enric Lucas on Annapurna, 1991 by Marko Prezelj and Andrej Štremfelj on Kanchenjunga South, 2005 by Vince Anderson and Steve House on Nanga Parbat, 2009 by Boris Dedeshko and Denis Urubko on Cho Oyu, and 2013 by Ueli Steck on Annapurna).

Structured coaching in competitive sports, and recently in sport climbing and bouldering, helps athletes learn how to train. This is not a part of alpine climbing's culture. Alpinists climb. We have been brought up to believe that to get stronger we must simply climb a lot. And with climbing, fitness will follow.

If you aspire to climb difficult routes on Patagonian spires and you have only been rock climbing for a short time, then you are best advised to spend a majority of your time climbing granite cracks—and do so as much as possible. No book can teach you how to lead a runout pitch. No story can show you how to bivouac. You can read a thousand accounts of leading a steep, difficult hand crack far above the Patagonian ice cap, but that will bring you no closer to actually doing it.

The fact is that you will gain the strength and endurance to climb a hard pitch much, much more quickly with a training regime plus climbing than by climbing alone. After learning the physiology explained in the early chapters of this book, you will also understand that the majority of your climbing is best done below your top limit. This is for endurance, as well as technique, and psychological progress. This knowledge will help you gain the strength and endurance, and from that strength and endurance the disciplined mind and the correct technique will flow more easily.

One of the fundamental concepts of training for any sport is that event (climbing) specific training must come on top of a very well-established base of conditioning. We acknowledge that climbing, and particularly alpine climbing, is a very highly skill-dependent sport requiring a broad range of knowledge, experience, and ability. It is exactly this need for climbing skill that tends to push alpinists (and all climbers) to "just climb" for training.

Consider that in the sport of running, the explosive power of a 100-meter sprinter and the dogged endurance of the ultra-marathoner are both running; yet the two are vastly different events. The surprise to many is that training for both of these events starts with the same general strength and conditioning to enhance basic physical qualities. As the 100-meter runner and the ultra-marathoner progress through their training plan, and through their careers, each will benefit from more and more specific training. This means that each will spend more and more time running distances and paces closer and closer to what they hope to achieve during their race. They know that the higher their level of basic fitness at the time they commence their event-specific training, the higher their performance will peak in their ultimate event.

For conventional endurance sports, such as running, the event-specific training makes up a smaller percentage of the total volume of training than you might imagine, both on an annual basis as well as during a lifetime. Depending on the development stage and the nature of the goals, specific training (meaning running a distance and pace approaching race distance and pace) can range from less than 10 percent of total training volume for young people and beginners up to a maximum of about 30 percent for world-class athletes.

Athletes commonly lose sight of the distinction between supportive basic training and the event-specific training and begin to overemphasize more event-specific training. The event-specific training and actual performances are the sexy stuff that makes impressive YouTube videos and exciting headlines that create the urban myths surrounding champions. Is there an alpinist who has not been inspired by the video of Ueli Steck soloing the 1938 Route on the north face of the Eiger in two hours and forty-eight minutes? One would have to be soulless not to feel motivated while watching the video of David Rudisha crushing his competition in the 800-meter Olympic final in the 2012 London Olympics as he set (yet) another world record. What you do not see as you watch these masters perform at the peak fitness of their lives are the countless hours of basic, non-event-specific, supportive training that went into their record breaking.

To shed more light on how conventional sport can inform training for climbing, we'll use some analogies. Take the sport of cross-country ski racing, which Scott has an extensive background in as both an athlete and a coach at the World Cup level. These events demand that the athletes be able to sustain power levels between 95 percent up to 120 percent of their VO$_2$ max for durations of up to several minutes at a time on gently rolling terrain to long, steep uphills. Then they need to recover quickly during the fast and often technically demanding downhill sections so that they can repeat the maximal efforts again many times over during a race lasting up to, or a little over, two hours. Technique is critical to success due to the large contribution economy of movement plays in determining speed. For the best skiers in this sport, approximately 80 percent of training volume is made up of non-event-specific training in such a way that the event (a ski race in this case) is broken down into its component parts and the training is focused on improving the athlete's abilities specific to those components. We can and will teach you how to apply this with climbing.

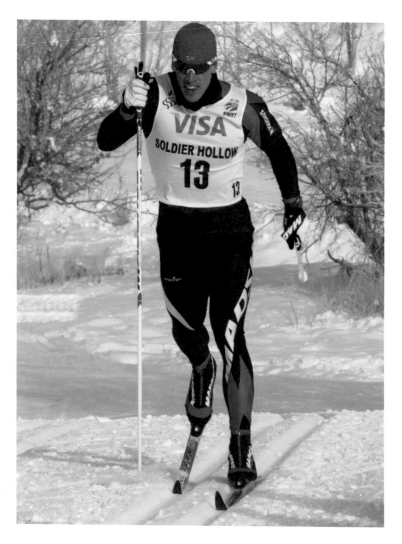

The long duration of Nordic ski races and the full-body nature of this sport are physiologically similar to climbing long technical routes.
Photo: Ian Harvey

In cross-country ski racing these components can be represented by strength and power training, various intensities and modes of aerobic base conditioning, technique drills, etc. Only 20 percent of their overall yearly volume is spent doing training that specifically models the demands of an actual race.

For the climber training for the Disappointment Cleaver Route on Mount Rainier the training will be fairly simple since the principal quality required for that event is aerobic endurance and technique is not a major factor. The non-climbing-specific work will include strength training but will mainly consist of hiking and running in the mountains. As the training progresses, it will include climbs of nontechnical peaks with snow or glaciers. It is easy to see how the nonspecific training of hiking up and down hills lends support to the more demanding Mount Rainier climb.

This translation to climbing becomes more complicated when the event becomes a technical alpine route, possibly at altitude. Start to think like a coach and it should quickly become apparent that the basic supportive training will encompass all of the Rainier climber's training with the addition of technically demanding routes of various lengths and difficulties that challenge several of the physical and mental qualities needed to succeed at the main goal. To extend the analogy, you wouldn't train on climbs that encompass all aspects of your goal, but rather component parts. It can happen that some of these nonspecific training climbs may be admirable accomplishments in their own right. Just as a conventional athlete racks up an impressive résumé of jaw-droppingly difficult workouts and race wins on his way to setting a world record or winning an Olympic gold medal.

One challenge for the alpinist with lofty goals is coming up with event-specific training. In other words, finding routes that combine components of the traits needed on the goal route. Alpinism has traditionally given lip service to this notion without fully understanding the context within which it fits. Climbers in North America have progressed from their home range to the Canadian Rockies to the Alps with perhaps a stint in the Alaska Range thrown in before heading to the Himalaya. Gaston Rébuffat in fact gave a step-by-step guide to this progressive approach in 1973 when he published *The Mont Blanc Massif: The Hundred Finest Routes*, which leads aspiring alpinists one step at a time through a progression of the skill-acquisition aspect of becoming an alpinist. But the message was not fully conveyed in terms of how this progression fits into the big picture of physically and mentally training for alpinism.

First Steps, Missteps

By Steve House

I take a deep gasp of air and swing a tool at the lip of the ice wall. I glance up at Marko Prezelj standing above me, waiting. I gasp and pull up, my legs feel like jelly, my shoulders burn for oxygen. I cock my tool back to make another swing, Marko turns and climbs off, rhythmically ascending the wind-scoured ice toward 22,967 feet (7,000 meters) on Nuptse's South Face. I allow a half rest, expel my breath hard as I swing, pull, and start after him, cueing my kicks to the staccato rhythm of his ascent.

In 2002, after a sixty-hour ascent of Denali's Slovak Direct and a twenty-five-hour climb of Mount Foraker's Infinite Spur under my belt, I thought I was ready to trade up to the big leagues; climbing in the Himalaya. Marko Prezelj, whom I'd met in Alaska, was the perfect partner: a veteran of over a dozen Himalayan expeditions with many alpine-style ascents to his credit. That spring, high on Nuptse, the wind seemed to pull the breath out of me. Despite my success in Alaska I was not fit enough to climb these great walls.

Back home, I attended the Nordic Ski Club workouts with Laura McCabe, a two-time Olympian. Nordic skiing is known as one of the hardest sports with some of the fittest athletes, and there I met my first coach, a Canadian Nordic skier who had recently finished her MS in exercise physiology. With the help of Patagonia, Inc., I hired my first coach, trading clothing for a training program with the goal of a new route in alpine style on 25,659-foot (7,821-meter) high Masherbrum.

By the time the snow flew I would wake in the dark to strap on Nordic skis and skate the local trails by headlamp before reporting to work at 7:00 a.m. at North Cascades Heli-Skiing, where I'd spend four of every seven days fulfilling people's jet-fueled quest for powder. I bought a heart-rate monitor that I used during each training session and tracked every minute spent in Zone 2, a low heart rate, steadily collecting endurance, hour by hour.

In June 2003, at Masherbrum Base Camp, Marko and I started up a little-known 21,000-foot (6,401-meter) peak to acclimate. Marko accelerated away from me like I was standing still. I had felt good that morning, so I decided that Marko must have played a trick on me by putting a rock in my pack. He's funny like that. I stopped in the middle of the couloir and emptied every single item out of my pack. No rock.

Home once again without success on Masherbrum, I stopped by to visit my friend Scott Johnston and we began talking about Masherbrum, which led back to my training that winter.

"*You were way overtrained,*" Scott told me. "*All due respect to your coach, but I don't think she understands alpinism; she trained you like a skier, and you worked like a mountaineer.*"

I admitted I had not recorded my hours of heli-ski guiding as training time. Scott scoffed in disbelief, "*That was stupid.*"

"*I was skiing downhill, Scott, with a helicopter to haul us up to the top of each run. You hardly count that as training.*"

What followed was a long and careful explanation from Scott of some basic training principles, the same ideas that form the foundation of this book. The same principles all top-level coaches and athletes subscribe to.

Since that day in 2003 Scott taught and guided me to most of what I know about training. This information is based on many decades of research done by a committed scientific community that studies human performance and by Scott's own years of competing at national and World Cup levels in both swimming and Nordic skiing. Add to that Scott's many climbing expeditions to Alaska, Canada, and the Himalaya, and he has acquired a set of knowledge and experiences that is, to my mind, unique in the climbing world.

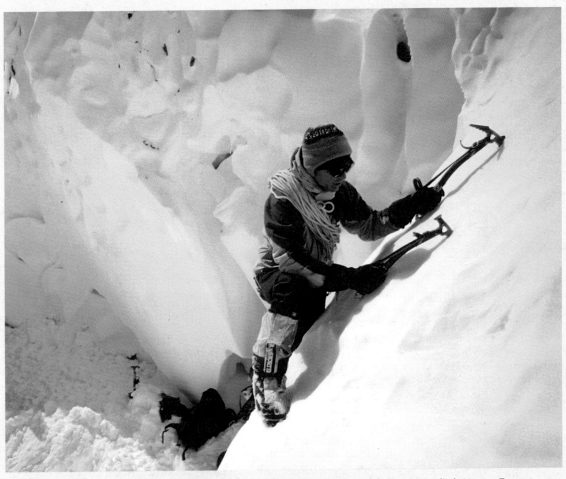

Steve House leaving the high bivouac on Nuptse's south face in an unsuccessful attempt to climb Nuptse East (25,603'/7,804m). *Photo: Marko Prezelj*

Steve has used the approach we advocate in this book by spending a prodigious amount of time on basic, supportive, non-event-specific training. He has then successfully built upon that with progressively more event-specific training on more and more demanding alpine routes. At the elite level it will be necessary to travel far and wide and plan long and hard to find appropriate event-specific training climbs.

Let's use another running analogy to make a point: Do you think Usain Bolt trains for setting the world record in the 100- and 200-meter track events by going to the track every day and running to break his old record? If you do, then you are vastly mistaken. He trains the many components that, when combined, allow him to be the fastest human ever. Only a tiny fraction of his time is spent actually running the 100 or 200 meters at race intensity.

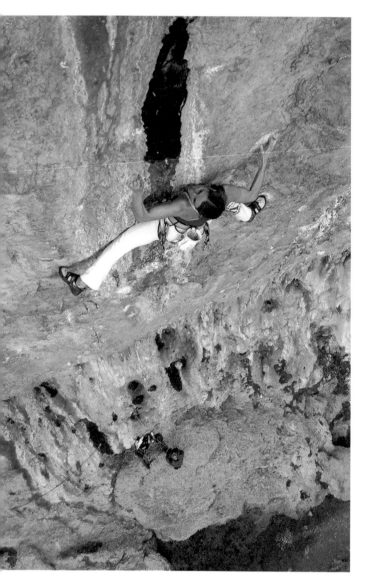

Look at one of the most quantifiable areas of climbing: sport climbing. Does it make sense that top-level sport climbers should spend the bulk of their time trying to climb right at their limit, working a project, with only a tiny fraction of their training volume spent climbing other, easier routes? Why don't top sport climbers like Chris Sharma climb new 5.15s every week? If he can do it once, he can do it weekly, right? Wrong. This would be akin to Bolt running 100s at race pace several days a week in hopes of improving the physical qualities that will allow him to break his record again. Top coaches and athletes in conventional sports abandoned this approach to training long ago.

The information in this book is strongly rooted in the science of human physiology, which draws upon decades of research and practice. We often look to other sports to learn what makes their best athletes. The best athletes, be they a runner, cyclist, skier, or football player, are not born with tree-trunk legs or greyhound lungs. Typically they train with a coach, probably from a very early age. Their bodies adapt to every workout, every meal, every rest, to slowly, additively, become

Martina Čufar redpointing Vizija (8c or 5.14b) at Miša Peč, Slovenia. *Photo: Marko Prezelj* incredible athletes. Who has followed this same path in alpine climbing? No one, yet. Those who execute on this path will be the ones to change alpine climbing forever.

Training for alpinism is different in some ways than training for other sports. The duration is longer, sometimes more than a week. The intensity is intermittent; cruxes come, and cruxes go. The event, the climb, can often not be put on your calendar months in advance—when the weather clears, you climb. Failure can be fatal; alpinism carries significant mortal risk.

Buhl, Messner, Bonatti, Habeler, Loretan, Scott, MacIntyre, Kammerlander, Kukuczka, and Kurtyka. These are the names of those who raised the bar of alpinism in the twentieth century. They mostly used climbing as their training for climbing, with Buhl, Messner, and Habeler being notable exceptions for their times. For those with talent equal to these legends, that will be enough. Steve counts himself among those with no special athletic talent. In alpinism, the most talented are unlikely to be those who will change how we climb. Talent can make you lazy. Innovation will be left to the hardest workers, training intelligently.

In the spring of 2004, Steve had completed his first single year of training under Scott's tutelage. In April, after a strenuous six-day climb of the north face of North Twin with Marko Prezelj, he navigated in a whiteout across the Columbia Icefield for fourteen hours while breaking trail through new snow. Steve was tired, but he retained the physical and mental reserves to put them in exactly the right spot after a twenty-mile crossing by map, compass, and GPS. Three months later in Pakistan he soloed a new route on K7 in forty-four hours round-trip from base camp. This was the first time in the history of alpine climbing that someone had climbed such a difficult route on such a high mountain alone—and survived. One year later Vince Anderson and Steve climbed what is regarded as the most difficult route established on an 8,000-meter peak climbing alpine style. The approach we've taken, and shared in this book, works.

And what of those climbers who have been alpinists all their lives without any need for records or firsts? What of Gaston Rébuffat's admonition for "self-discovery, deepening a little further with every climb: who we are, how far we can go, what is our potential, where are the limits of our technique, our strength, our skill, our mountaineering sense?" That is here as well. Training becomes an important path to your self-discovery; a part of your climbing.

Don't Epic— Keep It Under Control

By Ueli Steck

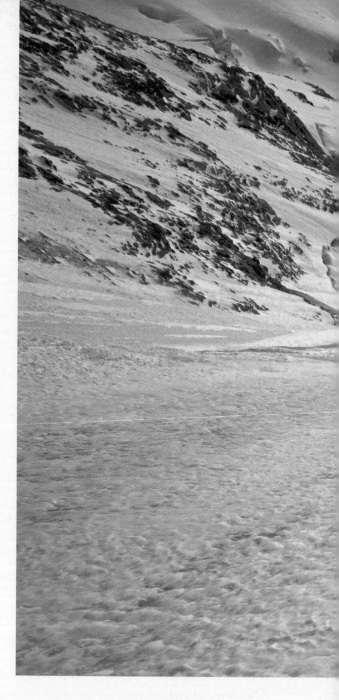

I am a control freak. Even in daily life I need a very strong structure. On the mountain I need to have the feeling that I have everything under control. I think this attitude keeps me alive. Fortunately I'm a coward; otherwise my ambition would have ruined me already.

I need a clear goal; I'm not the type of person who climbs a bit and then by chance goes for a run. I always need a goal, and that goal is the foundation for an efficient workout. There is a difference whether you want to climb an 8,000-meter peak, climb 5.13 free solo, or free climb El Cap. You have to accept that you cannot be your best all the time at every climbing discipline. If I want to free climb a route on El Cap, I don't run a marathon. I spend my time climbing because running takes the time and energy that I could spend on training for rock climbing. Also cardiovascular training like running needs to be adapted to my specific goal. I need a different kind of endurance to climb the north face of Eiger as fast as possible than I need for a Himalayan ascent. These details make the crucial difference. Exactly here it starts to get interesting. I have already lived my own experiences; I know exactly what it takes to get to this level of fitness.

Training needs to vary periodically. The body cannot run all year at the highest level. That's a big problem for many climbers; they feel pressure to always to be their best. Trying to peak all the time creates a plateau, and no more performance improvements will be possible until you break this cycle. With appropriate training you will reach peak periods that are much higher than this plateau. You only have to arrange that you peak at the right moment, and this requires a plan. I always train according to a plan.

For me, climbing is a continuous development. I always wanted to set a climbing speed record on the Eiger North Face. I've done it by optimizing my training for that route. The next step was to onsight speed climb an unknown route, and on the north faces of the Grandes Jorasses and the Matterhorn I realized that goal. With this knowledge

I've opened up new possibilities for myself. I know I can climb a wall of 1,000 meters (3,281 feet) in two hours and thirty minutes without knowing the route. For the Himalaya this opens new dimensions. I had one and a half days of nice weather on Shisha Pangma, and the south wall is 2,000 meters (6,561 feet) high. Climbing a wall like this in a weather window of one and a half days is what I was looking for. The route I was climbing was quite challenging, with steep, rocky passages: Ten and a half hours later, I stood on the summit.

A weather report for two days is always very precise. That means overall I have a big safety reserve on routes

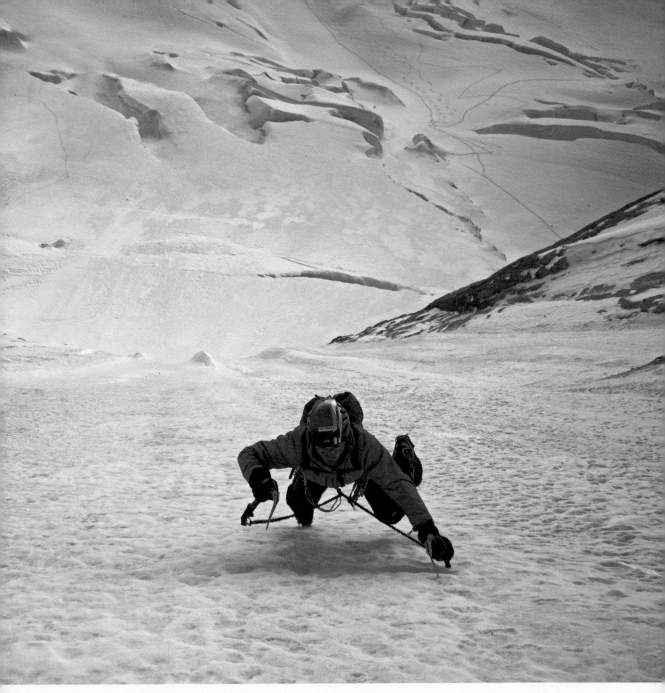

Ueli Steck en route to soloing the Colton-MacIntyre route on the Grand Jorasses in two hours and twenty-one minutes. *Photo: Jonathan Griffith*

like this, and this security comes from my physical fitness. I can calculate exactly, so I don't have any dangerous adventures, no epics.

The most important thing is that you come back—with or without summiting. You have to be honest with yourself that in the end no one really cares—you do it for yourself. Everyone must decide for him or herself how much risk he or she wants to take. Risk is not measurable and is always dependent on the individual.

You need to know that it is impossible to indefinitely push your limits: higher, faster, better. Eventually you reach a peak and then it goes back down. I believe it's important that you don't lose your passion and that you enjoy the outdoors and challenging yourself, no matter what your level is.

Swiss alpinist Ueli Steck's name is synonymous with training for alpinism. He is perhaps most famous for climbing the north face of the Eiger in two hours and forty-eight minutes.

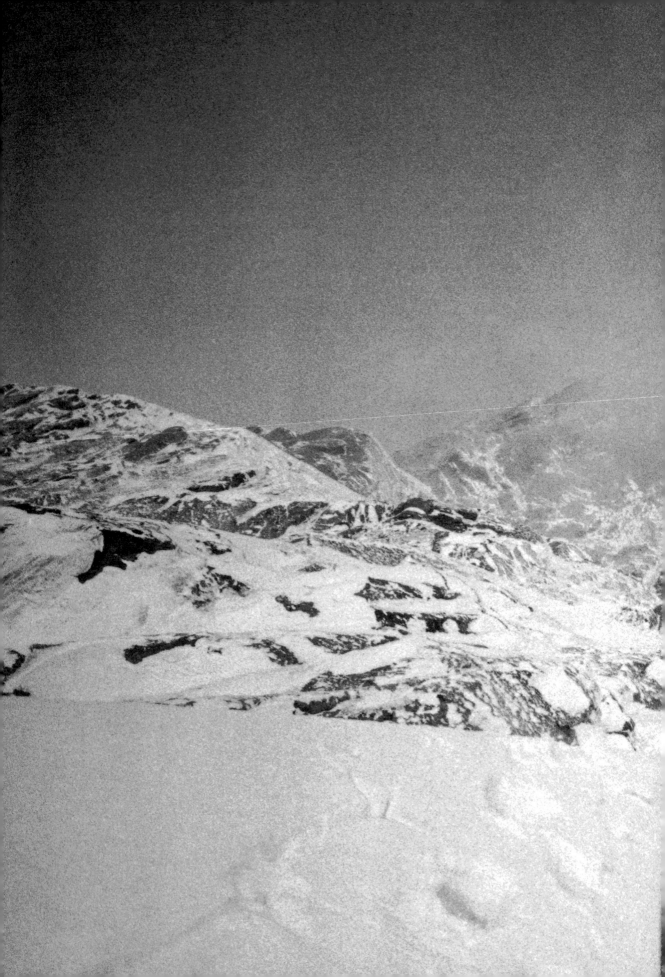

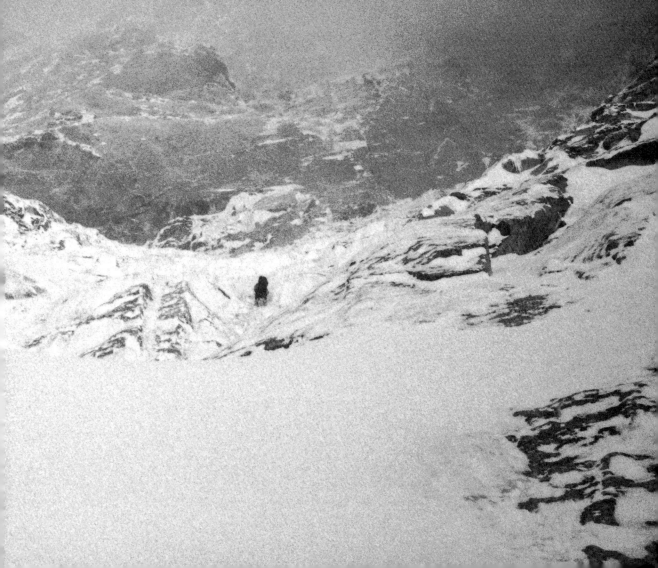

Section 1

The Methodology and Physiology of Endurance Training

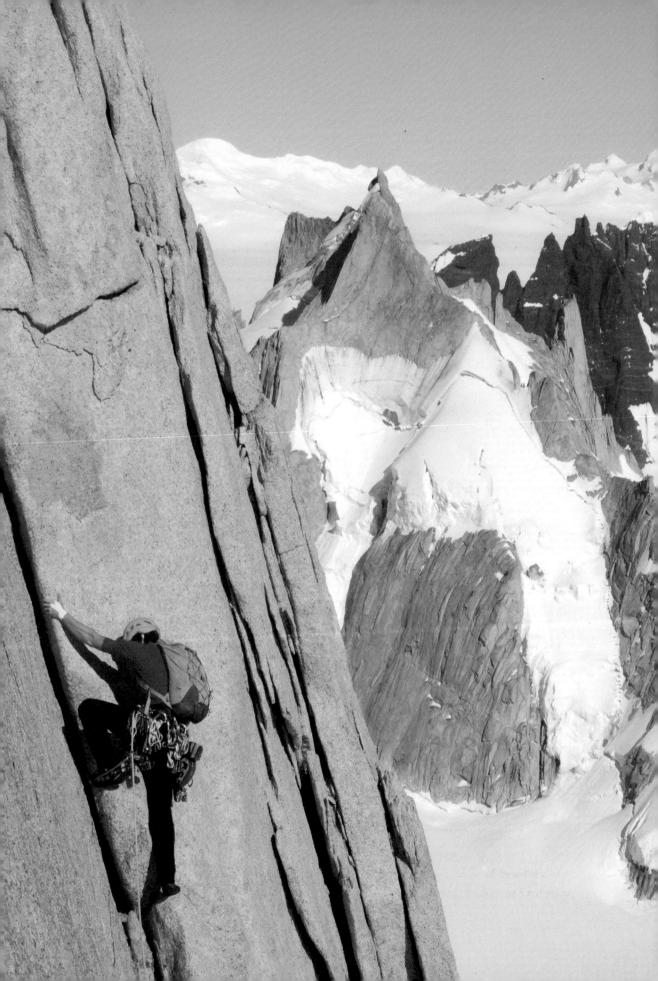

Chapter 2

The Methodology of Endurance Training

"Alpinism is the art of climbing mountains
by confronting the greatest dangers with the
greatest prudence. Art is used here to mean the
accomplishment of knowledge in action. You cannot
stay on the summit forever. You have to come down
again. So what's the point? Only this: what is above
knows what is below, what is below does not know what
is above. While climbing, take note of all the difficulties
along your path. During the descent, you will no longer
see them, but you will know that they are there if you
have observed carefully. There is an art to finding your
way in the lower regions by the memory of what you
have seen when you were higher up. When you can no
longer see, you can at least still know."

— RENÉ DAUMAL, from *Mount Analogue*

THE ALPINIST AS ATHLETE

Many would argue that alpinism is art, not sport. Alpinism places
unique demands on its practitioners. In no organized sport do the
participants have to endure days of struggle just to get to the starting

Opposite: Colin Haley climbing the
Kearney-Knight variation to the
Casarotto Route on the Goretta Pillar
of Cerro Fitz Roy during the second
ascent of the Care Bear Traverse.
Photo: Rolando Garibotti

Previous spread: Steve House
leading on the south face of Kunyang
Chish East (24,278', 7,400m) in the
Karakoram Range, Pakistan, during
an unsuccessful attempt on the then
unclimbed peak.
Photo: Vince Anderson

line of their event. The option to drop out of a race that is going badly does not exist for a climber halfway up a big route, and may entail more risk than pushing on. A team of volunteers will not be waiting with warm blankets and hot food at the next bivy ledge. When you reach the summit, having overcome the challenges that inspired you for months or years, you are not at the finish line. The race is not over. You can't relax and let your guard down like a normal athlete. The descent is often as much (or more of) a challenge as the climb.

We can respect the gulf that separates alpinism from a running race and still appreciate that the physiology that accounts for endurance is the same if you are running a foot race in the city park or front pointing up the second ice field on the north face of the Eiger. We climbers have much to learn from the training done in conventional sports.

Structured training for climbing is a relatively recent phenomenon. So far most of the literature and practice have been focused specifically on rock climbing. A half-century of trial and error has produced some excellent resources for those looking to apply modern strength training theory to rock climbing. Alpine climbing, on the other hand, is the last bastion of training luddites. Historically, many of the great names in alpine climbing seemed to have just gone climbing as training. In fact, the model alpinist has often portrayed himself in literature as a half-crazed nonconformist, living life on the edge every moment he's sober enough to climb. It is true that amazing feats of skill and daring have been accomplished using this rather random approach. For some climbers that "life on the edge" approach may be the only way they can accomplish these feats, but there are far better methods to prepare for the challenges of alpine climbing.

Even though Vince Lombardi used this quote for football, it is perhaps even more poignant for alpinism: "Fatigue makes cowards of us all." In the mountains, fatigue is the biggest controllable limitation that will come between you and success. You will never exploit your full technical capacity if your fitness remains a weak link. Conventional sports have undergone an evolution in training methods during the last fifty years. Curiosity and the inherent improvement brought about by competition have driven this evolution to a state of high refinement such that today's athletes have a very specialized approach to training at the elite levels.

On big routes in big mountains, speed equals safety. Traveling fast over complex technical terrain requires a high level of technical ability *and* the endurance to support it. These two quite divergent capabilities need to be developed over years of practice. Omitting either limits your potential.

Getting Results

By Steve House

In the autumn of 2003, upon returning from Masherbrum, I started into my new training program with Scott. At the time I was fresh off my first real success in the Himalaya, a solo new route on an unclimbed 19,685-foot (6,000-meter) peak in the Karakoram. In the next twenty-four months, between September 2003 and September 2005, I would succeed on a large number of significant alpine routes:

- The Talkeetna Standard, a new route on Alaska's Eye Tooth

- The second ascent of the Roberts-Rowell-Ward route on the east face of Mount Dickey

- The House-Prezelj variation to the Lowe-Jones route on the north face of North Twin

- A new route established alone on K7 in a forty-one-hour round-trip push

- An attempt to 24,278 feet (7,400 meters) on Nanga Parbat's Rupal Face with Bruce Miller

- Redpointing various rock climbs up to 5.12d

- Onsight three alpine rock routes (to 5.12b) at 17,000 feet (5,180 meters) on Peru's La Esfinge

- A new route with Marko Prezelj on the west face of Cayesh

- The first free ascent of the French Route on Taulliraju with Marko Prezelj

- The Anderson-House route on the Rupal Face of Nanga Parbat

To me, it is clear I was able to do those climbs because of the training. I was mentally focused and fully committed to alpine climbing, and that commitment played a big part in the success. But at the end of the day, I did those climbs because I was fit. I had a big base from a lifetime of athletics, over fifteen years of climbing and twelve years of guiding on top of a hyperactive youth. And the training refined that fitness. This is the identical approach that Scott and I share in this book: building a base and then refining that fitness for the objective at hand. Without that training, most of these routes would not have been realized.

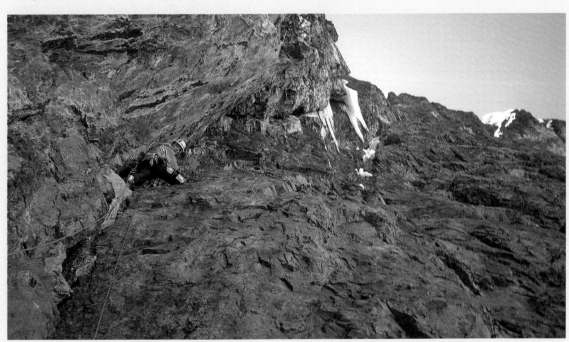

Steve House climbing a difficult mixed pitch during the one-day first ascent of the House-Prezelj route on the west face of Cayesh (18,760', 5,719m) in Peru. *Photo: Marko Prezelj*

Transitions

By Zoe Hart

I grew up in suburban New Jersey playing traditional sports. It was easy to stay fit as part of a team and with someone else to manage my training program. Half way through my junior year of college, soon after I found climbing, I gave up my spot on the Division I Big East championship softball team for climbing dreams.

The next several years I was acutely aware of the lack of discipline in my practice of climbing, and I missed the support of my teammates. I wondered how to train. How to stay fit? Everyone did something different, but the best answer always seemed to be just to climb. And so I climbed, but in between climbing trips I lost both my fitness and motivation.

When I finished university I was able to climb full time, and fitness came easily: climbing, learning, pushing grades. Eventually, I found work as a mountain guide and established more balance in my life, with some downtime, and a home base. I also arrived at a plateau in my training. With horror I watched my fitness ebb. A friend pointed out that it would be a shame to not see how far I could go in climbing if I were to train and live with discipline. It was then that I started to think about food as fuel, to think about what muscle groups climbing taxes and how to strengthen them.

I found my way past that plateau thanks to the help of a friend and personal trainer who helped me to develop a program. Finding a structure for my habitually haphazard training regime helped me to work through my weaknesses. Throughout the fall I balanced sessions in the gym with long trail runs and climbing days mixed with periods of rest. I found myself climbing strong and confident by the time the winter mixed climbing season came around.

That winter I led runout, heady mixed routes in Scotland and hard mixed climbs on the granite of the Northeast. I placed second in the Ouray Mixed-Climbing Competition and shared leads on Cryophobia, a long, hard mixed line in Alberta, Canada. With day-to-day discipline and hard work, I found that I could achieve goals I had previously seen as out of reach. Training gave me confidence in my body, which equaled confidence in my mind.

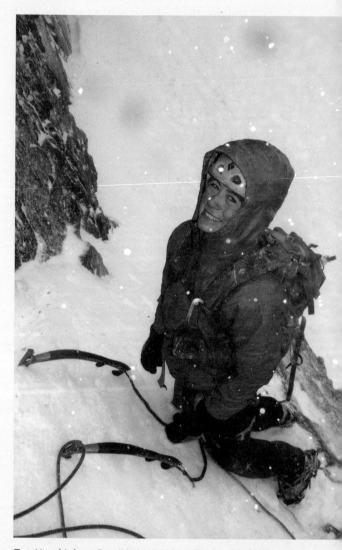

Zoe Hart high on Ben Nevis (4,410', 1,344m), Scotland, on her way to climbing a new route on the mountain during an international winter climbing meet in 2009.
Photo: Ian Parnell

Zoe Hart lives in France where she works as an IFMGA-certified mountain guide and professional alpinist. Her current transition is learning the balance of motherhood.

THE TWO TYPES OF TRAINING

There are really only two types of training for any sport.

1) The general conditioning that readies you for event-specific training.

This conditioning consists of a mixture of strength and endurance training and may not be climbing specific.

2) That training that prepares you in a specific way for the event itself.

This training consists primarily of climbing or workouts that model directly the specific demands of climbing.

It is important to understand that the role of nonspecific training is not intended to be of immediate benefit to your climbing, unless of course you have low fitness. Its purpose is to generate a base of support to do the specific workouts and the training for climbing.

Putting Some Numbers to It

How much you prepare depends completely on your training background and goals. Motivation, along with realistic time and energy allotments, is often the biggest limitation to the time you can allot for training. You can't coach desire, and no matter how fancy your training plan or how high your stated goals are, it comes down to getting out the door and doing the work day after day.

World-class endurance athletes spend a prodigious amount of time training for their races. At the highest levels it is truly a full-time job, allowing for only enough time and energy to rest and refuel between workouts. Here are some examples to put things in perspective. Running, being the least efficient and most stressful on the body, generally consumes the least number of dedicated hours for top athletes. In a week of training, around sixteen hours will be spent running. This translates to about 120 miles of running plus a couple of strength training sessions. Of all types of endurance athletes, cyclists can tolerate the most training. They need it due to the non-weight-bearing, seated posture and the efficiency of the bike. Many pros ride their bikes between twenty-five to thirty hours per week. Top swimmers can train in the twenty-hour-per-week range. World Cup cross-country skiers can surpass twenty to twenty-five hours with yearly volumes of 800 to 1,000 hours being normal for the top men.

Elite-level women in these sports generally train in the range of about 10 percent less than the best men. This is usually due to women competing at shorter distances than the men. However, in the marathon, Ironman triathlon, and ultra-marathon running events, the top women train at the same levels as the men; there is no reason they cannot do as much as their male counterparts. This will be the same for women alpinists.

Between 2003 and 2009 Steve trained in the range of 820 to 942 hours per year, which put his volume on a par with other world-class endurance athletes. When you read of his ascents, such as the Rupal Face climb, you are seeing what Dr. K. Anders Ericsson, the psychologist and world expert on excellence, calls the iceberg illusion: the end product of a preparation process measured in years. He had no special talents but had created a structure in his life where he could devote himself fully to climbing and train with Scott as his coach. When you watch or read about the accomplishments of any great climber, what you don't see is the thousands of hours of climbing and other training that have literally altered their anatomical and neurological structures so that they can accomplish what is otherwise impossible.

The point we hope to make with these figures is not to intimidate you or to suggest that you must train at this level to succeed. What we want to make clear is that your results will be proportional to the time you spend in preparation. Keep these figures in mind as a yardstick when considering what is humanly possible for athletes of any discipline that have spent years steadily increasing training loads.

Three forty-five-minute Stairmaster workouts a week will not allow you to reach your ultimate potential. But this may be a perfectly reasonable starting place for you given your personal constraints. The important thing is to progress, adapt, and in the process learn some valuable lessons.

A BRIEF DISCUSSION OF PHYSIOLOGY BASICS

While athletes do not need to be exercise physiologists, understanding the basics of how and why your body responds to training will be necessary for you to develop your own training plan. Very few of us have the luxury of a private coach. Without a coach, you need to have some means of guiding your own training. This guidance is best found in a sound application of current exercise science. These are principles that governed our training choices for Steve, and we have learned a lot from that experience. What we propose to do in these first chapters is to give you a simplified understanding of an extremely complex physical system. With this basic knowledge we'll lay out methods to apply this theory to your own training.

Opposite: Ines Papert climbs the Great Corner (M7+, 1,000′, 300m) on Senja Island, Norway. *Photo: Thomas Senf*

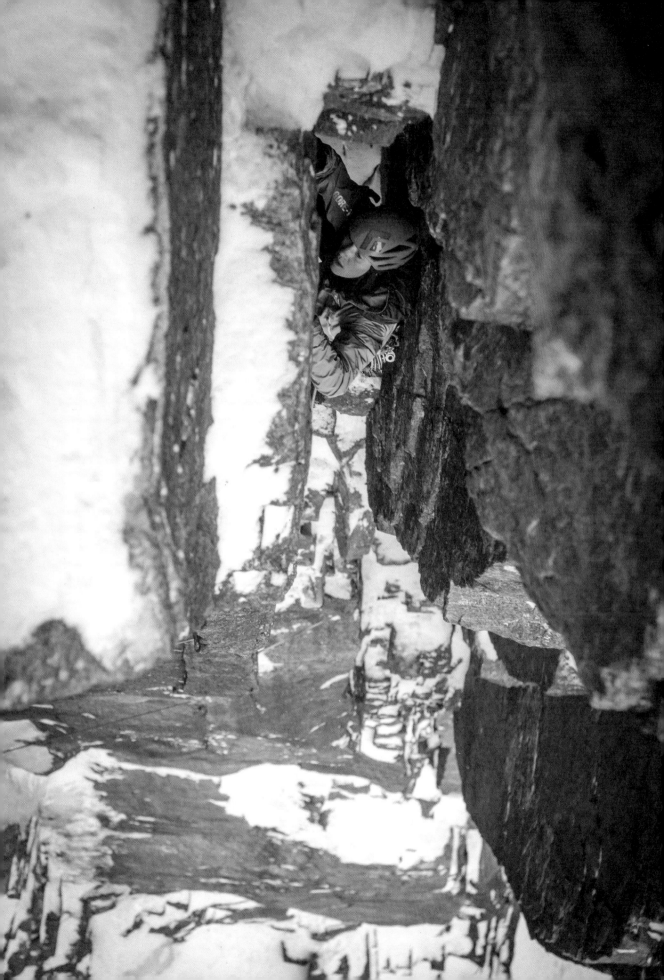

Climbing movements are the result of muscular contraction. Muscles require energy to contract. That energy comes from a chemical process called *metabolism*. We'll go into a bit more depth in chapter 3, but for now you can envision metabolism as a pathway of energy production. One of these pathways is *aerobic*, meaning that it depends on oxygen for the chemical reactions it uses to produce this energy for movement. The other pathway is *anaerobic*, meaning that the energy for movement can be produced in the absence of oxygen.

Ever since our single-cell predecessors crawled out of the primordial muck into an oxygen-rich atmosphere, much of life on Earth has developed an aerobic metabolism. Humans are very much aerobic organisms and can live only a few minutes without oxygen. However, like our simpler, very distant cousins—yeast and bacteria—we humans have also retained the capacity for anaerobic metabolism as well. Ironically, considering our reliance on oxygen for energy, we actually supply our maximum power output anaerobically, albeit for only a very short time. Using all of their anaerobic capacity, a few champion sprint track cyclists have been known to develop maximum power outputs in excess of 1,800 watts for a few seconds (Gardiner et al., 2007). But before you get too impressed, keep in mind that this is only a bit more than the power of a cheap blow dryer that you can hold in one hand! In reality, we humans are pretty puny when it comes to absolute strength and power.

On the other hand, our aerobic metabolism allows us to produce moderate power for very long periods. We call this attribute aerobic endurance and we will explore this quality in some depth throughout this book. A fit human can run down most other animals in a contest of endurance (Bramble and Lieberman, 2004.). A succinct definition of endurance is: The ability to resist fatigue, in both a muscular and cardiovascular sense (Costil and Wilmore, 1994). While this may sound like a vague definition—How much fatigue? For how long must one resist that fatigue? In fact it pertains directly to any activity you choose. Alpine climbing, where the efforts need to be sustained for a minimum of several hours, and often for days on end, demands one type of endurance. A sport climber redpointing at his limit, where the climber needs to sustain near-maximal efforts for a few minutes, needs another type of endurance. Thus the qualities that make up endurance and the training of those qualities varies depending on the application. This concept will take up the vast majority of our discussion in these early chapters.

THE ADAPTATION TO A TRAINING STIMULUS

While at the chemical level of metabolism, the efficiency of the different energy pathways is relatively fixed, with proper training you can alter the type of reactions *(lipolysis,* the metabolism of fats, or *glycolysis,* the metabolism of sugars) that are occurring. Whichever metabolic process your training promotes, through that training you prioritize that energy pathway and greatly influence the performance outcomes.

Certain *enzymes* that aid metabolism are produced because they are more practical when the body is not doing any athletic activity. So a sedentary person will possess a higher concentration of these enzymes in his muscle tissues. In other words, a lazy slug will have lazy slug enzymes that work very well for a lazy slug but not well for an athlete. The enzymes that help an athlete function more efficiently must be produced. And they get produced only in response to the body realizing, through repeated bouts of activity, that they are needed. These enzymes will not work well for the lazy slug. If this slug somehow had these athletic enzymes, they would never get used and the body would get rid of them since they are just taking up space. The body only builds, keeps, and maintains what is used and needed, which is why your training must be consistent.

In order to respond to or improve from our training efforts, both the body's functional and structural systems must be stimulated to do so. Training purposefully stresses those systems just enough so that the body "thinks" that the systems are at risk of failing their purpose, or are too close to injury for comfort. Your training must be stressful enough to stimulate change, but not so stressful as to damage your body. Obviously this is a fine distinction. Allow sufficient time for your body to absorb the training load and avoid injury. Understanding the training response cycle is critical to effective and safe training.

THE TRAINING EFFECT

"Training is not the work that you do, it is the value
and the cost of your body's response to that work."

— Legendary coach RENATO CANOVA
Canova's runners have garnered more world records, world championships,
and Olympic medals than those of any other running coach.

The human body has an amazing capacity to adapt to physical stress.
But it does this best if that stress is applied in a constructive, consistent, and progressive manner. To see progress in your fitness you need
to temporarily put some systems of the body into a crisis state and
allow the body to restore its homeostasis through its natural regener-
ative processes. This stress/recovery process results in what is termed
a training effect. If properly coordinated, these adaptive mechanisms
result in a process known as *supercompensation*, whereby your body
overcompensates and ends up at a higher fitness level than before the
stress of training was applied. Only the body's systems that experience
the stress of training adapt to handle future stress better.

If there is a new training stimulus applied while your body is still in
a supercompensated state, the resultant new level of adaptation will be
higher than the previous one.

In principle, this progression of load and adaptation is the goal of
all well-structured training. This consistent and progressive nature is
what sets training apart from simply exercising for health, and is one

Examples of the Training Effect

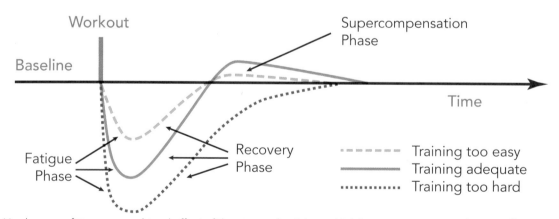

You become fitter as a combined effect of the stress of training, which has a temporary weakening effect,
followed by a recovery period during which your body compensates for the stress that has been applied to it.
Too much stress interferes with the body's adaptation. Too little stress does not elicit enough of a response.

Long-Term Training Effect

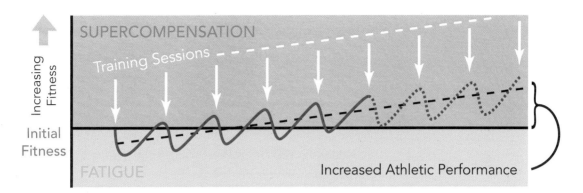

Ideal application of the stress of training during the supercompensation phase results in long-term fitness increase.

of the trickiest aspects to get right. The various changes that your body undergoes due to this training effect occur at different rates, and the restorative periods can vary from a few hours to several days depending on which body systems experience stress.

THE GUIDING PRINCIPLES: CONTINUITY, GRADUALNESS, AND MODULATION

These three words embody the principles of all successful training programs. A solid understanding of them will help you build your program from general to more specific conditioning.

As mentioned earlier, correct training places one or more of your body's systems into a crisis state. These stresses impact the body's structural and functional systems. By structural, we mean the actual protein structures of your body (muscle, capillaries, mitochondria, etc.). By functional, we mean the metabolic, enzymatic, hormonal, and other physiological functions that exist within the structures. The myriad numbers of processes that occur to both these systems take place at varying rates. Some of these adaptations occur on the order of hours; others occur over the course of days, weeks, or even years.

A failure to adapt (known as stagnation) can occur, and if unaddressed can lead to overtraining, which results in a diminishing level of fitness. It takes time for the body to adjust to the training load you impose. A reapplication of another similar training stress will not give you the benefits you seek if your body's structural and functional systems have not sufficiently adapted to your current training load.

Continuity

Continuity in training refers to maintaining a regular schedule of training with minimal interruption. You have to be motivated and disciplined to fulfill the requirements of the plan you lay out. Obviously, there needs to be some flexibility to account for the unexpected. Lapses in training do happen. They can be managed, but they cannot be overlooked. If you miss a week of training due to work, travel, or sickness, you can't pretend that you actually did all that training and progress to the next part of the plan. Your body will not be adapted to the next step, and you'll be likely to have setbacks.

How you manage this discontinuity depends on its length and the reason for it. Occasional breaks of a couple of days are not much of a problem as long as they do not diminish the training load by more than roughly 5 percent in a month, but frequent or prolonged breaks from training that amount to more than 10 percent of the monthly volume do create a need to adjust your subsequent training.

Gradualness

Gradualness is an acknowledgement of the body's limited capability to adapt to the training stimulus. As inspirational as the movies may have been, Sylvester Stallone violated this basic principle repeatedly in the Rocky series. Hollywood allows that sort of fantasy. Real life does not. Occasional bursts (or lapses) of enthusiasm and motivation that result in big jumps in training load are a common approach to training by beginners and dabblers. The results from this sporadic exercise (we can't call it training) will never lead to good results. Your body's numerous systems require time to adapt to the various stresses you apply with a training load. Gradualness is a virtue that cannot be overemphasized.

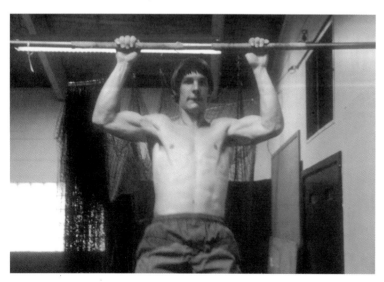

Steve House began training for rock climbing as a teen by doing numerous pull-ups.
Photo: Marty Treadway

A gradual progression of the training load means different things for different athletes. Beginners and those with a low annual volume of training can progress faster than those with many years of training who are closer to their ultimate potential fitness. As a general rule, beginners can increase training volume by as much as 25 percent per year and up to 50 percent during a three-week training cycle. Advanced athletes will be unable to make such jumps because they are already operating much closer to their body's capacity. For them, a 10 percent jump in yearly volume should be considered a maximum. Elite-level athletes often make no change in overall annual training volume, instead seeking gains by juggling the amount of higher-intensity and specific training.

Modulation

Modulation is the undulating level of training stimulus that allows your body a chance to recover its *homeostasis* (biological equilibrium in living organisms) after that crisis period. But it will also allow you to overload those intended systems and then put them into the next and higher crisis state with the new, higher training load. Depending on the systems you intend to stress, this modulation can follow a cycle measured in hours up to one measured in days. It can take three weeks for some significant changes to happen in the structural and functional systems. With care, an athlete can modulate his training to allow several systems to adapt at the same time.

Through empirical processes, coaches have come to realize that adaptation occurs in roughly three- to six-week cycles. During the first three weeks, your body rapidly adapts. During the next three weeks, if the training load is held constant, it begins to yield diminishing results as your body structurally and functionally adapts to that training stimulus. During these second three weeks many of the adaptations begin to consolidate, creating a base upon which to build the next step upward on the fitness ladder.

Once your body is adapted to the stress of the current training load, what used to be a crisis state will no longer be enough to cause your body to keep adapting. Some creative changes to the training load need to be implemented for the next three-week cycle or progress will stop as you become adapted to this new level of crisis. These changes vary according to the qualities that the athlete hopes to develop. For a quality such as endurance, these adjustments are simple and involve mostly an increase in the volume of training along with the concurrent increase in speed at the individual's aerobic threshold pace. For the simultaneous training of different qualities such as speed and endurance or power and endurance, even more elaborate training systems need to be implemented, which is beyond the scope of this book and must be administrated with care and finesse, usually by a coach.

SPECIFICITY

Only the systems that are stressed are going to see the training effect. That being said, beginner endurance athletes and those with long lapses in their training history can make good gains in fitness initially by doing any prolonged endurance activity. As your fitness improves, your gains in climbing-specific fitness will become more elusive unless you shift to activities directly related to your intended activity. For example, at this stage in his career Steve won't see much benefit to his climbing speed from swimming laps or paddling a canoe for hours on a lake (for him these can be very beneficial recovery workouts). However, a person with very limited endurance training background will see an improvement in overall fitness from these general exercises, which will translate into improved climbing performance. This principle is known as the *Specificity of Training*.

By *specificity*, we mean that the most effective training will be specific to the movements done, and at a similar speed and intensity of climbing. To a very large extent, elite-level swimmers principally swim for training, champion cyclists ride, top runners run, and world-class skiers ski. A general sport like alpinism can include more nonspecific modalities than these traditional sports, especially in the early base-building period and for less athletically mature individuals. But the biggest benefits will come from preparing for and modeling the demands of alpine climbing as closely as possible. This is the reason top climbers spend so much time climbing.

As an alpinist seeking to improve your endurance you should give priority to weight-bearing exercise. This means running or hiking, especially uphill, which will be more specific training than swimming. Cycling is also a great general exercise. However, bikes are very efficient modes of transportation and this makes them less effective training tools from the time versus benefit standpoint. The sitting position on the bike means that you do not have to support your full body weight, which greatly reduces the energy cost of the exercise and the muscle mass used to propel yourself. Being strapped to a machine limits the range of motion, the coordination, balance, and variability of the footing required while climbing. You should not rely solely on cycling as a training mode. We have known some hard-core athletes who have gone so far as to remove the seat to avoid the temptation to sit down.

Swimming is another great exercise that has little carryover to alpine climbing. The prone position in swimming makes it so the heart has

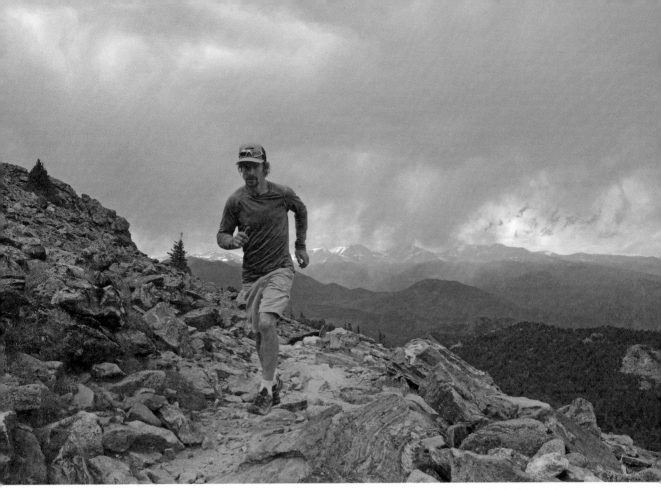

Running in Rocky Mountain National Park. *Photo: Eva House*

to work much less to pump the blood. The water also keeps the body cool, leaving more blood available for the working muscles. If this is beginning to sound like running and hiking should be emphasized in your basic preparation time, then you are getting the picture.

PREPARATION FOR SUCCESS

While the authors are fully aware of the value of lessons learned in the school of hard knocks, we have written this book in an attempt to help you chart a more direct path to your own alpine success.

We stated in chapter 1 that you can't learn to lead thin ice or poorly protected pitches of rock from the pages of a book, but you can prepare for success in a rational way. This will not only give you a better shot at tagging that summit, but also allow you to minimize the risk while you do it.

As we've discussed, athletes in mainstream sports train the component parts of their event many hundreds or thousands of times so that when their big day arrives it is merely a matter of putting those well-practiced components together. This gives them the physical skills as well as the mental confidence necessary to succeed.

Alpine climbers need to do the same thing. If the first time you lead a long runout pitch on loose rock is on your goal climb, you have not set yourself up for success. If carrying a heavy pack while dragging a sled to the 14,000-foot (4,267-meter) camp on the west buttress of Denali is the hardest day you've ever spent in the mountains, then you are very likely not going to have the physical and mental stamina to continue another seven days to the summit.

THE INDIVIDUALITY OF TRAINING

The individual nature of each athlete's response to training has made many a coach's hair turn gray. We are not machines who all respond the same way to a given input. Training prescriptions are not cookbook recipes, where mixing the same ingredients in the correct proportions will result in a perfect cake. Athletes are not cakes. Each of us has unique qualities we bring into this venture that results in our own unique response to it.

To paraphrase Renato Canova: The one thing we can be certain of if we apply the same training to a group of athletes, is that each individual will get a different response. The wisdom of this simple statement is lost on many coaches and athletes, but we will stress its importance. It is the basis for your critical analysis of every aspect of your training program. Since very few alpinists have the luxury of a personal coach, it will be very useful to know how best to regulate your own training to avoid the pitfalls that cause setbacks and lack of success in meeting performance goals.

This individuality comes from numerous sources: genetic predisposition, training history and athletic background, time constraints, age, gender, life's daily stresses and how you deal with them, your current fitness and health. All of these elements have a significant effect on your response to training. The modern popularity of spreadsheet-type training plans—along with the Internet gurus who espouse them—that list what workout you will be doing on a particular day two months from today, show a lack of understanding of this notion of individuality, and of gauging the training to match the body's response. These spreadsheets have an emotional appeal: They look so planned and neat and tidy, how could they not be a road map to excellence? If your body was a simple machine like a car, that road map might prove useful.

UNDERSTANDING THE LANGUAGE OF INTENSITY

The intensity of training determines the energy systems involved in producing the movements you are making. It also determines what types of muscle fibers (discussed in chapter 3) get recruited to do the work. Therefore it is important to understand and monitor the intensity of your training.

At any given instant, your metabolism exists somewhere along an energy continuum. Higher-intensity exercise requires a greater contribution of anaerobic energy supply than does lower-intensity work. These anaerobic energy pathways cannot be sustained for as long as aerobic metabolism; we'll discuss this in detail in the next chapter. High intensities feel harder. Low intensities feel like you can go for a long, long time. Think of sprinting full-out (high intensity) versus jogging slowly. By controlling the intensity of the training, you control both which types of *muscle fibers* get trained and which energy pathways are used.

The endurance required for alpinism, with its long duration of low-to-moderate-power outputs, is almost completely determined by the limitation of your aerobic metabolic processes. The implication of this important fact is that alpinists need to devote the vast majority of their training time to long duration, low- to moderate-intensity work that will enhance these aerobic qualities. Having a way to gauge intensity is a valuable training tool.

Speed, power output, and perceived effort are all ways of gauging the intensity of your training. Perceived effort is highly subjective and, as such, an unreliable way to gauge training intensity, although it is the most commonly used one. Speed monitoring is handy if you are running around a track. Power metering devices are great gadgets for cyclists. Unfortunately, neither speed, nor power measurements fit neatly into the constantly variable terrain and conditions of the alpinist, and perceived effort is not easily or accurately measured.

Other methods have been developed that can prove useful for the training we propose. In the next pages we will explain some of the various methods for determining training intensity along with their relative merits. Each has its place and its adherents. In the end they all are attempts to relate subtle, if not insensible, metabolic shifts to something you can perceive.

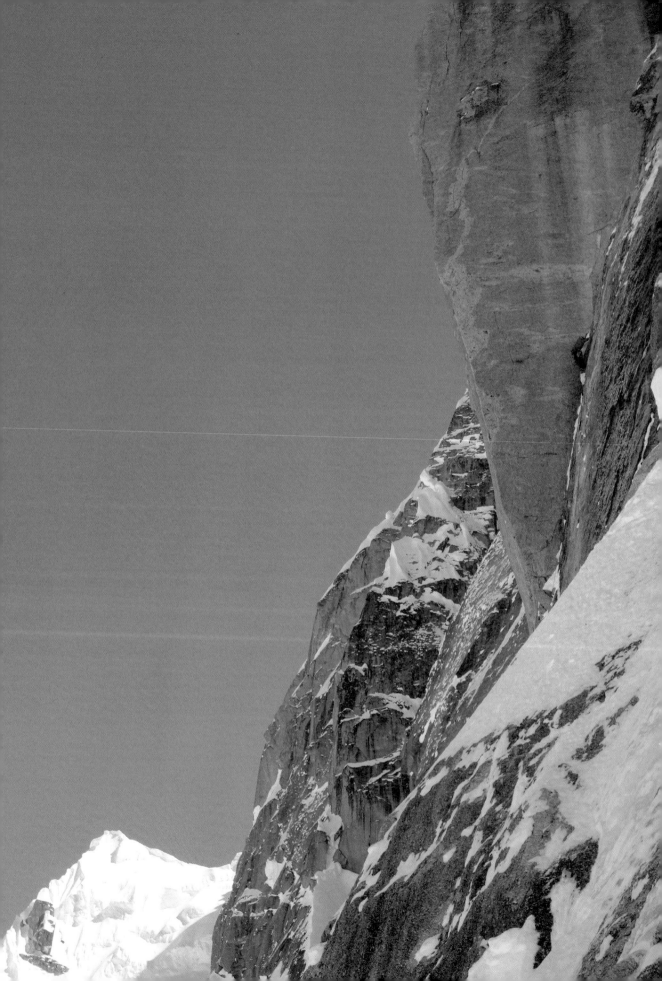

Heart-Rate Monitoring as an Intensity Guide

A simple way to gauge and quantify effort that does not put any burden on you to be observant is to use your heart rate. While not a 100 percent accurate reflection of intensity, heart-rate measurement is very useful because of its portability (by using a wrist-mounted monitor), adaptability to a variety of terrain and modes of training, and ability to give instant feedback. These all make heart-rate (HR) monitoring a valuable biofeedback tool. Even using the cheapest HR monitor will allow you to begin to recognize and relate to your body's subtle feedback system in a quantifiable way. You might surprise yourself when you begin to use an HR monitor and find out that what you had assumed was an easy effort is not so easy after all.

Heart-Rate Zones

Using percentages of maximum HR gives a reasonably good approximation of intensity for most athletes. This is the standard way of expressing intensity when other more accurate methods (such as a treadmill step test, which measures your blood lactate and oxygen uptake) are not available. The zones are defined as a percentage range of each individual's maximum heart rate and are described in detail in the next section. They range from Zone 1 for the lowest intensity aerobic training through 5 for maximal effort. It is important to recognize that these zones are highly individual depending mainly on your previous training background and genetics.

If you have spent most of your training time at medium to high intensities, your Zone 1 will be relatively low and small while your Zone 3 will cover a larger range of HR. This is more indication of the individuality of training.

Heart-rate zones were originally described and utilized by Scandinavian cross-country ski racers in the early 1980s, when wrist-mounted HR monitors were first developed and manufactured by Polarelectro of Finland. These handy devices allowed the skiers to monitor their

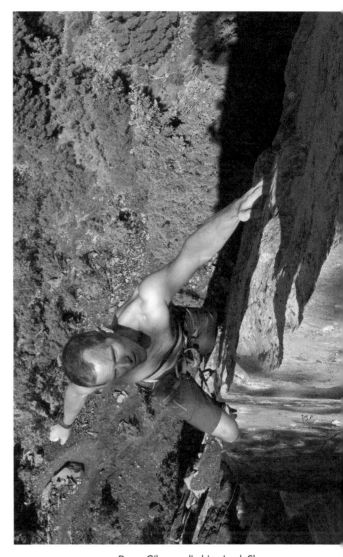

Bryan Gilmore climbing Look Sharp, a 5.11 route on the Pool Wall above Ouray, Colorado, while wearing a heart rate monitor to help him keep his intensity in check. Bryan is a very advanced rock climber and alpinist whose base fitness will benefit from climbing a stack of 5.11 pitches at a moderate heart rate. *Photo: Eva House*

Opposite: An unknown climber ascending the Prow pitch of the Bibler-Klewin route on Mount Hunter (14,573'/4,442m), Alaska. *Photo: Steve House*

training intensity in a way that had never been available before. Other endurance athletes, such as runners and swimmers, had long been able to control the intensity of training based on their speed. Because every track and pool is a known distance, most variables that affect training could be controlled. The coach could assign training intensity based on the athlete's current level of fitness, assessed from recent race or time trial paces. Because of the cross-country ski racer's use of variable terrain without any uniformity of distance or conditions, the control enjoyed by runners and swimmers was not available to ski coaches. The nature of climbing in the mountains more closely mimics that of cross-country skiing in terms of variability than it does running on a track, making a heart-rate monitor a useful training tool for alpinists.

Since the 1980s, the zone system (sometimes in a slightly modified form) has gained nearly universal acceptance as providing good, basic training guidelines for endurance sports. While you can indeed rely on your perception of effort, as mentioned before, this has proven to be a very poor indicator for most people, and we do not recommend relying on it for controlling training intensity. We encourage you to use a HR monitor for a least some of your training.

More (or harder) is not better. Use the full range of each given zone. Don't think that you must always be pushing the top end of each of these percentage ranges in order to get the benefits. For most of us, the typical prescribed 10 percentage point range will translate into a maximum of twenty beats and more likely in the seventeen to eighteen beat range. Allowing the intensity of your training to float around in each zone will hit all the physiological targets we are aiming for.

Recovery Zone (roughly 50 percent or less of max HR)

Below Zone 1 lies an intensity that plays a minor role in improving aerobic fitness. But this zone plays a major role in speeding recovery from the more demanding training sessions. You should feel better right after or within a few hours of completing one of these. It can be almost any form of light exercise and you may benefit most from a modality different than your primary one. One of our favorites for hammered legs is going for a swim. No specific duration is given in the accompanying charts because this is so individual. For some, a fifteen-minute walk before bed will be perfect. Some will use daily foam rolls or yoga. Others may find a one hour slow jog does the trick. Heart rate for recovery workouts should be roughly 20 percent below the upper Zone 1 heart rate.

Wearing an HR Monitor While Climbing

If you routinely rock climb, in a gym or at a crag, it can be interesting to wear an HR monitor while climbing. You will quickly identify what types of routes and what difficulty level elevates your heart rate to which zone. On routes near your limit, you will see your HR spike as you approach and execute the crux. You can also teach yourself how low you must bring your HR while resting at a good stance before launching into more difficult climbing. This is a valuable training modality if you incorporate technical rock climbing in your training plan.

Heart Rate Zones

INTENSITY	APPROXIMATE % OF MAX HR	FEELING	VENTILATION
Recovery	<55%	Very Light	Conversational
Zone 1	55–75%	Easy Breathing	Conversational
Zone 2	75–80%	Medium	Nose Breathing
Zone 3	80–90%	Fun Hard	Short Sentences
Zone 4	90–95%	Hard	No Talking
Zone 5	N/A	Maximum	N/A

Your heart rate is a very good indicator of the intensity of exercise and is easily monitored while you train. While the percentage of max heart rate is statistically accurate, it may or may not best reflect your individual fitness state. Ventilation, on the other hand, will always give immediate and accurate feedback as to the state of your metabolism. Learning to recognize the subtle shifts in your breathing can be useful and rewarding.

Zone 1: Basic Endurance (roughly 60–70 percent of max HR)

This is easy-paced training. The distinction between the top of Zone 1 and bottom of Zone 2 is nebulous. We use 10 percent below the top of Zone 2 (the aerobic threshold which is defined below), as the upper limit of Zone 1.

We will delve into more detail on this subject later but in the meantime consider these two simple facts:

- Harder is not better when it comes to the development of your aerobic threshold. Intensity is not a substitute for duration when it comes to increasing this capacity, and in fact an overreliance on intensity can diminish aerobic capacity.

- Zones 1 and 2 are the intensities you will spend the vast majority of your time in. Improving your aerobic base will pay bigger dividends in alpine climbing than time spent improving any other fitness quality because it allows you to sustain higher submaximal climbing speeds for longer times. It also speeds recovery from hard climbs and workouts. Ultimately, your pace will be faster for a lower energetic cost.

There are several important training implications from these facts that will become more and more evident as you read on.

The world's elite endurance athletes spend more than 85 percent of their training volume at these low intensities (Zones 1 and 2); do not let these zone's ease fool you into thinking that they do not offer significant training benefits. This is the work that does the most to establish the endurance base, which will be explained in detail in chapter 3. This zone has the least reliance on specificity so a variety of training modalities such as climbing, approaching climbs, hiking, and running can be used with decent results. This allows for increased volume without overuse and boredom. The benefits of this aerobic endurance training are best accrued from frequent long-duration training sessions at this low intensity.

For some of you Zones 1 and 2 will be the hardest zones to train in. You may find that you can barely jog, or can only hike uphill very slowly, before you must begin mouth breathing or your speech becomes disrupted and your heart rate starts to climb right through Zone 2 and into Zone 3. This situation arises more often that you might think. We call this phenomenon Aerobic Deficiency Syndrome, these people are forced to rely on the contributions of their anaerobic energy pathways even to do slow-paced work. We have seen many such athletes. If you

Ski mountaineering, being weight bearing and mimicking the environment and motions of mountaineering, is great alpine-climbing-specific training. Julian Alps, Slovenia. *Photo: Marko Prezelj*

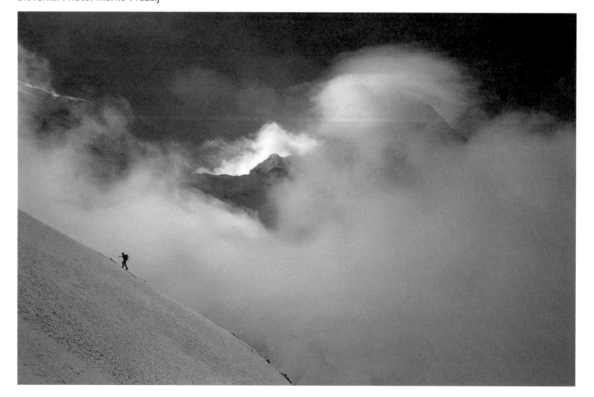

find yourself short of breath at low intensities and low heart rates, or if you are unable to carry on a conversation while hiking up the approach trail, then you really need to read Mark Twight's essay "TINSTAAFL" and understand chapter 3. There is a cure; we'll give you a prescription for it in this book, but it takes time and patience.

Zone 2: No Man's Land
(roughly 70–80 percent of max HR)

This is often referred to as a "conversational pace." You will be able to speak in complete sentences with your training partner, and the pace should feel relaxed and easy. To find the upper end of this zone, start by exercising slowly while breathing through your nose only. As you increase the intensity/speed gradually, note the point at which this nose breathing becomes noisy and labored or continuous conversation becomes impossible. This is the upper end of Zone 2.

This reference point corresponds to what exercise physiologists call the aerobic threshold (AeT). For reference: during a blood lactate test this would be the point at which the level of blood lactate concentration would have risen 1mMol/L above its baseline amount. Aerobic threshold power output is the single most important measure of a person's aerobic system. Thus it is the most important measure of endurance for an alpine climber.

For the well trained, this intensity is sometimes referred to by coaches as "black hole training." For the fit, this intensity is too hard to be easy but not hard enough to elicit the positive effects of high-intensity training. It carries with it a burden of fatigue unworthy of its benefits. Zone 1 will therefore make up the bulk of your base training if you have a very strong background of aerobic endurance training.

However, for those with little aerobic training history (referred to as Aerobic Deficiency Syndrome) this zone can be used for virtually all aerobic base training. The reason is that the pace at this intensity will be quite slow and therefor there will be little accumulation of neuromuscular fatigue and this effort level won't even feel like training. Your perceptions here will often belie the intensity. With increasing aerobic capacity Zones 1 and 2 grow as the aerobic threshold moves upward while Zones 3 and 4 narrow in terms of HR and metabolism

Intensity versus Duration

The most common refrain used by amateur athletes about including larger volumes of easy training into their programs is that they do not have time. They have a limited number of hours to train per week. With this limitation, they are easily tempted into the thinking that they can make up with intensity what they are not doing with volume. Of course, adding intensity does improve your fitness quickly. However, without a strong base of aerobic support, training at higher intensity will never allow you to maximize your fitness potential. Our goal with this book is to explain how to maximize your fitness, not give you a quick-fix prescription.

Long ago, coaches recognized the impressive results that high-intensity training had on their charges. Like most of today's acolytes of intensity, they thought, "If a little is good, more must be better." In other words, why waste our time training slow when we could train fast in less time? Competition, especially at the world-class level, is unforgiving and provides the ultimate test of training theory. The final outcome of these battles of training ideology has been that athletes who supplemented a huge base of aerobic endurance training with event-specific high-intensity work had much better outcomes than athletes who relied on a steady diet of high-intensity training. A historical review of the improvement in times that have occurred in the distance events in rowing, swimming, and running during the past fifty years is a powerful demonstration of the evolutionary nature of training theory. These sports make good case studies because of their simplicity and the minor equipment improvements during that period.

In the parlance of our time: Endurance training has already "Been there, done that" many times over. The test results, verified in the competitive arenas of the world throughout much of the twentieth century, tell the same story: An endurance athlete cannot achieve maximal performance on a diet of high-intensity training.

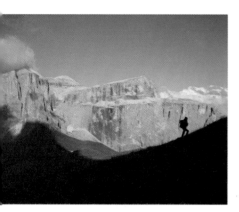

Approaching the Langkofel (10,436', 3,181m) in the Dolomites of South Tyrol, Italy. *Photo: Steve House*

and are squeezed into the remaining higher heart rates as the athlete becomes aerobically more powerful.

To be clear: Low intensity does not mean slow in well-conditioned athletes. Those who have spent the time to maximally develop their aerobic capacity can maintain prolonged high speeds (in conventional sports, typically 80–85 percent of race pace) at their aerobic threshold. A high aerobic threshold will allow you to make a strenuous approach with a heavy pack at a nice, fast pace while easily carrying on a conversation with your partner. It will mean arriving at the base of the route without spending much of your precious energy reserves, you will arrive in a refreshed state, rather than already being tired before you set foot on the actual climbing route. Long slow distance (sometimes called LSD) is a misused phase that does not describe the kind of training we are proposing here. A different term long easy distance (LED) fits this training philosophy much better.

Zone 3: Uppermost Aerobic Training (roughly 80–90 percent of max HR)

While still considered aerobic training, Zone 3 is of a different nature than Zone 1 and 2. At this intensity, the increase in speed requires the muscles to up their game. Glycolysis becomes the dominant source for ATP, both in the slow twitch muscle fibers and as more fast twitch fibers get recruited. Lactate levels begin to rise more sharply with the increased pace. Lactate accumulation remains at levels sustainable for up to an hour in well trained athletes with no performance degradation. Because of the high energy demands to sustain these speeds and the duration that can be sustained at this intensity both the aerobic and glycolytic systems get a hefty training stimulus from Zone 3 training. For the less well trained, this intensity will have a strong muscular endurance effect because the limit to this endurance is imposed by the aerobic capacity of those fast twitch fibers needed to sustain this output.

The upper end of this intensity zone is defined by the lactate threshold (the speed at which lactate begins to accumulate faster that it can be removed). Beyond the lactate threshold every athlete is operating on borrowed time and will be forced to slow the pace. Most athletes very quickly develop an intuitive sense for what this feels like. In Zone 3, you should still feel like you have another gear that you could shift into to go even faster at any time should you desire. At the upper end of this zone your breathing will still be rhythmic and controlled but become much deeper.

Many people see Zone 3 training as the magic intensity, the one stop shop of endurance training. They assume that since this zone has such a powerful training effect it can be used almost exclusively to make endurance training more time efficient. Tempting as this may be we strongly caution you to not overutilize this intensity because it puts you into the utilization training modality, with all the pitfalls associated with that. Zone 3 training is seductive because it will give an immediate boost to anyone. This intensity should typically make up no more than 10 percent of the total annual training volume. For those with Aerobic Deficiency Syndrome, over use of this intensity can easily lead to a performance decline.

Zone 4: The Anaerobic Zone (roughly 90–100 percent of max HR)

In this zone your metabolism will have shifted to one where a significant contribution of energy is coming from anaerobic metabolism. This mix of hard aerobic and anaerobic training is sometimes referred to as VO_2 max training because studies have shown that, for well-trained endurance athletes, this intensity can have the most beneficial effect on improving the maximum aerobic power. Make no mistake, this is hard training and the pace is sustainable only for a few minutes before you will be forced to slow down. An interval method of training is usually used since it allows repeated efforts at the hard intensity necessary to affect the desired adaptations. If the pace drops below the desired intensity due to fatigue, then the training effect will not be the one that was hoped for.

While it does give the maximum aerobic stimulus to your body, it also gives a significant stimulus to your anaerobic system. As you will learn in chapter 3, this can have a real downside in terms of your aerobic base if sustained for too long or done too often—especially if you do not maintain a large volume of aerobic base training at the same time.

Your breathing in this zone will not allow more than a word or two being gasped out, and when you stop you'll be breathing about as deeply as you can. The classic pose for athletes having finished an effort like this is bent at the waist with hands on knees supporting the upper body and breathing very deeply and rapidly. This posture frees up the breathing muscles to pump air in and out of the lungs. It also lowers the head to the level of the heart, reducing the required blood pressure the heart must supply to get blood to the brain. For even top endurance athletes, this hard training makes up perhaps only 2–6 percent of their yearly volume.

For this zone to produce its best results in terms of increasing your aerobic power, many top coaches carefully limit the amount of high-intensity (Zone 4) training they prescribe until they see their athletes' aerobic threshold pace come to within 10 percent (or even 5 percent for world class athletes) of the pace they can sustain at their personal anaerobic threshold. Only then can they be assured that the aerobic system has the base to support this higher-intensity work. Bear in mind that the sports these coaches and athletes are training for have much shorter events using much higher intensity work than does alpine climbing. While there definitely can be some benefit to include a small fraction of Zone 4 training for a well-conditioned climber with a high aerobic threshold, the moderate intensity of long days in the mountains do not place much of a premium on VO$_2$ max. For the alpinist, the time and energy spent on this type of training is likely to result in insignificant gains in fitness. That time would probably be better spent doing Zone 1, 2, and 3 training, or spent on strength training or specific climbing training.

If you are getting the idea that this type of training is not a priority, then you are right. For events lasting less than two hours it is key to

Interval Training

Training at Zone 4 intensities are often referred to as *hard aerobic training*. Conducted properly it will be quite exhausting. But it can provide a valuable stimulus to developing muscular and cardiac endurance and should be included, especially during the later periods of an advanced athlete's training. Like any other training the adaptation to it is a result of the duration of the training load. The problem is that due to the exhaustive nature of this hard training it is not possible to do much of it at one time.

Intermittent training has been around for over a hundred years in various forms but we owe the popular modern variation of it to one man. In the late 1930s German track coach Woldemar Gerschler coined the term *interval training* when describing his method of intermittent training where high-intensity work bouts were separated by intervals of rest. His theory was that it was during these intervals of rest that the most important changes to the heart muscle occurred. By repeating relatively short bouts of high-intensity training separated by rest intervals the athlete could accomplish a high volume of high-intensity training in one session. Doing so resulted in unique

adaptations, and this gave birth to the modern use of this intermittent training method.

The basic principle of interval training is that you go hard, then rest and then repeat over and over again. Of course there are many variations of how many repetitions, how long each repetition is, how hard the intensity is, and how much and what kind of rest to use during the recovery interval to get the best effect. Hundreds upon hundreds of studies have been done on interval training to determine what works best. The ultimate answer to the questions posed is . . . it depends. It depends on:

- What training effect is desired.
- What training background the athlete has.
- When in the training cycle the interval training occurs.

What you need to understand about interval training is that it is an important component of training. It is a very effective use of the training time. It will yield its best results when imposed on a solid aerobic base and done in conjunction with a moderately high volume of purely aerobic training. But most importantly, it should not be considered a shortcut to fitness, nor a stand-alone method of training.

improving performance. For events like an alpine climb that will last at least six to eight hours, its contribution to performance drops to near zero; we explain it here primarily for completeness and to give you a broader perspective on aerobic training.

Zone 5: Maximum Effort

This is maximum effort, which can only be sustained for perhaps twenty seconds to one minute. Heart rate plays no part in monitoring this zone because the shortness of the effort means the cardiac response will not be in proportion to the intensity. For this zone you just go as hard as you can. It is a very effective way to build strength, power, and power endurance in the big muscle groups used to go uphill. A good example of this intensity is climbing a route's crux for several moves at your maximum ability—as is common in bouldering. As we explain in chapters 4 and 5, even endurance athletes can benefit greatly from training in this zone to increase specific strength and power.

Determining Your Maximum Heart Rate— Not for the Faint of Heart (Literally)

One of the more common ways of defining intensity zones is to use percentages of one's maximum heart rate. We prefer a more individualized approach to determining zones and several options are discussed in great detail on Uphillathlete.com. But, here's a way to go about determining your own max HR.

First, forget the commonly espoused method of subtracting your age from 220 to get your maximum heart rate. These simple equations come from statistical analyses of large populations and represent an average value for the population at large. While this method may give a good indication of your personal maximum (if you happen to be average), don't count on it. These formulas do not reflect individual variability, but have gained popularity due to their simple application and the fact that a person does not have to endure the pain of the actual test.

The only way to find your actual max HR is to do a max HR test. A max test is not to be taken lightly, as it requires severe physical stress to elicit a maximal HR response. You must be healthy, well rested, and very highly motivated.

The test involves a gradual warm-up that starts very easy and becomes progressively harder over the course of fifteen minutes. The last two or three minutes should have you sweating and breathing moderately but not hard. Your perception at the end of this warm-up should be that the effort was moderate, leaving you with a feeling of vigor (not fatigue and dread).

Without stopping to rest, run hard for two minutes up a hill with a grade steep enough (usually about 6–10 percent) to allow you to run but not so steep you are forced to hike. The last twenty seconds should be run as hard as you can will yourself to go to the point of complete exhaustion. If you collapse at the end, you have probably gone hard enough to elicit a maximum cardiac response. At the end of this two-minute test check your HR and it will be within five beats of your maximum heart rate.

Failure to achieve a maximum in this test is most commonly attributed to starting the test in a fatigued state (possibly from too hard a warm-up). If your muscles are tired and you have not recovered from previous efforts, the muscles will not be able to make maximal demands on the heart to supply oxygen. If this is the case, the effort will feel extremely hard, but the cardiac response will be submaximal.

Unless you are very well trained as a cyclist or have a low fitness level, it is very unlikely that you will be able to elicit a maximum cardiac response by cycling unless you stand up while peddling. This is due to the efficiency of the bike and the smaller muscle mass recruited for the work.

Other Forms of Monitoring Intensity

Lactate Monitoring

Much like the elaborate but common heart-rate monitors that can measure things previously only measured by doctors, a handheld device now exists that can give a snapshot of your intensity of effort at a level that twenty years ago required expensive and sophisticated physiology lab equipment.

This device is a portable blood lactate meter. In chapter 3 we'll discuss the metabolism of the muscle cell in some detail, but for now understand that lactate is a form of sugar that is a metabolic product of higher-intensity (anaerobic) energy production. It is produced when the energy demands of the muscle become too great to be met by purely aerobic metabolism. There is a direct correlation between the intensity of exercise and the amount of lactate in the bloodstream. Using a portable blood lactate monitor, it is possible to get a very good idea of the metabolic state inside the working muscles and determine just how hard you are working.

While these devices offer accurate measurement and are readily available, at $400–$500 each they are price prohibitive for most athletes not belonging to a team or club. They are mentioned here for the sake of completeness in our discussion rather than to overweight their importance for amateur athletes.

Breath Monitoring

The stimulus to breathe is largely a product of your autonomic nervous system, meaning that it is somewhat out of your control and luckily goes on without conscious thought. We tend to think of breathing as the inhalation of oxygen but the exhalation of CO_2 serves a very valuable purpose in balancing your body's pH (acid-base balance) level, which must be maintained within fairly narrow boundaries. The rate and depth of ventilation gives real-time feedback as to what metabolic processes are going on inside your working muscles. As explained in the above discussions on Zone 1 and 3 intensities, there are two important ventilatory markers for judging exercise intensity. While these are subtle and are best determined

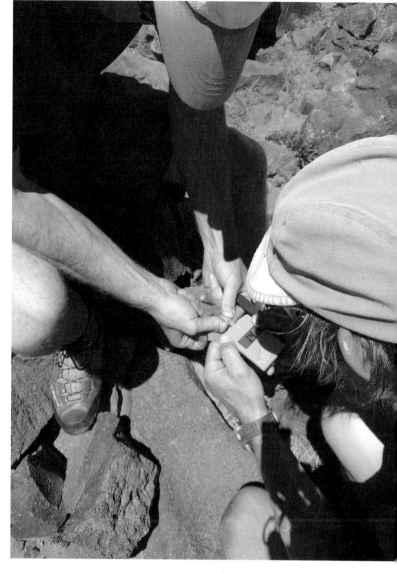

Measuring blood lactate after a climb of Mount Bachelor in Oregon.
Photo: Steve House collection

during a laboratory treadmill test, the astute athlete can sense and make use of them to give insight into the metabolic processes that are driving his muscles. See our discussion of intensity zones earlier for a more complete explanation of these ventilatory markers.

TRAINING CYCLES

Proper training is cyclic. It follows the principle of modulation: Harder training is followed by easier times, which are again followed by harder (stressful) times. This is the two-phase cycle of easy/hard.

Some other variations of modulation are: easy/medium/hard or easy/hard/medium. The main concept is training and recovery. Simple. All of the coaching and science is just to make it work faster, better, and safer. (And to be more fun too.)

You will notice that these cycles follow at all levels. From second to second: muscle contraction/rest cycles. From minute to minute, day to day, week to week, and month to month. This is the basic concept. The body needs stimulus to move away from its place of rest to improve, then it needs a time to make the changes that allow it to adapt. That is the bare bones of training.

These cycles require time. If you do not mentally prepare yourself to stay the course and allow your body the time it needs to change and restructure itself, you will fail in your efforts—either by force (an injury or stagnation) or by disappointment and the resulting lack of motivation.

Each period supports the one following it, and is supported by all the periods that have preceded it. Each period must be viewed in the context of fitting into the overall plan. Shortcutting or rushing any of them will likely leave you unprepared for the stresses of the next period.

When you are training, you are not just training your body, but you are also, maybe even primarily, training your mind.

PERIODIZATION

Coaches use the term *periodization* to describe the phases of a full training cycle. The more advanced the athlete and the loftier the goals, the more important it becomes to periodize the training—break the training cycle into discrete segments, each with its own focus. This allows you to emphasize specific training in an additive process where the training that has gone before supports that which is about to be undertaken.

The structured and cumulative method can be compared to the more normal approach among climbers of training everything all the time in no particular order. This random approach can provide good results when used by climbers of lower abilities. Just as a person looking to run her first marathon and hoping to break four hours can do just about any sort of training at any time and see benefits from it, a beginner looking to climb his first mountain can use almost any training approach to enhance his performance on the climb. But when a top marathon runner looks to improve her time she must very carefully target specific mental, physical, and technical shortcomings to have a good chance of improving. Using a random approach will not give her the best result. If you are an experienced and capable climber looking to continue advancing in your abilities, you need a focused, structured approach.

The complete cycle for alpinism will usually be annual due to the seasonal nature of the main climbing season. The value of periodizing your training has been understood since the time of ancient gladiators, but we owe much of its current refined state to the work of Soviet and Eastern Bloc sports scientists. They were the first to lay out in detail the periodization schedule for track and field athletes during the 1960s. Periodization allows you to focus on shorter-term goals of training by breaking the long term down into segments, each with its own focus and physiological function. There is a good deal of room for overlap of these periods in a sport like alpine climbing, with its heavy reliance on basic endurance and strength. This has the further advantage of more variety and less routine in your training.

There are traditional designations for these training periods. In chronological order they are: Recovery, Transition, Base, and Specific.

Training Periods

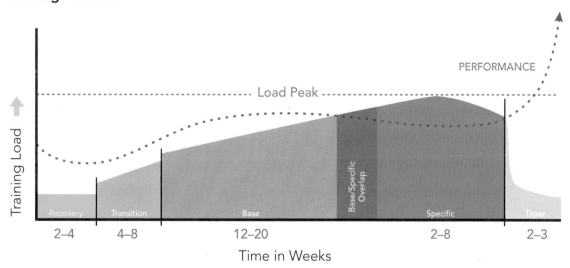

This graph illustrates the guiding principle of progression in training. It takes time for your body to absorb the training load and adapt to the stresses imposed on it by training. If you give it a chance to adapt, what once seemed impossible can become routine. The performance curve lags behind the training load curve, and it is not until the load is reduced that the true benefits of this gradual and progressive nature of training will come to full fruition.

Below are general descriptions of each period. How to structure and execute each of these periods will be discussed in later chapters. We will also break these periods down into shorter pieces that help you plan your daily and weekly workouts.

Recovery Period

Alpine climbing at a high level is very physically, psychologically, and emotionally taxing. It is critical that you are well recovered from any previous serious and demanding climb(s), even if unsuccessful, before you embark on either another hard climb or a new training season. The fatigue of the central nervous system is one of the hardest to sense and often takes the longest to recover from. The length of this recovery is determined by the demands of the climb(s) that have gone before it. Take a break from climbing. Do other recreational activities at a low level. Have fun. This can all be difficult for the Type A athlete who's jonesing to get back into the next training cycle for the next big objective. Taking this necessary short break of at least one to three weeks refreshes both body and mind before starting the next cycle. If you are normally driven to be active but feel lethargic, there is probably a good reason and that reason may be an underlying fatigue.

Transition Period

When beginning a new yearly training plan, especially if you have not been following any sort of structured program recently, it is important to give your body a chance to accustom itself to the routine and stress of regular training. If you are a seasoned athlete, this period can be as short as two to three weeks. For beginners or those coming off the couch after a long break, it should be eight weeks. If you are in great shape from a previous season and only need a short recovery break then it can be shortened to six weeks or in some cases even four weeks among the well conditioned.

In this phase, you'll spend your time gradually becoming an athlete again. Many people struggle with this period because they come into it highly motivated, rested, and hungry to get back to training. They have new goals, renewed energy, a new training plan, and are stoked from recent success. This can lead to prematurely ramping back to full-fledged training loads before their bodies are ready. Even though the workouts will be somewhat unstructured and quite general in nature, the training load must still be progressive and gradual in nature. You may not even train daily in the beginning of this period, but you are still setting the stage for some real training ahead. The strength plan you follow will be the General Strength Routine detailed in chapter 7.

Base Period

"Train your weakness. Race your strength."

— EDDIE BORYSEWICZ, renowned cycling coach

The purpose of this period is to build a general resistance to fatigue by increasing the capacity of each of the fundamental physiological qualities that contribute to your alpine climbing success, and most importantly your aerobic threshold.

This is the period where you put the money in the bank. It is the longest and most important training period. The bigger your bank balance is, the more hard work you will be capable of in the specific workouts to come; this will, in turn, take you to a new, higher fitness level and offer you the best chance of success on your primary objective.

The adaptation of the aerobic systems necessary to maximize your oxidative energy resources is one that responds to gentle, frequent coaxing rather than infrequent, brutal flogging. During this phase, volume is the key. The more you train, the bigger the base you have to work from. The intensity needs to be kept low to moderate on most workouts, or you will not be able to achieve the necessary high volume.

If you are a mountain professional, such as a guide, or you are a very active amateur alpine climber who has spent one hundred-plus days in the mountains each year for the last several years, you are off to a great start. You've already developed a substantial base of aerobic training. Your basic aerobic and strength capacities are probably already high, which will allow you to move to a more advanced training regimen. For less-active amateurs who get out for long, full days of climbing fewer than six to seven days a month, you will need to pay particular attention to this phase since your basic endurance and strength is likely underdeveloped.

Dealing with the Fatigue

A low but somewhat persistent level of fatigue is not only likely, but to be expected through much of this Base Period due to chronic glycogen depletion. Training while a bit tired from time to time during the Base Period will enhance the training effect. Just don't expect to perform record-breaking times on workouts or climbs during this period. You'll likely be a bit flat through most of it. Nonetheless, you should see a general improvement in your basic fitness at the low-intensity levels. If you do intend to engage in a harder effort or challenging climb, you can restore your energy by taking a couple of very easy days before the effort.

The Importance of the Base Period

For the less-experienced alpine climbers and those without much of an endurance sports background, this will be not only the main training period, but it may be the *only* training period you use to prepare for the big climb. For those climbers, this type of training, despite its mundane and repetitive nature, will yield the best return on time invested and help you develop the base needed in the future that you will require to handle higher training loads and achieve bigger climbing goals. For most alpinists, this key period will last twelve weeks at minimum. For the very fit who have several years of serious training under their belts and who are coming off a successful previous season of training and climbing, it can be as short as eight to ten weeks. For those with minimal to no structured previous endurance training, or heading off on an extended expedition, it can last sixteen to twenty-four weeks. Essentially, you cannot overdo this period. Your bank account can never be too big.

To emphasize just how important this phase is to *all* endurance sports, consider the 800-meter track event. This is an event that world-class male athletes contest in about 1:43. That is one minute and forty-three seconds. Hardly what most of us would consider a very long time in terms of endurance. The 800 meter is considered to be the track event most reliant on a high level of anaerobic/glycolytic energy supply. Yet, for decades successful 800-meter runners have followed a training prescription that has a heavy emphasis on the Base Period with training volumes as high as eighty to one hundred miles of running per week. During this phase, 90 percent of these miles are run at less than the athlete's lactate threshold (LT); in other words in Zone 3 or below. So even for this short endurance event with its heavy reliance upon anaerobic energy sources, the best 800-meter runners in the world spend many, many hours training their aerobic system. If an 800-meter runner needs that much aerobic training, does it not stand to reason that an alpine climber, whose event lasts many hours or days, needs it even more?

How Can I Tell if It's Working?

The results of the training you do during the Base Period will be slow to accumulate and subtle to detect. Don't expect to see or feel any significant fitness gains before four weeks. After twelve weeks, you will really begin to see and feel the effects of a consistent, gradual, and progressive training plan with its big volume of low-intensity training. This slow adaptation is due to the structural changes that are going on at the cellular level in your muscles. The protein synthesis necessary to grow new capillaries and increase mitochondrial mass takes weeks for measurable changes to occur, and will take years of consistent training to maximize. Each year can build on the previous ones. During this phase, your heart rates will be mostly in Zone 1, with some training in Zone 2 and occasional sessions of Zone 3. Athletes with several years of solid training will be able to use more Zone 3 intensity because they have a more well-developed aerobic physiology to support these harder efforts. The strength training will also be periodized according to the details laid out in the strength chapters. Train well through this phase and you will be setting yourself up for success. Eliminate or shortcut this phase and you'll never reach your potential.

Specific Period

Toward the end of the Base Period and phasing into the beginning of this period, we start to add in special workouts that create a more sport-specific training load on the structural and functional systems directly related to climbing. In these, we put some of the fundamental qualities we have been developing together in one workout to simulate physiological stress and conditions you will encounter while climbing. This means we may begin to combine uphill interval training with carrying water jugs, or combining uphill interval training with alpine climbing on a route that is easy for you. This is very demanding training, both mentally and physically, and will give the best results if undertaken after extensive preparation during the previous periods. Adequate recovery before and after the principle workouts is essential.

The Specific training period can have some overlap in time with the Base Period to allow for a shift in emphasis from general volume to more focused sport-specific volume. As the special workouts progress to become more challenging, the interim workouts will become less intense and serve the function of maintenance of basic endurance as well as recovery. Near the end of this period will come the final tune-up training in which you put all the individual components you have worked on together into some test climbs. The better your preparation and the bigger your aerobic base, the more specific training you can handle and benefit from.

It is this period where the concept, popular among many top alpinists, of using only climbing for all their training, gets its physiological justification. These seasoned climbers have a high enough level of basic fitness and skill level from their years spent in the mountains that they can focus their training in a very specific way and see great returns. They are actually adhering to sound training periodization theory. Their basic fitness supports this higher specific training load. The more advanced the athlete in any sport, the more he needs specific training to improve. Again, those who do not have the years of accumulated fitness and that have more conventional working lives will benefit greatly in the long term from giving a priority to establishing a solid base upon which to add Specific training.

FATIGUE AND RECOVERY: HOW THEY ARE RELATED

Training makes you weaker, not stronger. It is during the recovery that you become stronger.

Before delving too far into the nitty-gritty of training we need to establish a common understanding about the importance of rest and recovery in the overall scheme of training. From the earlier discussions and the figures on the training effect (pages 46–47), you know that your body's initial reaction to the stress of training is to become weaker. Then, after a recovery period you achieve a higher level of fitness than before the training bout. But just what goes on in this recovery period? Is it bed rest? Is it reduced volume or intensity? How long do you need to recover before the next workout?

These important considerations dictate that correct training is a balancing act. Later, when we address overtraining, you will see through Steve's unfortunate experience that while many people are capable of writing a training plan for you, the trick is the successful implementation of that plan so that you arrive at your highest level of fitness at the correct time. This is where so many athletes get it wrong and what we hope to help you avoid.

The most underestimated component of a training plan is the recovery. Some level of fatigue will be your nearly constant companion when training. Fatigue is your body's feedback to you about the training. Learning how to interpret that feedback and respond appropriately will be fundamental to successful training.

Causes of Fatigue

Fatigue affects several of the body's systems and manifests in a number of different ways. Some of these fatigue symptoms resolve themselves almost immediately when you reduce the intensity of exercise. Others require several hours to complete the restoration process and still others may take several days to fully resolve. Without going into too much depth on the subject, the various forms of fatigue originate from:

- An accumulation of metabolic by-products in the active muscle cells

- A depletion of key catalytic elements within muscle cells

- A depletion of intramuscular glycogen stores

- A depletion of the neurological components that effect the transmission of nerve impulses that create muscle contractions

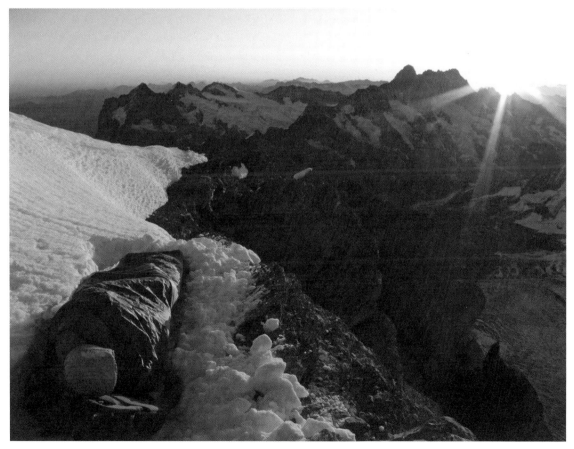

Richard Petersen getting in some recovery after climbing the Eiger North Face. *Photo: Steve House*

Response to Fatigue

The one thing that all the symptoms of fatigue share is your body's response. The response to all fatigue is a reduction in power output: You slow down and, in some cases, dramatically. This is the result of a reduced motor output from the central nervous system (CNS). When your brain receives the sensory input indicating an advanced stage of any of the various forms of fatigue, it responds by reducing its stimulus to the muscles. So that burn you feel in your legs is a symptom, but the cause of your slowing pace is your brain's response of reducing the activation signals it is sending to the muscles. This may seem like a silly distinction in the real world but in fact it holds a key to both your body and mind's adaptation to training.

Many studies have pointed to the anticipatory nature of this deeply ingrained self-preservation instinct. A dramatic disruption in your body's homeostasis triggers a poorly understood but well-documented CNS response to protect the organism against irreversible damage. By repeatedly upsetting this homeostasis with training stimuli, the CNS begins to raise its threshold of alarm, which then allows you to push new limits in your training with a less-dramatic CNS reaction. The brain is the most powerful tool in your training arsenal.

Of course it is essential to create fatigue through training in order for the training effect to occur. And, it is most likely that the fatigue you create will be a mix of some or all of the above-mentioned forms of fatigue. All of these forms require a recovery period of reduced stress to the involved systems in order for them to adapt, repair, and grow stronger.

Earlier in this chapter we looked at the cycle of fatigue and adaptation that makes up the training effect. The following chart puts into perspective the idea that the various systems affected by training adapt at different rates.

Recovery and How to Enhance It

Adaptation is the process through which the body restores its *homeostasis* (the state of internal biological equilibrium). It does this through a number of processes, not all of which are well understood but many of which seem to be enhanced by adopting certain recovery strategies. The term *recovery strategy* refers to the process of actively aiding the body's restoration of its homeostasis and therefore its adaptation to the training load. All this is done with the end result of allowing you to return to training sooner than would be possible without recovery.

Fatigue

The study of the causes of fatigue in athletes makes up an entire branch of exercise science. The work started in earnest during World War II when Harvard researchers began to seek a better understanding of fatigue to help those exposed to the rigors of war. Decades of research now allow us a much better understanding of the complexities of fatigue. For those interested in further pursuing this fascinating look at what limits human performance, we recommend first and foremost the bible of endurance training: *Lore of Running* by Dr. Tim Noakes, a pioneer in the study of fatigue and originator of the central governor theory. Another great source of information about fatigue is the website Sportscientist.com.

Recovery and Supercompensation

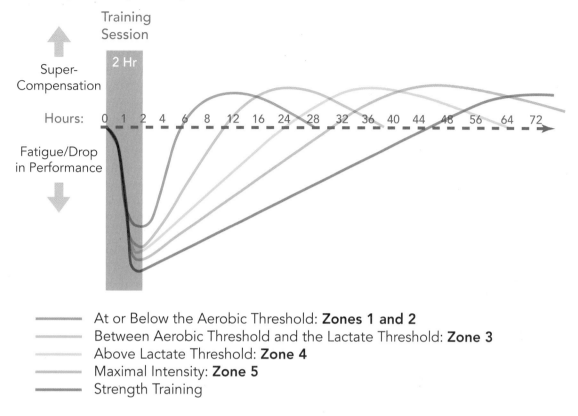

- At or Below the Aerobic Threshold: **Zones 1 and 2**
- Between Aerobic Threshold and the Lactate Threshold: **Zone 3**
- Above Lactate Threshold: **Zone 4**
- Maximal Intensity: **Zone 5**
- Strength Training

Recovery and supercompensation times after a two-hour training session of various intensities. The vertical scale is purely qualitative but the horizontal scale is in hours. While there is some interpersonal variability to these numbers, the originator of this scale collected data on hundreds of swimmers over many years to arrive at these values. It has been your authors' experience that these values hold quite well. Reproduced from *The Science of Winning* by Jan Olbrecht, courtesy of F&G Partners Publishing.

For athletes who are pushing the limits of the training load that their bodies can absorb, recovery strategies become an integral part of the overall plan. For beginners and those who are time limited in the amount of training they can fit in during a given week, recovery can still be a useful tool, but may not be so essential.

The following is a list of some of the simplest and most common methods used to enhance recovery.

Diet

Food is fuel, and athletes need high-octane fuel to power their Ferrari-like metabolisms. You need to eat with an eye toward recovery. What does this mean? Realize that heavy and prolonged exercise has a depleting effect on your nutritional stores. The sooner you can begin to get these building blocks into your system, the sooner they can start

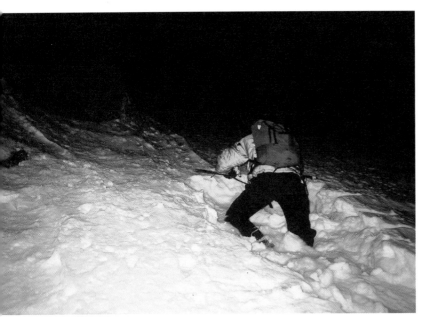

Vince Anderson breaking trail through waist-deep snow at 24,500' (7,500m) on the sixth and final day of climbing the Central Pillar of the Rupal Face of Nanga Parbat (26,660', 8,126m). Learning how to recover well during your training will teach you how to facilitate your recovery at bivouacs; an important component of success in multi-day alpine style climbing. *Photo: Steve House*

to repair the damage and depletion done by the training bout. For endurance sessions lasting longer than one hour we generally recommend carrying water mixed with a sports drink; this will reduce glycogen depletion during exercise.

A more complete discussion about eating for recovery is found in the nutrition chapter.

REM Sleep

We all have a general sense of how a good night's sleep or lack thereof affects our energy and outlook the next day. There is solid science to back up your seat-of-the-pants feeling.

Quality sleep is vital for the recovery process. A lot of important stuff happens during *REM* (rapid eye movement) *sleep* that aids your body in repairing damage inflicted by training. Much of that rebuilding comes about as a result of various hormones released during sleep, which then trigger certain genes to begin producing the proteins needed to make you stronger. REM sleep is a critical phase of sleep that is not definitively understood but we do know that it occurs in bouts of 90–120 minutes throughout the night and it involves a state of very deep relaxation that aids the recovery process. Studies have shown that two of the best stimulators for the release of your body's natural growth hormone, known as *Somatotropin* or GH1, are REM sleep and vigorous exercise. GH1, produced in the pituitary gland, is the principal signal to the genes responsible for muscle growth. Growth hormone is one of the body's primary tools for adapting to higher training loads. Enhancing its production is an easy and smart way to become a stronger climber.

Anything that gets in the way of REM sleep is going to have a serious impact on your recovery. Ever spend a fitful night on a cramped bivy ledge? How recovered did you feel the next morning when it was time to tackle the rest of the climb? But getting even an hour of deep sleep during a break or bivy can have an amazingly refreshing effect. If these experiences ring true for you, then you know what we are talking about. And those who can fall asleep easily anywhere have a valuable gift to use for alpine climbing.

Massage

Stiff and tight muscles are often the most obvious sign that you have been working your body hard. Endurance activities involve many repetitions of the same or very similar movements. This repetition often results in acute inflammation of the muscles, which you perceive as stiffness. The inflammation actually stimulates some of the adaptations to the training, but it can be too much of a good thing. Massage by a skilled practitioner increases the blood circulation in tired muscles. Improved circulation speeds the replenishment of vital nutrients, reduces this muscular inflammation, and speeds recovery. This is the reason professional bike racers use massage after heavy training and between stages on multi-day races. It works! You may feel lethargic after a massage; we recommend drinking extra water after your massage and avoiding heavy training for the next twelve hours.

Recovery Workouts

These workouts should not be considered in the same way as normal training. While they do have a maintenance effect on aerobic qualities, their main use is to speed the recovery process. While it may seem counterintuitive that more exercise will do anything other than deplete your already-taxed reserves, these very low-intensity sessions improve circulation and flush the muscles as well as increasing aerobic enzyme activity.

Keep in mind the following when using recovery workouts:

- The intensity must feel very easy. More discussion of this is found in the section Understanding the Language of Intensity in this chapter.

- They are most commonly used by athletes who are stacking workouts as closely together as possible, usually twice a day, but can be helpful after an especially tough day in the mountains.

- Alternate modes of training such as cycling, paddling, and especially swimming will give needed relief to overused legs.

- Even a gentle walk can be a good recovery workout if you are really tired or feeling a little sick.

- Light exercise beats being sedentary for aiding recovery.

Ice Baths

This may sound more like punishment than recovery, but dunking tired legs—or even better, your whole body—into ice cold water has

Forty Years of Climbing

By Christophe Moulin

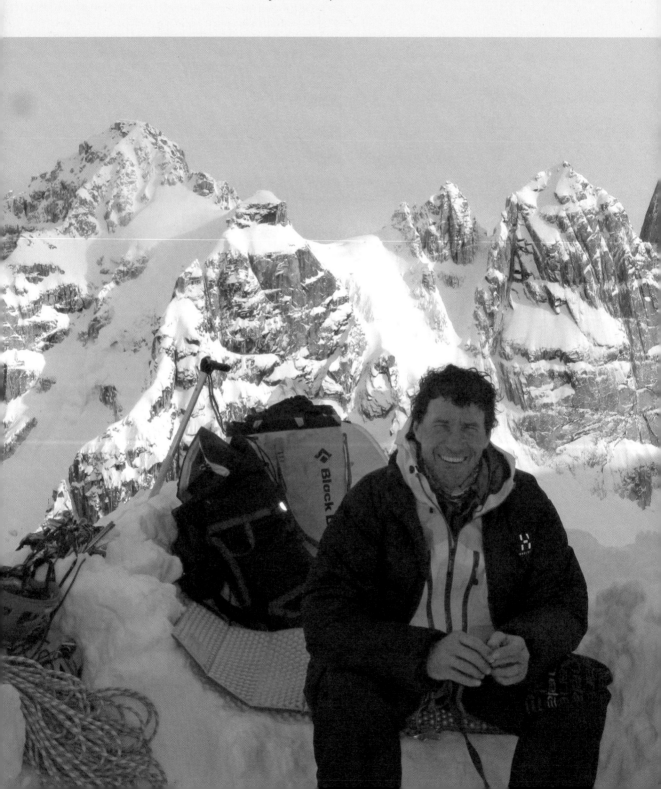

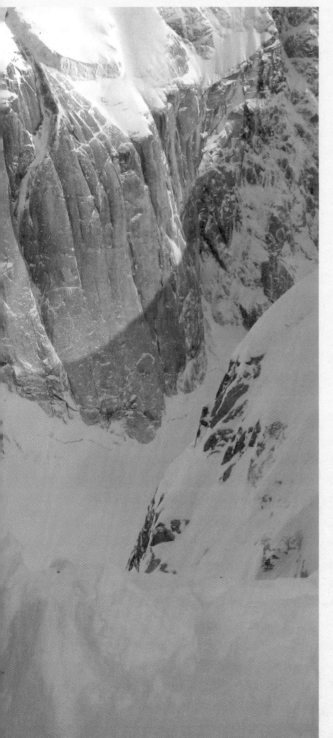

am fifty-four years old and I've been alpine climbing since I was fourteen. When I was in my early twenties, I spent lots of time partying and going to nightclubs with girls. When I wasn't partying, I climbed with my brother. When we'd climb, our day would take two or three times longer than the guidebook's projected time. We often returned to the valley late and exhausted.

Then I read an amazing book that changed my life: *The Seventh Grade* by Reinhold Messner. From that day I started to train. As my fitness improved my days in the mountains became easier and easier.

In 1993 I was on an attempt of the south pillar of Nuptse with Patrick Berhault, Gérard Vionnet, and Michel Fauquet. Patrick and I were super fit. In France, the day before we left for Nuptse, we headed out for a final training run. The result of all this training, and in fact overtraining, was detrimental. Our base camp was located at 5,100 meters (16,732 feet). Patrick only lasted three days before returning to France. I spent the whole week sleeping, or trying to sleep, with the worst headache imaginable.

While I was suffering at base camp and with Patrick on his way back to France, Michel was doing the work of carrying our gear to the base of the pillar, 400 meters (1,312 feet) above base camp. I wasn't able to help at all.

When Michel and I decided to head for the summit, as a team of two climbing alpine style, he was already exhausted; I was just starting to feel better. At the end of seven days of climbing, 300 meters (984 feet) below the summit, we abandoned our attempt. We had climbed all the most difficult sections. I will always have a bitter taste in my mouth from this failed attempt because I know that I didn't manage my training in an intelligent way, and this left us short of the summit.

Today I train younger climbers to become top alpinists. I am the director of the Groupes Excellence program of the Club Alpin Français. I try to teach them how to train technically and physically, but I never forget to emphasize two facets that are essential to me: rest and mental strength.

Rest is the foundation of training. It is essential to balance periods of training or climbing with periods of downtime.

I have learned to integrate mental training in a manner that is somewhat unconscious. Determination, motivation, visualization, courage, stress management, and channeling emotions must be concretely managed. These facets must never be considered as secondary priorities. Today 60 percent of what I teach young alpinists is management of the mental aspects of performance. That is to say, it is imperative to rest the body and the mind.

Christophe Moulin works as the director for the Club Alpin Français Groupes Excellence program, a mentorship program aimed at technically proficient young alpinists. He himself has completed many difficult alpine-style ascents throughout the world.

Christophe Moulin at the first bivy of a new route on the Mooses Tooth in Alaska in 2012. *Photo: Christophe Moulin*

an anti-inflammatory effect. A study published in the July 2008 *International Journal of Sports Medicine* found that an ice bath or contrast bath (moving from cold to warm water) was significantly more effective for recovery than simple rest. We have used this method for years with many athletes, and our anecdotal evidence suggests that it is helpful. So avail yourself of the nearby icy stream for quick wade after the next hard day in the mountains and start to see the benefits of this simple method.

Compression Clothing

Several companies produce compression clothing, which are tight-fitting garments that provide a gentle, uniform pressure to the skin. This pressure aids in the venous return of your blood to your heart. Normally venous return is helped by activity, but these clothes can be worn during rest periods and seem to improve recovery by enhancing circulation. Although most commonly worn as knee socks and tights, shirts are also available. When traveling and sitting still for many hours (such as during long flights or drives) many athletes wear the socks and/or tights so that they do not arrive at their destination with heavy legs. Pneumatic compression leggings are another step up the recovery ladder as an aid to circulation by introducing a massaging effect to the compression. Even lying down with legs elevated will help in this regard.

Electro-Stim

This subject could fill an entire book but we'll just briefly mention it as a recovery tool.

Artificial electrical stimulation of muscle fibers has been around for years, having been developed in the 1800s, but perfected for use by athletes in the former USSR. Years of study resulted in effective methods for using E-stim for building strength and endurance in muscle fibers, both of which found applications in the medical world of rehabilitation from injury and in the sports world for additional nonvolitional muscle training.

Several brands of E-stim machines are currently available that include multiple programs you can select from. Our experience indicates that the most beneficial program feature these devices have for athletes in training is the recovery program. It acts like a massage without the therapist. Professional bike racers swear by these tools as a method to help them get ready for the next day's hard race.

MONITORING YOUR TRAINING

It should be apparent that the higher your goals, the harder you will have to work and the more you need to monitor your training in order stay as close to that delicate training-stress/rest balance point as possible without stepping over it. The dramatic wasting effects of overtraining need to be treated with respect as the training loads become higher.

High is a relative term. A beginner's high training load might barely be a maintenance load for a world-class athlete. There is no one-size-fits-all training prescription, which is why we've created a book that teaches you how to train rather than doling out a prescription. Thoughtful application of sound training principles accompanied by attentive monitoring will give you the best outcome.

First and foremost, adhere to the principle of gradualness in the progression of your training load. Except for rare instances of premeditated over-reaching, give yourself a chance to absorb the previous load. This will give you the best chance of staying clear of overtraining.

Take an active part in understanding the effects that your training is having on your body. This involves learning to interpret the subtle signals your body is sending you. Some of these signals are so subtle that without sophisticated monitoring equipment it can be very difficult to sense them. Here are some of the ways of monitoring training.

Morning Resting Heart Rate

At the low-tech end, some people advocate checking your morning resting heart rate and tracking this on a near-daily basis. It is often suggested that when this resting HR is elevated by more than 10 percent for a couple of days in a row, you should begin to suspect that your body's sympathetic nervous system (see chapter 3 for details) is kicked into high gear as a result of overstimulation from excessive training load. It may also be due to an infection or impending sickness, or some other stress in your life. But whatever the cause, you need to be watchful and monitor your response to training more closely over the next few days to see if the HR deviates even more or if it begins to return to a more normal level.

Years of attempts with many athletes to make this simple system work has made us skeptical to recommend it as a surefire method. Most athletes' results will be spotty with this resting HR method.

There are too many other variables that control resting heart rate to make it an accurate predictor of fatigue. This is not to say that you should disregard an elevated morning pulse, but it should be weighed with other factors.

Heart-Rate Variability (HRV)

While expensive laboratory tests of cortisol and lymphocyte levels can be very informative, they are impractical for almost all athletes. The best personal monitor of your recovery and preparedness for more hard training is a heart-rate variability test. This measure of the time interval between the electrical pulses of your heart is known as heart-rate variability (HRV). Just to be clear, this is not the same as your heart rate, and this inter-beat variability cannot be detected without some pretty sophisticated electronics.

Since your heart rate is controlled by the autonomic nervous system, HRV gives a good look at the balance between the parasympathetic and sympathetic nervous systems. It turns out that well-trained athletes have relatively high HRV when resting. Sedentary, unfit people as well as tired but fit people have lower HRV at rest. When an athlete's HRV is low, it is an excellent indicator that the autonomic nervous system is out of balance due to fatigue. Along with the endocrine and immune systems, the autonomic nervous system is the first to show your response to training. While a visit to the doctor's office for an Electro Cardiogram (ECG or EKG) is a good way to get a look at your HRV, getting a full EKG presents serious financial and logistical barriers.

Luckily, modern technology can now put this test within reach of amateur athletes via consumer-level devices that measure it, along with the software to interpret those results.

Finnish exercise physiologist Heikki Rusko developed a simple test protocol, orthostatic testing, to assess an athlete's preparedness for more training. Later, working in conjunction with the Finnish heart-rate monitor company Polarelectro, he helped develop the technology to do these HRV EKG measurements using a Polar heart-rate monitor.

This same technology has been commercially available to consumers at a cost of a few hundred dollars for several years in select Polar models. Polar markets this software in several models as the "OwnOptimizer" program. Recently other companies have jumped on the HRV bandwagon and offer their own recovery-monitoring HR monitors.

Polar's program uses the EKG results in conjunction with the heart rate's response to a simple five-minute test to make a very accurate assessment of your state of recovery from training, after which it recommends an appropriate training load for the day. This may sound outrageous, but after testing this device on four national-level and world-class athletes, Scott is convinced of its efficacy especially when combined with a qualitative assessment. The real beauty of this test lies in its predictive quality, allowing you a forward look at subtle changes in your body that can't be detected by your senses alone. This can be a good forewarning of impending problems with absorbing a future training load. This tool will be most useful for climbers executing a demanding training plan.

Grading Your Workouts

An additional useful and simple tool we often use for monitoring training progress is to give each workout a letter grade, just like you got in school, and record this value in your log. Training logs are discussed in more detail in chapter 7. Using this grading method in conjunction with the any of the several HRV recovery monitoring tools will give you the best control outside of having your own private physiologic lab staffed with scientists.

An "A" means you felt like a superhuman and had plenty in reserve.

A "B" means it was a good workout. You completed the task with no problem.

A "C" means you did the workout but felt "flat" or "off."

A "D" means you could not finish the planned workout or had to reduce it.

An "F" means you could not train that day due to fatigue or illness.

By grading each workout this way, you can make a quick scan of your log over the past few weeks and see trends. A good rule of thumb is that if you have more than two Cs in a row, or a C and D within two days of each other, you need to stop and assess what is going on. For some reason, you are not absorbing the training: the load is too high for your current fitness state, or the recovery is insufficient.

Not every workout is going to be an A, but if you keep having poor grades, then your body is trying to tell you something. You may be getting sick and not have any symptoms yet. If you continue without changing something, the Cs will become Ds, and will begin to fill the pages of your log. At this point, you are no longer adapting to the training and headed toward overtraining.

RETURNING TO TRAINING AFTER A BREAK

Breaks can be planned or unplanned. Life has a way of getting in the way of the best-laid plans. Illness, injury, school, work, family, lovers, and friends can sometimes thwart your resolve to stick with your plan. Often the best strategy is to accept the minor setbacks with equanimity and try to learn something in hopes of not having to repeat them in the future.

Fatigue

This is perhaps the most common reason for unplanned disruptions in a training plan. It is only natural that when you are exploring the limits of what your body can handle, you may occasionally step over that limit. Earlier in this section we discussed in detail ways to monitor for fatigue. In general, short-term tiredness goes with the territory. Also in general, it is short term because you recognize it early and deal with it by reducing the training load for a day. This is almost always sufficient to restore your energy levels and get you back on track again.

Recovery Times

Let's suppose that you are tired from the previous day's exertions. Given that it takes between eight and seventy-two hours to restore intramuscular glycogen and fat stores, it is usually enough to just delay the next heavy training bout for several hours up to a day or two. Endurance training has a dramatic effect on the amount of intramuscular energy stores, with better-trained athletes having much larger stores than the untrained. That means that these recovery times between workouts are highly individualized. However, this is somewhat balanced out by the fact that the better trained will usually be training harder and for longer, so in the end rough guidelines do present themselves.

It has been our experience that high-intensity exercise and strength training require the longest recovery times of two to three full days before you'll be prepared to absorb the next similarly high load. Low-intensity endurance workouts of two hours or less will normally be recovered from in eight to twenty-four hours. Long duration (over two hours) training at even low intensity may require twenty-four to forty-eight hours for the restoration of glycogen stores. Refer to the figure on page 75. Eating during and within thirty to sixty minutes after these long workouts is vital to reduce the time needed for recovery.

Illness

Probably the second-biggest reason that people get derailed from their plan, illness is one that usually carries with it the most potential for long-term damage. Many people attach a stigma of weakness to illness. Not wanting to admit to weakness, it's common for them to assume a state of denial about their illness. We have often heard, "Oh, I'm not sick. It's just a cold. I can train through it." This denial can result in that simple cold becoming a sinus infection, upper-respiratory infection, or even pneumonia, all of which could take at least several weeks to fully recover from.

A simple cold is a viral infection. You have this cold because your body's natural defense mechanisms were not able to ward off this virus, and now it is flourishing inside you. It is entirely likely that you are sick because you are training hard. While light to moderate training loads can boost natural immunity, heavy loads (either high intensity or long duration) will cause a drop in immunity, especially during the first hour immediately following the workout. Hence, the age-old admonition from coaches to change into dry clothes at the end of a hard workout and wear a hat in winter. Your body is especially vulnerable to infection during this window of time, and these extra precautions don't take much effort and really can pay off.

Our recommendation, after dealing with many athletes over many years, is that when the first signs of an illness show up, STOP TRAINING. Your body and its limited energy reserves are fully engaged in producing antibodies to fight the infection. Additional stress caused by imposing a training load on a sick body will only delay or negate the desired healing, as well as potentially open the door to additional bugs already lurking inside your body. Especially, do not train if you have a fever. This simple but effective method guarantees that you'll be able to get back to effective training in the least amount of time.

After the Illness

So what about after this cold or other minor illness? What is a good way to get back to regular training? You might still have some head congestion but your energy levels have come back up. Even a common head cold is going to take two to three days to shake off. Do not expect to jump right back to where you left off on that third or fourth day. In chapter 3 we'll explain why even a few days without an aerobic stimulus has a negative effect on the aerobic qualities you have developed.

To immediately engage in the same heavy training load you were doing before you got sick will usually be a letdown. Your perceived exertion

Compulsion to Train

Letting a compulsion to train overpower the advice not to train when sick often results in the following pattern. See if this sounds familiar:

Day 1 Illness symptoms arise but you keep training normally for the first day.

Day 2 That night the symptoms worsen and so the next day you train lightly thinking this will be enough to get over it.

Day 3 The symptoms are a bit worse so you take a day off.

Day 4 There is no change in the symptoms, but you get restless and go for a run.

Day 5 You are still not feeling great but some friends are going climbing so you go too.

Day 6 You are feeling a bit worse so you take the day off. You're going to shake this thing.

Day 7 Your symptoms are a little better, and you're back to training. Hard workout. Yahoo!

Day 8 Feeling really sick now, you take the day off.

Day 9 You have a hard time getting out of bed.

Day 10 Chills and fever.

Day 11 Still weak.

Day 12 A little better. No training.

Day 13 Got to do something! But had to cut the workout short—no energy!

Day 14 Back in bed with bronchial infection. On antibiotics now.

Without continuing to belabor this point, you can see how easily two weeks can slip away ineffectively trying to continue to train and ending up with an illness that will derail training for another ten days or so. What could have been brushed off in a week will now linger for the better part of a month. The result is that it will take a good deal of time to regain your previous strength.

will be higher as you are forced to rely on more anaerobic metabolism for energy. This will restrict the quality of the aerobic training you do during the first few days back. **We have found the simplest prescription for quickly regaining the flow in your training is to give yourself one day of easy training for every day you have been sick and away from training.** If you do this you'll feel the improvement in aerobic capacity from day to day as it returns to normal. You can very gradually increase duration and intensity during these few days. This method has worked well in many real-world applications. In most cases of minor illness, if you use this approach, within a week you will feel like your old self again.

Planned Breaks in Training

Travel, family, and work will occasionally come between you and training. If you have the chance to anticipate an upcoming break in your schedule it is possible to boost the training load for a short period, say a week, going into the trip. Then if you get only a few sporadic short, easy workouts during the trip, you can think of it as a recovery period. This sort of planned break following an overload period can be very beneficial to boost you to a higher level in the following days and weeks.

Just try to incorporate this into your plan a couple of weeks ahead of time so you can build into the hard week. This can remove the anxiety that often comes when missing training. You've planned for it, and you are using this break while visiting the parents or travelling for business as a chance to rebuild before tackling the next training block.

OVERTRAINING

Athletes who try to extract their maximum potential will most often be in a delicate balancing act, precariously close to the physiological edge between supreme fitness and utter physical collapse. The higher the level of the athlete, the narrower that edge will become, and the harder it is to balance there. Increasing fitness only comes as the result of increasing stress to the body. The elusive goal of every elite athlete is to find the proper balance between stress and recovery. Not enough stress and you will not achieve your potential for this training cycle, perhaps by a few percentage points. On the other hand, too much stress and you risk crashing hard, so hard that you will not reach your potential by a huge margin.

Over- versus Undertrained

It is far better to be a little undertrained than to be overtrained. This is an important training axiom to keep in mind. If you are undertrained

Overtraining and Lack of Recovery

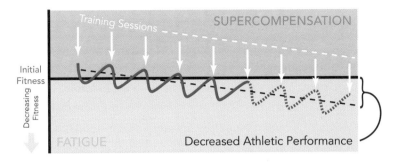

Repeated training sessions without sufficient recovery time can easily lead to a long-term decline in fitness. This condition can take months to recover from if not recognized and corrected early.

and well rested, you can always draw a bit deeper from the willpower well. If you are overtrained and tired, no amount of willpower can conjure strength and endurance from an empty well. You are likely to be exhausted, sick or injured, and lose it all.

Motivation versus Compulsion

Everyone involved in high-level athletics is driven to excel. Many climbers fall into this category. These people typically adhere to the "More is Better" school of training philosophy. Willpower, perseverance, drive, whatever you want to call the fire that burns hot inside your soul is, without a doubt, the most important attribute you have as a climber athlete. It can also be your worst enemy when it clouds your judgment and becomes a merciless taskmaster. Overtraining is not merely getting stiff and sore from a hard workout or needing a couple of days to recover from a particularly demanding climb. In the sport science world, that sort of short-term fatigue is called over-reaching and is a normal part of the training cycle. When chronic over-reaching develops into overtraining, a physiological bridge has been crossed that can be difficult to re-cross unless the athlete takes drastic action.

Acute overtraining can, in its simplest form, manifest itself as an injury. But an insidious and demoralizing side effect of overdoing structured endurance training is the failure of the body to adapt to the training stimuli. A negative training effect can occur whereby you become less fit even though you are training at the same or higher level than before. In mainstream endurance sports, overtraining is responsible for more failed athletic goals and it shortens more careers than any other factor besides injury. Some athletes suffer from it with several years of stagnation.

Endurance athletes find themselves at the highest risk for overtraining due to the high energy demands involved in their daily training

Deep Fatigue
on Kunyang Chish East

By Steve House

The red-and-white umbrella casts a meager shadow over my path, puffs of hot dust lift from each footstep as I lengthen my stride across the flat ground. Around this next corner, after weeks of travel and three days of hard walking, I will finally see the unclimbed summit of Kunyang Chish East.

Kunyang Chish Main is the twenty-first-highest peak in the world. With an elevation of 25,761 feet (7,852 meters), it's a giant by any standards. Its ridgelines have etched the north horizon for days, defining the boundaries of some of the largest nonpolar glaciers in the world. Kunyang Chish East, at 24,278 feet (7,400 meters), is the apex of the easternmost of those spiderweb ridges.

It is one year after Vince Anderson and I climbed Nanga Parbat, and it seems appropriate to go far off the beaten track and attempt a great, steep wall on an unknown summit. We both want to be far from the busyness and occasional competitiveness of 8,000-meter peaks. We have visions of pleasant climbing up long sheets of ice; short, difficult mixed sections; and secure bivouacs. We are drawn to this mountain's warm south face, which has the added benefit of clearing most quickly after storms.

Two weeks later I lead across a snow-covered rock slab and up to a small stance below a ridge. Above me skyscraper towers of black rock march up along the toothed ridgeline, the snow sags limply from every surface; a misty, damp fog masks the afternoon sun. Vince climbs up, looking past me as he stops at the belay and saying, "*That doesn't look easy.*" We had hoped this route, climbed to the main summit by a Japanese party, would provide an easy way to acclimate.

"*Yeah,*" I reply, "*it looks hard and dangerous.*"

An hour later we were retreating, aware that this sets back our acclimatization plans.

Six days left in our expedition, I wake to a canopy of stars. I feel lazy, limp, like I want to go back to sleep. I shake myself awake and reach for my boots. The climbing starts easy with moderate ice slopes we can steadily churn away at. Climbing unroped we each go our own pace; I go fast for a while, to see if I can find a spark. When I glance back, Vince is uncomfortably far away, and I wait for him.

"*Rope up?*" I ask as he climbs up to the protective rock I've snuggled up against.

"*Sure.*"

We tie in and Vince leads off, keeping an ice screw clipped to the rope between us as we climb. We don't say another word all day until I climb over the lip of the ice cave and see Vince grinning. "*Amazing!*" I say, swinging my pack onto the nearly flat floor.

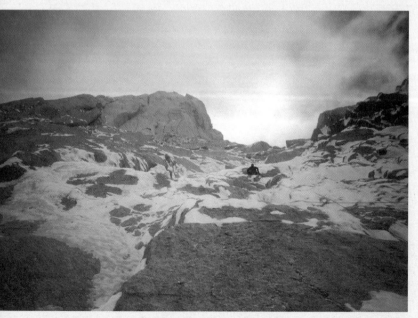

Vince Anderson leading difficult mixed ground at 23,000' (7,000m) on the south face of Kunyang Chish East (24,278', 7,400m). *Photo: Steve House*

"*Couldn't be much nicer. Safe too.*" He pokes the solid ice roof with the spike of his ax and I start to smooth out the floor for sleeping.

The third day, Vince leads several pitches of steep and runout mixed climbing far above the deck. I'm gasping to follow with the heavy pack; fearful of slipping, hoping the belay is good. I'm impressed; we are higher than the summit of Denali and he is onsighting insecure M6 pitches with two good pieces of pro on the pitch. I arrive at the belay, calves spent, and breath heaving.

Two hours later we crest the face and climb together up deepening snow to a fine, flat ridge. Nanga Parbat had been an eight-day marathon; this was going to be a comparatively easy four days up, one down. We pitch our tent on a perfect flat knoll of snow—the views of the Himalaya are indescribable, peak after unclimbed peak swells out to the horizon.

In the morning it is frostbite cold, and we haven't slept well. The lassitude we've been accumulating for six weeks seems to collapse onto our shoulders all at once. Stubbornly, I sit up and start the stove, nearly freezing the tips of my fingers in the process.

It's past noon now. Vince pushes an energy gel into his mouth, takes a swig of water, and passes the waterbag to me. He looks beaten down and tired. I feel worse than he looks. I open the one-liter bottle of meal-replacement shake. Maybe I only need calories. I tip the bottle and drink half: 2,000 calories, down the hole. Vince looks up and recognizing my effort, says, "Nice."

I smile and swallow some water before fishing for a hard candy in my parka pocket. Man, that stuff tastes bad. *"OK, man, let's see how badass this mountain is!"*

Vince's head jolts up, he smiles, and I reach over to put him on belay. He leads out, slowly. The snow is knee deep and a cornice looms to our right; after fifty feet (15 meters) the ridge steepens. He's shoveling the snow with his hands, trying to make some progress.

I feel it, knowing what's about to happen, and kneel in the snow. The energy drink comes up. I vomit at my feet, wipe my mouth, and try to kick some snow over the stain.

Vince has turned around, *"You OK?"*

"Oh yeah, just a little cramp. I'm OK."

"How's it look up there?" But he doesn't reply, he turns back and continues his attempt to climb the steep snow, but can't.

Ten minutes later, we turn around. Disheartened and now shivering with a sudden chill, we start down, reaching the tent at dusk.

Back home I search for answers. I review my training from that year and find that I've actually trained significantly less than pre–Nanga Parbat. Why then, was I so tired? Looking closer, I see that I started training again two months after Nanga Parbat. Probably too soon.

I'd never go back for those final three hundred plus feet (one hundred meters) of corniced, unstable snow climbing, but I feel an odd mix of shame and pride that we didn't climb Kunyang Chish East that year. Shame that we

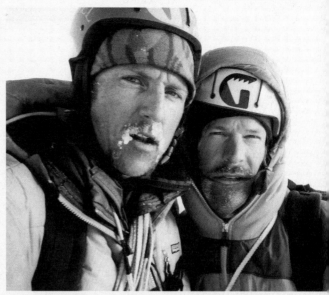

Steve House and Vince Anderson at their highpoint on their Kunyang Chish East attempt. *Photo: Vince Anderson*

didn't have it in us. Pride that we were able to turn back so close, that we had the strength to say no when the warning signs were telling us to retreat. On Kunyang Chish East, we were unfocused, tired, and undermotivated. We never properly completed the nasty, necessary task of acclimating. What is more, we were not recovered, physically or mentally, from the huge effort on Nanga Parbat twelve months earlier.

This is a common, and often fatal, mistake that many alpinists have made. Success reaps reward and reward feels good. Naturally we quest for more success on bigger projects. Eventually, if you follow this cycle long enough, you'll climb yourself to extinction. Many alpinists have; most of the Peter Boardman and Joe Tasker generation of British mountaineers did just that.

Frankly, we would have been better off going to lesser mountains or taking a vacation from alpinism. An effort like we produced on Nanga Parbat takes more than eight weeks to recover from. Hindsight isn't perfect, but knowing what I know now, I wish we'd taken more time off from hard alpine climbing to recover, physically and mentally. I wouldn't prescribe doing nothing; I'd climb, bike, run, ski, have fun, but I wouldn't go to the big mountains for at least a year. Unfortunately my ego wouldn't let us take a break.

regimen. These can exceed 7,000 kcal/day during heavy training. Unfortunately, most athletes don't intuitively recognize overtraining. In many cases, overtraining takes so long to acknowledge that by the time it is properly diagnosed, it is usually too late for anything but the most draconian measures.

Early Signs and the Common Response

The first and most common sign of the early stages of overtraining is repeated shortcomings in performance accompanied by a feeling of flatness or low energy. The athlete's typical assumption is that this performance decrease relates to a lack of fitness.

The response by most of the self-coached will be to immediately add more training of some sort. The thought being that the program lacks some key ingredient, and if they just add more of this or that, their lost fitness will return. After they increase their training with no improvement and usually a further decrease in performance, they continue to seek solutions that involve more training. Thus begins a dangerous downward spiral that can ultimately lead to where Steve found himself in 2003 before he came to Scott seeking help with his training.

Overtraining is more easily measurable if you race 10,000 meters on foot, and your times drop off. It's much harder to recognize in climbing where the track is different every day. This is one reason that we will advise having benchmark climbs or workouts you can do to check for progress or regression in your program.

Symptoms

The earliest effects of overtraining impact the sympathetic nervous system (refer to chapter 3 for a discussion of the nervous system). It starts with the immediate effect of raising the heart rate for every level of exertion compared to your normal heart rate for the equivalent level of exertion. You just don't have your normal pep and vigor and feel flat in training. The levels of the stress hormone cortisol begin to stay elevated between training sessions, although this takes a trip to the doctor to determine.

If nothing is done to mitigate the early overtraining, it can progress to a much more debilitating type involving the parasympathetic nervous system. When the parasympathetic nervous system gets involved, there are more negative hormonal effects and a *lowering* of the heart rate for all effort levels compared to normal rates. When this occurs, the athlete will know by any one or a number of these unpleasant symptoms:

- Persistent, deep fatigue

- Prolonged elevated cortisol levels (requires a blood test)

- Lowered testosterone levels (requires a blood test)

- Decreased heart rate variability (requires a special HR monitor or EKG)

- Irritability

- Depression

- Weight loss

- Absence of menstruation

- Insomnia

- Lowered libido

- Loss of enthusiasm and motivation

The profound state of deep neurological fatigue reached at this point necessitates, at the minimum, several weeks of complete rest and only then a gradual reintroduction of easy exercise. Sounds grim, right? It is a condition to be avoided at all costs. The best way to avoid this condition is to monitor your response to training by using methods described earlier in this chapter. The cost of overtraining and under-recovering is so much worse than undertraining, it is far better to err on the conservative side.

OVERTRAINING CAN LEAD TO OVERUSE INJURY

If a muscle is exposed to a new training load on a routine and consistent basis before full recovery from the previous training session has occurred, at the very least, no training adaptation will be seen. More likely, however, is that the cumulative effect of this premature stress will perpetuate small injuries that will further weaken the muscle. The muscle/brain connection will then self-inhibit the ability to contract the muscle in an attempt to protect that muscle from further damage. A dedicated athlete can easily overcome this pain and suffering and manage to maintain the overuse, but soon a minor tear will turn into a major inflammatory cycle leading to overt injury and scarring. Chronic tendonitis or worse—full tendon or muscle rupture—will occur.

While these injuries are not necessarily an indication of overtraining as discussed above, they do point out that the adaptation we seek through training is not occurring. This lack of adaptation can be a good indicator that you are on a collision course with overtraining if some remedial steps are not begun.

Take these warning signs for what they are: your body's red flag attempts at getting your attention that things are amiss. Rather than get caught up in numbers and times, etc., just understand what is going on and pay attention to the bigger picture of your body's responses to the training.

WHAT SHOULD YOU FEEL?

You should feel a little tired immediately after the workout, but not severely so. More often you will feel energized. You should feel good the next day—not sore or beat. By the time your next training session arrives, you should feel stronger and psyched to do it again. If instead you are exhausted and/or very stiff and sore for a day or two, you overdid it, and your body is telling you in the only way it can. A lack of motivation to train especially after a good warm-up is a strong indicator that you are not recovered and that you need to shorten or skip your planned workout.

If you do not feel a progressive increase in energy, strength, and overall fitness from week to week, you are almost surely either training too hard, not allowing enough time for recovery, or your active recovery sessions are too intense. Granted there are always a few burnout days here and there, but if the general trend is down, not up, you need to address the situation. See the earlier section of this chapter for a discussion of recovery techniques.

Far too many times we have had climbers come to ask us training questions after they have become injured or overtrained. And invariably, when we explain the above-mentioned concepts, their response is, "Oh, I guess I was definitely overtraining or under-recovering." By the time they ask, "Now what do I do?" it is often too late for all but the most drastic measures.

SUMMARY: TRAINING PRINCIPLES

Training should be viewed as the structured and progressive application of physical stress on your body followed by periods during which your body is allowed to regain its homeostasis.

Training is distinct from fitness activities in that it has a goal of raising certain physiological qualities in a coordinated and predictable manner in order to produce a planned-for increase in performance.

Training is not what you do, but how your body reacts to what you do.

Understand the physiological effects of each training zone:

- Zone 1: 55–75 percent max HR. Basic aerobic. This is the key component of a big motor. It is done at or below your nose-breathing limit.

- Zone 2: 75–80 percent max HR. High-end aerobic. Used by advanced athletes with years of base.

- Zone 3: 80–90 percent max HR. Max aerobic effect. Fun, hard.

- Zone 4: 90–95 percent of max HR. Strong anaerobic component. This zone is used sparingly even by the best.

Monitor your training.

- Ventilation is a great physiologic-feedback mechanism to track intensity.

- Use a heart-rate monitor for daily training. Using this tool lets you monitor your level of intensity. Certain types of these monitors let you evaluate your level of recovery.

- Keep a log, but avoid letting data drive your training. A log enables a progressive approach and helps you monitor your body's response to training. A log also lessens your likelihood of overtraining.

- Periodize your training to help with progressivity. Each period and each workout builds on the previous ones and prepares you for the next step.

- If you don't feel like training that day, that is your subconscious telling you to take it easy.

TINSTAAFL: There Is No Such Thing As A Free Lunch

By Mark Twight

Periodically people ask me specific questions about training for endurance, and specifically my experience with using short, high-intensity cross- and circuit-training to improve it. My answer is based on the twenty-year period I spent climbing mountains, as well as more recent experiences with ski-mountaineering racing, bike racing, and decades of experience training others for similar events.

Folks usually don't like what I have to tell them.

When someone asks about what I now refer to as the *free lunch* method of improving endurance performance, or any intervention whereby a time-crunched athlete tries to achieve a particular result by means of a shortcut, I first refer them to an article I wrote about my two-year test of this concept. The article is archived on the Gym Jones website, but I'll summarize it here:

No top-performing endurance athletes achieve their results on a diet of short, hard intervals and circuit training in the gym. Instead they build hours and hours of baseline fitness and then temper the foundation in races, and with a very small percentage of high-intensity interval training. Do you imagine that a bicycle racer who rides 20,000 miles per year isn't looking for a way to achieve the same results without having to spend so much time in the saddle? Or that someone has invented a shortcut, a method to end-run all the effort and time and suffering, and that no one else had previously tried it? I thought I had found the shortcut. I was wrong. Others think they have found it. Some are even selling it. The true professionals are not convinced. And they are not being beaten by anyone taking shortcuts.

When I was drunk on CrossFit punch I kept trying to force the square peg of high-intensity circuit training and heavy lifting into the round hole of endurance performance simply because I liked training in the gym. I was addicted to the endogenous opiates produced by hard effort and wanted to continue getting high. But I also wanted to run and ride—long distances for long hours. So, being human and weak, I tricked myself into believing the work that got me high could also give me the results

I sought. And in the grips of that high I ignored my performance on the mountain, preferring instead to point out my performance in the gym, my performance compared to others, my fast time on some contrived circuit that means nothing outside of the narrow context of the weight room.

If you train long-endurance exclusively you'll be weak and slow though able to go forever. To go long and fast your training program must also include strength training plus high-intensity intervals and speed work—each introduced at the appropriate time—to sharpen the large foundation of endurance that we presume exists.

The actual story is longer than the conclusion and its details aid understanding. After eight years of following the training program detailed in my book, *Extreme Alpinism—Climbing Light, Fast and High* (The Mountaineers Books, 1999), which had worked quite well, I began testing some different ideas.

In early 2003, I finally understood that machined-based movements limit range of motion and neglect supporting, stabilizing musculature so the transferability of the results to sport performance is limited, and can actually increase the risk of injury. However, movements done on foot, using free weights (dumbbells, barbell, kettlebells, etc.) require three-dimensional stabilization, balance, and sport-like muscle-firing sequences and timing that is easily transferable to sport-specific performance.

So-called functional training—and I use the term *functional* to describe artificial training that has a high degree of transferability to sport performance—can increase strength in both muscles and connective tissue, which reduces the risk of injury. Muscles trained this way need not be re-educated outside of the gym because the movements, loads, intensity, and duration may be easily tuned to match sport-specific actions. So instead of doing quad extensions and seated leg presses I began doing back and front squats and deadlifts, and eventually lunges and weighted step-ups because these looked and felt a lot more like what I did in the mountains.

Later that year I attended a CrossFit seminar to learn more about the modern manifestation of circuit training.

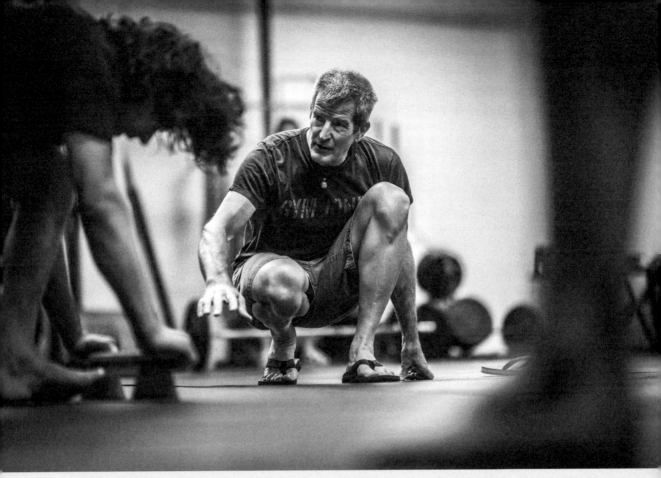

Mark Twight coaching Brazilian Jiu-Jitsu competitor James Gardner at Gym Jones. *Photo: Clay Enos*

I went there in shape for my sport but was destroyed by the varied fitness challenges that were presented. I had worked long and hard to become and remain fit for the mountains and when I was actively climbing I was one of the faster, more fit guys around.

The CrossFit argument and its presenter were quite convincing. I was susceptible to the easier way, the cure-in-a-bottle way, and my anti-establishment personality wanted the experts to be wrong, so I fell into the trap of thinking there might be a free lunch—a shortcut to improved endurance—even though it went against everything I had learned over the previous twenty years.

Using the concepts taught at the seminar I designed a program and a test, then dove in headlong. For fifteen weeks my average workout lasted no longer than fifteen minutes. I trained artificially, in the gym. I executed a variety of whole-body movements with and without weight at an intensity that caused huge cardiorespiratory demands. During the final three weeks of the work-up I did some sport-specific training to sort out my equipment for the test, which was the 2004 Powder Keg ski-mountaineering race, though only two or three workouts lasted as long as I predicted the test would take.

In the end I placed eleventh of sixty-six in my division after 2:21:19 of racing, but I was twenty-five minutes slower than my division's winner and almost fifty minutes slower than the overall winner (Rico Elmer, the 2004 world champion). On the scale of great-good-shitty-sucks, I sucked, but I convinced myself the test results proved that short-duration, high-intensity circuits in the gym, combined with high-intensity intervals are indeed very good preparation for endurance and power-endurance efforts despite the brevity of the workouts.

My mistake was to believe that these workouts and the entire test took place in a vacuum when, in fact, I used a fifteen-week-long sharpening period to fine-tune a twenty-year endurance base gained by training and climbing at intensities specific to long-endurance effort. The same training program would not produce a similar result in an athlete who did not have the same foundation. Or for someone without similar understanding of pacing (energy management) and the nutrition and hydration strategies, which can only come from long, individual, trial-and-error experience such as I had done during my climbing career. Having missed the tree and the forest, I pushed my deluded self deeper into the rabbit hole.

Convinced of the truth of my experiment, I lined up at the North American Ski Mountaineering Championships in Jackson Hole one week after the Powder Keg. A single, moderate workout done midweek was enough to stall my recovery progress, and I blew up halfway into the race and then struggled to the finish next-to-last. It has become obvious since—and should have been then—that recovery must be trained. In other words, recovery adaptations to the training load and duration occur just like the compensatory muscular and endurance adaptations to imposed athletic demands. I had trained myself to recover from efforts of a particular intensity and duration. The Powder Keg cut deeper than my ability to recover. I started the race in Jackson Hole with my tank a quarter full but without a gauge I had no idea it would be empty within an hour. I based my pace on how I felt at the start line, having not yet heard Scott Johnston's wise words, "Everyone feels good at the beginning of a race." When my tank ran dry I went out with whimper, not a bang.

In response to this experience I began adding one long effort to my free lunch training program every seven to ten days. This appeared to improve recovery from longer sessions so—in my bubble—I kept trying to force the training means I wanted to use to produce the results I wanted to achieve. And I interpreted those results by putting the best possible spin on them when they did not match my expectations.

During my infatuation with the free lunch method of improving endurance I argued it to Scott Johnston with the fervor of a born-again fanatic. Being a friend, he was nice enough to listen, and even tolerated the spittle. Eventually he countered by writing, "I still stick by the tried-and-tested methods I have described [in our correspondence]. Not because I know so much, but because I have seen them work, and work well for many years on both myself and many, many others. They have produced world champions and top national results."

He was nice enough to treat me with kid gloves when he stated, "To say that one anecdotal experience convinces you that your way is better seems hasty. It seems

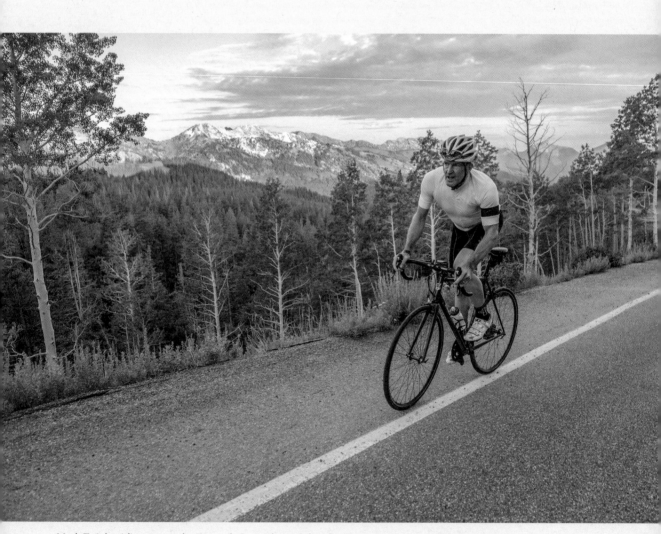

Mark Twight riding across the Wasatch Crest above Salt Lake City, summer 2013. *Photo: Clay Enos*

unlikely that all these great athletes have been wrong in their approach and that you have stumbled on some secret training method yet to be discovered. Because, if your way could give the best results then the best athletes would have adopted it; especially if it could be done in less time."

When I opined that so-called elite athletes were finishing well in endurance events on a diet of twenty-minute workouts and less-than-800-meter runs, he replied, "I have seen this phenomenon many times in younger skiers but also in Masters racers who, because they didn't have much time to train, did a majority of their training in Zone 3 and 4. Basically they were looking for a shortcut to fitness. In every case that I have personally seen or been involved in coaching, when these skiers (from ages twenty to fifty) went to a more conventional Zone 1–2 regime followed by well-timed and administered Zone 3–4 workouts, their results improved."

This fell on deaf ears because I wanted badly to be right—the same way every time-crunched athlete wants to believe that he can compete in (not merely finish) a marathon or ultra-distance event on a training diet of six hours per week by doing 3x20 minutes in the sub-threshold sweet spot three times per week. It is easy to confuse hard with effective. And it is tough to argue with experience earned on the national and international level, but I did.

I kept training short and racing long. I wasn't fast. I didn't recover well. I didn't progress from year to year. Surely I was doing something wrong because the program itself couldn't be flawed. So I tried harder. When greater intensity didn't work, I increased the frequency of my over-distance efforts, and modified and tested, and continued racing to the same results. When I tired of that I began looking at the definitions, and the general sameness of the intensities, and I discussed the causes of fatigue and my lack of power with various coaches, trainers, and thinkers.

Scott clued me in to the relationship between volume and recovery. "In XC skiing the shortest normal man's race (before the advent of the sprint format) is forty minutes while the longest can last a bit more than two hours. A World Cup (WC) skier will compete in forty races in a season though not all are WC events. My biggest year was forty-five, which included eight fifty-kilometer races. We were racing three days per week, sometimes four. A big base seemed to be what allowed us to recover quickly from one effort and be sort of rested for the next. Note: there was no training during competition phase, only racing and rest so volume would drop a lot. At least that was the theory we were sold on and practiced, and all the big guns seemed to prove it. Hence a big training volume for a WC skier would be 800–1,000 hours per year. This included hard training too, but probably 90 percent time-wise in Zone 1–2. My guess is that alpinism is closer to XC skiing than it is to swimming or rowing in terms of duration and the need to recover quickly." I had used examples of rowing and swimming and sprint triathlon results to bolster my position on the subject of high-intensity training. Then I read this:

Back in the early and mid '60s the Germans' training approach [placed] a greater emphasis on high-intensity intervals. What they found was that, to a great extent they did reach high performance levels with this training program. But they were not seeing progressive improvement from year to year among their elite athletes. Every year they came up to the same level, fell back down in the off-season, and repeated the process the next season. Then they changed the composition of the training to higher volume, lower intensity (fewer killer intervals at max speed) and the long-term progress began to occur. (By Stephen Seiler, in an article on the website www.time-to-run.com)

I realized how badly I'd swallowed the hook, and how hard I had hit the ceiling of anaerobic development, at the expense of other capacities.

In my experience, the distribution of training in the free lunch training context is exactly opposite of that shown to be most effective at improving endurance performance. During my experiment, before I began tweaking by adding longer efforts, my average total training time per week was three to four hours and roughly 70 percent of that was done at very high intensity, defined as 90–95 percent of VO_2 max. I did the remaining 30 percent of the work at low intensity in warm-up, cool-down, or recovery phases, or while practicing technique. This ratio alone shows very clearly why the free lunch could not, as a stand-alone program, possibly improve my endurance.

When I mined my old training logs I realized I'd done my best climbing in the mountains during the years when I averaged between 800 and 1,000 hours of volume annually. I asked Steve how much he was averaging per year. Over the first six months of 2008 he accumulated more than 600 hours of training volume to prepare for Makalu later in the year. During the eight weeks prior to setting the record on the Grand Traverse in the Tetons (six hours, forty-nine minutes), Rolando Garibotti hiked and climbed and ran 125,000 feet (38,100 meters) of elevation gain. The final week of his preparatory program, which included the actual record-setting traverse, totaled 31,700 feet (9,662 meters) of vertical gain. Of course, he covered many, many miles as well and this took many, many hours. My best season of bike racing (2010) coincided with the greatest volume of training: 8,100 miles on the bike and 510 hours total training volume, an increase of 25 percent in mileage, and about 10 percent in total volume from recent yearly averages. To me, all of this indicates that an entry fee—in this

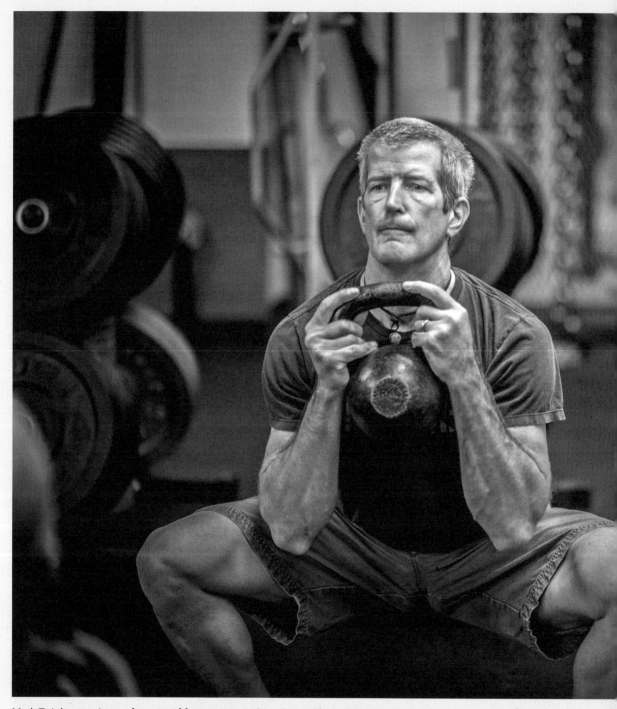

Mark Twight warming up for a set of front squats at Gym Jones. *Photo: Clay Enos*

case, a certain amount of training volume—is required to perform at every level and the higher the level, the higher the fee. Expectations must match investment, and rules govern the game.

I broke the rules but expected an equivalent or better outcome. Eventually I paid. Eighteen months of nothing but short, hard efforts cured my endurance. Sure, I could go hard, sometimes for two to three hours, but hard is relative and doesn't necessarily mean fast. I couldn't recover when I did go long, and the old days when I could move for twelve to twenty-four hours nonstop were a distant memory. Thus ended

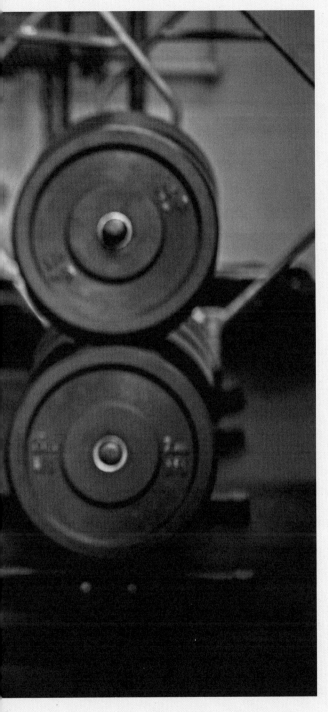

It took a long time. Every day I cursed myself for having sacrificed the hours and days and years I had worked to build a twenty-year base on what was obviously a pipe dream. I trained 435 hours in 2006 but spent too much time in the gym. I could have spent those 57 hours on more relevant work. In 2007, I trained 475 hours, with only 29 in the gym. In 2008, I averaged 40 hours of training per month, very little in the gym and my lactate threshold bumped eleven beats per minute higher (BPM) over 2005. As a percentage of VO_2 max it was within two to three BPM of the highest levels I achieved in the mid-90s. I could put out reasonable power for about four hours, and keep going for eight or nine. By 2009, my fitness was good enough to climb Denali in thirteen days round-trip, and to be present in the field sprint at the end of the 206-mile Logan-to-Jackson road bike race, where I finished four seconds off the winner. In 2010, I was second in my category at the Tour de Park City after 150 miles of racing, sixty of them in a hard breakaway with five others. I was happy to be back.

I recovered my endurance fitness faster than one could create it from scratch because my body remembered its former condition and I hadn't lost my ability to manage fueling and hydration, temperature regulation, and pacing. I recovered movement efficiency and economy, and quickly rediscovered the psychological state that allowed me to enjoy sustained suffering. All of this factors into performance. I recovered my endurance when the balance of training information and experience, combined with the realities described in my training log overcame my conviction that there was an easier way. There is an order to follow. There are rules. It's not random. It's planned and executed and tested and modified along the way because there is no such thing as a shortcut or a free lunch—and no way to evade hard, intelligent work.

Mark Twight's climbing had a major influence on American alpinism, and he authored two important climbing books, Kiss or Kill *and* Extreme Alpinism. *Mark is the founder and owner, with his wife, Lisa, of Gym Jones. www.gymjones.com*

my love affair with short-duration, high-intensity "cross-training" to the exclusion of other forms. After failing to overhaul the method itself, and failing to create a hybrid, I decided it was time to rehabilitate my own fitness by returning to the basics, by following the rules.

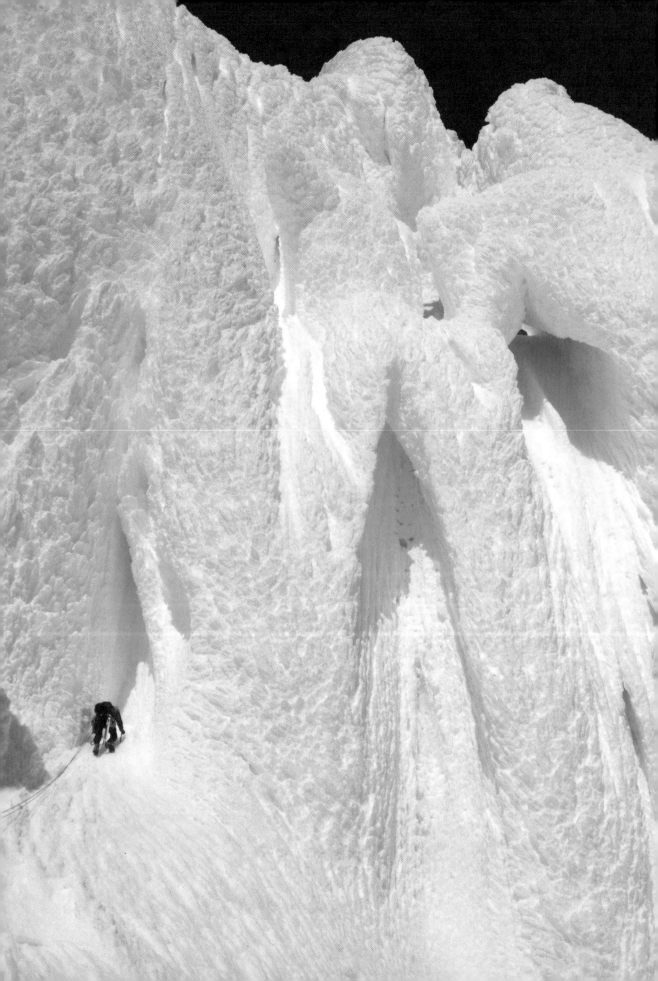

Chapter 3

The Physiology of Endurance Training

"I would say that the need to climb comes from that tough, lonely place of searching for your dignity. You know, that place—where we actually choose to confront our own weaknesses and fears, where we rebel against the terror of death—is really about dignity. That's why alpinism is not just the act of ascending a mountain, but also inwardly of ascending above your self."

– VOYTEK KURTYKA, from an interview
in Alpinist #43, Summer 2013

THE EVOLUTION OF ENDURANCE

According to one popular theory of evolutionary biology, early hominids in equatorial latitudes exploited their aerobic endurance and lack of hair (which allowed them to avoid the overheating fate of their prey) to run their next meal to the point of exhaustion. This subsequently helped them rise to the top of the food chain despite their physical weakness. It was by virtue of their staying power that our predecessors could get close enough to kill an otherwise much more powerful

Opposite: Colin Haley about to climb into a 160-foot long natural tunnel on the Ragni Route, west face of Cerro Torre, during the first ascent of the Torre Traverse, Patagonia. *Photo: Rolando Garibotti.*

animal after the prey became too weak to defend itself. The theory goes on to say that the high-protein diet resulting from successful hunts allowed increased development in brain capacity and complexity, which in turn led to all the subsequent cultural advances and evolutionary traits we have inherited. The mere fact that you are able to read these printed words is the direct result of our species' inherent endurance. (Liedenberg, 2008; Billat et al., 2003)

THE AEROBIC BASE

This term *aerobic base* gets tossed around a lot in the literature of endurance sports, with most practitioners acknowledging the importance of it when it comes to performance. But what exactly is it? When we speak of someone with "a big motor," what do we really mean? We will answer these questions in this chapter.

We humans are genetically predisposed to endurance activities. But what is it that makes some humans more capable of processing larger amounts of oxygen, doing larger amounts of work, and producing higher power outputs for longer periods before fatigue sets in?

It is simply the result of that aerobic base and the training that maximizes it.

The term aerobic base refers to a well-developed aerobic energy production system in the working muscles as well as the ability of the heart to pump large amounts of blood along with the oxygen it carries. It allows for the enhanced ability to do prolonged (from two minutes to many hours) periods of moderate work without incurring so much fatigue that you have to slow down or stop the exercise. **The better developed the aerobic base, the faster you can move for these extended periods**.

The VO_2 Max Myth

Exercise physiologists have their own language for describing this aerobic base idea. The aerobic base is composed of two main components: The first is maximum amount of oxygen that your body can process and sustain for several minutes (known as VO_2 max). The second is the percentage of that maximum that you can maintain for a long period (this length can vary depending on who is measuring it and for what event, but it is generally from twenty minutes to one hour). The first component, VO_2 max, is often referred to as aerobic power. The second component is often referred to as aerobic capacity or the fractional utilization of VO_2 max and corresponds to the anaerobic threshold and endurance.

In the lay press the VO_2 max term has taken on a hallowed meaning beyond its usefulness as a predictor of performance. Since it is a quantity that you can maintain for only a short time it does not reflect the endurance factor we know is mainly responsible for performance in events lasting longer than about ten minutes. **Your VO_2 max shows what your maximum potential is, while the fractional utilization, or anaerobic threshold, is the percentage of that maximum you are capable of maintaining for long durations (over thirty minutes.)** It is the combination of these two elements that determines a person's aerobic endurance capacity. While VO_2 max is trainable to some extent, especially among untrained individuals, it responds poorly to training among elite athletes who have several years of consistent training under their belts.

In fact one of the authors (Scott) once coached a very talented World Cup cross-country skier who had previously been the subject of a five-year-long attempt by his National Team to raise his VO_2 max. In other words a large percentage of his training volume was made up of workouts designed primarily to improve his VO_2 max. This approach had taken a vast amount of financial and human resources in terms of coaching, training, and testing. When viewing his multiple tests, Scott was struck by the fact that the variation in his VO_2 max test results could best be explained by the randomness that occurs from test to

The Role of the Genetic Gift

We are not all created equal, and there are inherited genetic attributes that will enable some individuals to have a higher potential for developing aerobic endurance, just as there are those among us who are genetically predisposed to excel at music or math. However, as with any genetic predisposition, the line that separates nature from nurture is fuzzy at best. One may have genes that favor a particular adaptation, but you must still stimulate those genes to express themselves through many hours of practice.

Early in human evolution, people with poor endurance either became prey or were out-competed for food and other resources. Endurance was critical to human survival, and those who had it lived to pass it on to their progeny. Because of its role in survival, evolution has been perfecting our endurance trait for many millennia so the genetic variation in the population as a whole is smaller than the genetic variation for some other characteristics such as explosive power or mathematics, that have played a smaller part in ensuring the next generation's survival.

While a few of us may be genetically gifted, the impact your genes have on your performance is not worth concerning yourself with. Unless you are one of the extremely lucky (or unlucky) outliers, your genetics are not all that different from the genetics of most of the better athletes in the world. What is most important is how well and how frequently you practice and train. As Anders Ericsson, the psychologist and researcher on expertise wrote: "When the human body is put under exceptional strain, a range of dormant genes in the DNA are expressed and extraordinary physiological processes are activated."

The history of endurance sports, as well as the more general study of people who excel at anything, has shown convincingly that motivation and perseverance far outweigh genetics until one is vying for the top spots among the world's best. The ultimate message here is that, for 90 percent of the population, genetics is no excuse. Motivation and intelligent training are much more important.

The North Face of the North Twin

By Steve House

Marko is standing, watching me because there isn't enough room for us both to sit on the ledge at the same time. This is where we will spend the night. Space is tight. I just rappelled down after filling a pack with snow as there is no ice or snow here; just a tiny rocky ledge the size of an office chair. We need to start the stove and make some water.

"How long since we had water?" I ask.

"Ne vem," replies Marko. He speaks Slovene; I, English. It's an unusual arrangement, but we understand one another. He can't remember either.

"What time is it?" It's dark, and we are two days and thirty pitches into climbing up the north face of North Twin. This 4,000-foot (1,219-meter) wall is seventeen miles by foot off the Banff-Jasper Highway and has been climbed only twice, and never in winter conditions. Marko doesn't answer my query about the time. His thoughts are elsewhere. It was dark when I built the anchor 150 feet (46 meters) above me and rappelled back here, to this, the best ledge we've seen all day. First I want to change into dry socks, put my boots back on, and then make water, soup, and dinner.

I start to pull the shell of my double boot back onto my foot. I feel a jolt and see that the cord I've tied in the back of the boot has broken and in my hand—a small loop to keep my boot safely clipped to me during maneuvers like this is all that remains. The boot appears to hover in the beam of my headlamp for a moment. I don't have time to reach for it. I shout; it's gone.

The next day Marko leads, I follow wearing one boot with a crampon on my left foot and my right inner boot wrapped in athletic tape on my right foot. I went through our garbage and pulled all of the plastic bags we had over my sock before lacing up the inner boot that morning.

Opposite: Marko Prezelj climbing the short traversing pitch to the ice in the exit cracks of the headwall. North face of the North Twin, Alberta. *Photo: Steve House*

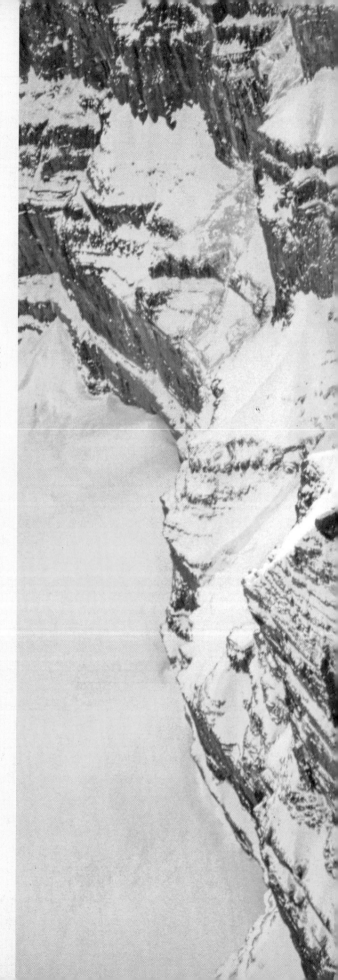

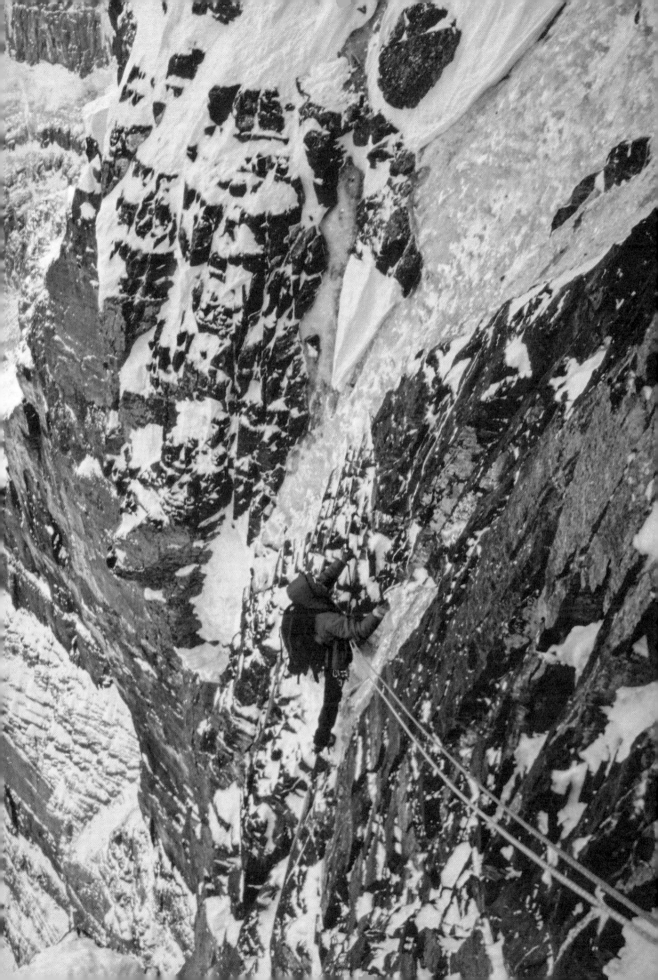

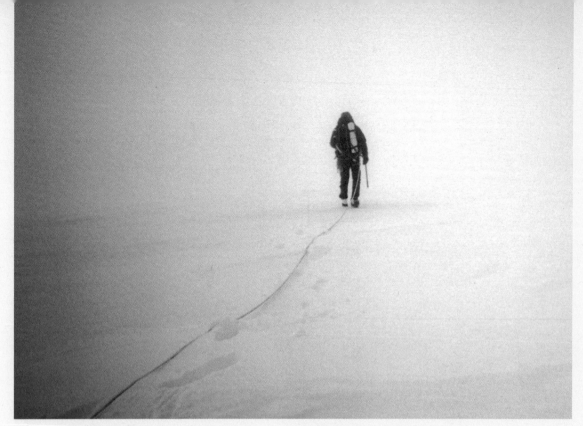

Steve House navigating across the Columbia Icefield in a storm. *Photo: Marko Prezelj*

I want to keep my sock as dry as I can; I don't want to lose any toes.

I begin to follow a complicated traverse that had taken Marko sixty minutes to lead. As I climb toward a small wire nut, the tension on the rope pops it out and I take a thirty-foot (nine-meter) swinging fall. One of our two ropes is cut to the core. At the belay we use the last of our tape to try to repair this damage, and then Marko leads off again, another short traverse, and finally a small success when he shouts back that he has ice screws for the belay. Ice means we're in the exit cracks, and getting closer to the end of the difficult climbing. The fourth lead of the day ascends an icy corner, a huge, left-angling crescent crack. I follow as Marko keeps a strong, tight belay. I can enjoy the climbing, though the snow is starting to fall, the first precipitation we've seen in four days.

Hours later and we're on the summit. The wind flings sharp flecks of ice into our faces that sting as we kneel in the snow digging a trench: Marko uses a shovel blade with no handle, I use our pot. For shelter we carry a five foot by eight foot (roughly, two by three meters) tarp that stuffs down to the size of an orange. We're underneath the east side of the summit cornice of North Twin, but the wind is blowing from the south and the strong gusts and blowing snow threaten to fill in our trench as fast as we dig it.

"*Kot na pokapolišču*," Marko says. A dark joke about grave digging that I don't acknowledge as I pull one edge of the tarp taut to the edge of the trench. We stake the corners with our ice tools and wrap slings around our crampons and bury them to lash the tarp down firmly. Still

it flutters like a torn sail behind a tempest-broken mast. Our trench is too wide and snow follows us in and settles on us lightly as we crawl inside our one shared sleeping bag and I turn on the stove.

At first light I make calculations with a pencil stub in the margin of the map. I plot waypoints on the map and enter ten-digit strings of numbers for each coordinate into the handheld GPS.

"*Concentrate*," I say to no one. Marko brews tea. We have no food. He is kneeling, facing away from me, away from the storm. I sit on a foam pad with my knee pinning the snow-covered map. We're both wearing all our clothes, my right foot is already cold. We cannot afford a mistake.

Many hours later my back hurts sharply from walking fourteen miles across the glacier—navigating by GPS the whole way—with one leg effectively two inches shorter than the other. We begin to descend, the glacier dips into the cloud. Dropping under the clouds for the first time in ages, I stop.

"*The pass!*" I yell at Marko through the wind that's screaming toward us. He looks up, sees the pass that leads us down a glacier and out to a highway. He keeps one hand on his hood to keep it from blowing off. He ducks his head down further, facing into the wind, and raises his ice ax with the other hand.

Victory.

He keeps walking.

test, and that no trend, either up or down, could be detected. These vast efforts had produced no measurable improvements and his skiing results had stagnated despite them. If, instead of this near mono-directional approach, an equal amount of time and effort had been placed on training several of the other qualities he needed to compete at the very top level, it is likely that this skier would have been a world champ.

The fractional utilization of VO_2 max (anaerobic threshold), on the other hand, is very trainable among all athletes and is one area in which both beginner and elite endurance athletes can make solid gains. For our purposes in alpine climbing, increasing this essential quality is the primary goal, and will be the principle training goal of the programs you design.

FUELS FOR ENERGY

Your body's movement requires energy. This energy comes from a fuel. The fuel used in the muscle cell is provided by the breakdown of the food you eat first by digestion in the gut and later by way of the process we referred to as metabolism in chapter 2. The energy of this fuel is stored in the chemical bonds of the fats, carbohydrates, and proteins contained in your food. Energy is released when chemical bonds are broken during the metabolic processes. In this chapter we will only consider the metabolism of carbohydrates and fats, since they provide the bulk of the fuel for muscle contraction.

The metabolism of fats, known as lipolysis, requires a lot of oxygen (aerobic metabolism) and is a relatively slow process. It proceeds by an entirely different chemical process in your muscle cell than that of carbohydrate metabolism. Both processes result in the same end product, a molecule called adenosine triphosphate or ATP, which is the gasoline of the cellular engine. In well-conditioned endurance athletes, fat supplies most of the fuel for producing ATP at low-intensity activity, especially when that activity lasts many hours. We'll look more closely at this crucial ingredient of endurance shortly.

The metabolism of the sugars that come from carbohydrates is called glycolysis. It is a faster process (about twice as fast) than the metabolism of fats. This higher-rate metabolism allows for more rapid ATP production and hence more muscle power for faster and more strenuous activity. Glycolysis can occur either with oxygen (aerobically) or without oxygen (anaerobically).

Your body's store of sugars is very limited, no more than approximately 2,000 calories depending on the individual and their diet, and can provide only enough energy to last a bit over an hour of moderate- to high-intensity exercise. Fat, on the other hand, is stored in large quantities, especially within the muscles of the well-trained endurance athlete who, though slim, likely carries around 100,000 calories. Fat contains about twice the energy, ounce for ounce, of sugar. One of the most beneficial results of aerobic training for alpinists is the adaptation of the muscle cells to prefer fats for fuels at a relatively higher intensity, which before training would have required glycolytic metabolism (the breakdown of sugars) with its inherently very limited fuel supply. Fat can provide a vast source of energy for the well-trained alpinist. By well trained, we mean your body can produce energy from fats at the rate required to sustain moderate power outputs for hours on end.

THE PHYSIOLOGY OF ENDURANCE

The molecule ATP is continually being produced and broken down within in the muscles to provide the energy used for movement. For endurance activities, the bulk of this ATP synthesis takes place in the mitochondria of the muscle cells and is driven by aerobic mechanisms. Science does not yet completely understand the complex way in which the mitochondria produce energy, but for our purposes it suffices to say that the mitochondria contain special enzymes to aid this process. Enzymes are biological catalysts. Catalysts act to speed up chemical reactions but are not consumed in the reaction, so they can be utilized over and over again. These enzymes help to produce the energy from the food we eat to build the ATP molecules.

ATP is a form of chemical energy that every cell in your body needs to survive and, most importantly for our discussions, powers muscular contractions. ATP must be continually resynthesized (which requires energy) in the cells after having been broken down (which releases energy) into its component parts during metabolism. It is this continual process of breaking apart and then resynthesizing the ATP molecule that sustains life. Since muscle contraction is what moves us, this is the energy we rely on for alpine climbing.

ATP (adenosine triphosphate) Production

Your aerobic work capacity depends on the rate at which your working muscle cells can produce ATP using aerobic metabolism. Therefore, more and faster ATP production yields more and faster work. This directly results in increased endurance and speed.

Fitness, Fat, and Fuel

By Scott Johnston

Colin Haley and I heard the commotion of jangling hardware from deep within our cozy sleeping bags and tried to block it out to sleep a few more hours. With a forecast for a perfect-weather June day, we saw no reason to rush out into the cold. We hunkered deeper to await the sun. As preparation for a planned single-push ascent of the Cassin Ridge, we had come to the 14,000-foot (4,267-meter) camp on Denali's West Buttress for some acclimatization. So far we'd mainly skied around, making runs from just below the fixed ropes on the west buttress and from the base of the rocks on the west rib before venturing higher on foot. The snow had been nice powder and could have entertained us well enough, but we were eager to get higher.

By 10 a.m. the sun hit us and we left camp. We calculated that we'd be able to get up and down the west buttress with light packs and that by staying in the sun all day we wouldn't need much extra clothing or camping gear. We set off with nothing more than a couple of liters of water, some snacks, and puffy jackets in our packs. As forecasted, the day remained perfect. The western routes on Denali have a spectacular view, and allow for an early warning of changing weather as well as late-evening sun for climbers. Except for a thin pall of smoke blowing in from massive Siberian fires, the sky was clear and bright.

We moved at a good clip but maintained a steady conversation between ourselves and with the climbers we passed along the way. As was our intention, we never hurried or pressed the pace but moved continuously, aside from a little crampon bouldering session at 16,500 feet (5,029 meters) and a short break to chat with a guide friend of mine at his camp at 17,400 feet (5,304 meters). By 3 p.m. we stood on the summit, wearing all our clothes as we hammed it up for a few photos. Our descent took us right back down the buttress and to our camp at 14,000 feet (4,267 meters) by 5 p.m., just in time for dinner. With the beautiful weather, light packs, and good fitness this had been a fun day out in the mountains rather than the epic test of will it turns into for so many ill-prepared Denali climbers.

What made our climb so casual? I was fifty-two. Five years previously, I had had open-heart surgery to correct a birth defect that had restricted the blood pumped to my lungs by 30 percent. What allowed an old man like me to keep pace with a twenty-year-old top-flight alpinist like Colin?

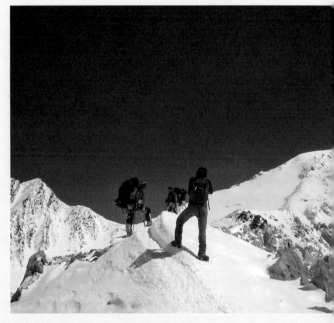

Colin Haley chatting with some more heavily laden mountaineers at 16,700' (5,100m) on Denali's West Buttress Route. *Photo: Scott Johnston*

Despite me being in the twilight of my alpine career and nowhere near the fitness of my twenties and thirties, I could still hold my own. For a period from my mid-thirties till late forties, I'd been working very long hours in my own business, which greatly restricted my climbing. Despite my largely weekend warrior status I knew how to train and carefully maintained at least some vestiges of the base fitness acquired through my younger years. I applied many of the principles you will find in this book to whip my aged body into shape.

What was it that enabled Colin and me to make this fast climb on McKinley so easily? Well adapted to long duration exercise at moderate power output, we could produce almost all of the power we required using fat as fuel and still go at a pace that an untrained climber could not maintain without dipping heavily into his limited glycogen. These same principles should lie at the heart of any successful training program for alpinists.

Aerobic Energy Pathway

The aerobic energy pathway is the alpinist's engine. This aerobic metabolic process is known as the Krebs cycle after the chemist who discovered it. During the Krebs cycle, thirty-eight ATP molecules are produced from each fuel molecule. Unfortunately, this is a relatively slow process (known as oxidative metabolism) due to the multitude of individual reactions needed to break down the fuel. The slow speed of this energy production limits the amount of power the muscle cells can produce. However, this type of oxidative metabolism allows for many hours or even days of continuous movement due to the use of fat as the primary fuel and the vast stores of it that we carry. The duration, power, and speed of this low-intensity work depend to a large extent on how big the previously discussed aerobic base (aerobic endurance) is.

Remember that this capacity is highly trainable; the higher the aerobic power you can sustain means the faster and longer you can move on the mountain. The difference between a high- and a low-aerobic capacity is the difference in going from 14,200 feet (4,328 meters) to the summit of Denali and back in a short day with a good weather window versus struggling to get from 14,200 feet to the 17,200-foot (5,243-meter) camp in the same time, only to be pinned down in a nasty storm for two days and have the summit snatched away.

Anaerobic Energy Pathway

The second method of ATP generation is known as the anaerobic pathway (glycolytic metabolism due to its reliance on glycogen for fuel). This takes place outside the mitochondria and the Krebs cycle, does not require oxygen, and can produce ATP much more quickly than can the Krebs cycle. As a result of this increased rate of ATP production, when muscle cells use this glycolytic pathway, they can produce more power. Think of it as a higher gear for faster movement.

This sounds like a way better deal than the slow Krebs cycle, so why don't our bodies rely on glycolysis for all the energy? As you might have guessed, there are a couple of good reasons.

Lactate: A Measure of the Intensity of Exercise

As the intensity of exercise increases, more and more ATP is supplied via glycolysis. A product of glycolysis is a molecule known as lactate. As lactate levels in the muscle cells increase beyond the ability of the muscles to re-metabolize this form of sugar it begins to leak into the blood and circulate through the body where is taken up and used as fuel by the heart and liver as well as remote skeletal muscles. Devices, called lactate monitors, exist that allow for the easy measurement of the lactate concentration in the blood. Because lactate rises in step with glycolysis, its measurement gives a snapshot of the intensity of exercise at the time the blood is tested. Coaches and physiologists can use these measurements to monitor the intensity of an athlete's training. The accumulation of blood lactate is not a linear process. As the athlete nears his limit of endurance the lactate levels rise very rapidly in synch with the rates of glycolysis as shown in the following figure.

Intensity versus Lactate

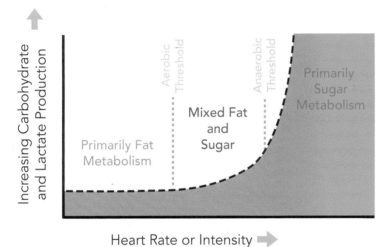

Increasing exercise intensity is fueled by increasing sugar metabolism (glycolysis) and a correspondent drop in the percentage of fat used for fuel (lipolysis). The process of glycolysis results in an increase in muscle cell acidity along with an increase in lactate production. A high rate of glycolysis cannot be sustained for long periods.

The High Cost of High Power Outputs

The impressive power production of glycolysis, the metabolization of sugar, comes at a cost to your body. Hydrogen ions (H+) are produced during glycolysis. These ions result in an increase in acidity (measured as a drop in pH) that upsets the body's delicate balance and leads to fatigue. Sure, you can produce much more muscle power with high rates of glycolysis, but you will fatigue quickly and be forced to slow down or stop to allow your body to restore its homeostasis. We are all familiar with this sensation when we push the pace too hard: that burn in the muscles and the associated hyperventilation that will bring even the strongest to their knees if kept up for too long. In alpine climbing we rely almost entirely on the sustainable, aerobic energy production. Because we are on the go for many hours at a stretch, producing too much power by way of glycolysis is a recipe for failure.

The improvement we seek with correct training is the ability to produce more and more power with less reliance on glycolysis and its attendant drawback of unsustainability. Mechanisms do exist that enable the muscle cells to deal with these glycolytic by-products, and these will become central to our discussion toward the end of this chapter. The training mechanism, however, is covered in the following section.

BOOSTING YOUR AEROBIC POWER

Since ATP provides the energy that powers movement, and since aerobically derived ATP will be the most efficient and sustainable, we need to consider how best to develop the ability to aerobically produce ATP. How do we produce more ATP faster? This is what training for the aerobic base is all about.

To understand how best to aerobically produce ATP faster, we need to examine the factors that contribute to more ATP being produced aerobically. **There are three principle adaptations that result in increased ATP production in the muscles:**

- **Increased mitochondrial mass**

- **Increased aerobic enzymes**

- **Increased capillary bed density**

Luckily, mitochondrial mass, enzyme production, and capillary density are all improved by using the same training methods. We can stimulate all three adaptations with one workout. **For the alpinist the best stimuli for all three are the duration and frequency of the training load; the intensity of training is not as important.**

Mitochondria as a Determinant of ATP Production

Mitochondria are tiny (even by cellular standards) organelles inside every cell in your body and are literally the engines of life. Inside the mitochondria, fuels from food and body stores are combined with oxygen. In the middle of the last century it was discovered that certain types of athletic training have a pronounced effect on both the size and the number of mitochondria in a muscle cell. It was also discovered that the more mitochondrial mass in a muscle cell, the more sites that are available for aerobic metabolism to occur, leading to more ATP synthesis and hence more aerobic muscle power. **The direct outcome**

More Mitochondria Equals More Aerobic Capacity

MORE MITOCHONDRIA => MORE ATP => MORE AEROBIC POWER => *MOVING FASTER*

of an increase in mitochondrial activity is increased aerobic power. The muscle can contract with more force and do it longer with less fatigue. Voila! More endurance! The adaptation of mitochondria takes place on a short-term scale of days to weeks but can continue, with proper stimuli, for several years.

Mitochondrial Biogenesis

Mitochondria undergo a process called *biogenesis* (an increase of mitochondrial mass in the cell) by becoming larger and by multiplying using mitosis. In case you don't recall that term from your high school biology class, it means that they split into two identical copies. The trigger for biogenesis comes from a physical stress, which causes certain genes within the mitochondria to express themselves and start the process of biogenesis. **The biogenesis response by the mitochondria begins to occur within minutes of the training stimulus and ceases within about twelve hours after the stress of training is removed and can result in a longer term doubling of mitochondrial mass.** (Davis et al., 1981) In your training, the most effective way to trigger this response is to induce an aerobic stress to your system, which is of sufficient duration and repeated with sufficient frequency. Of course the term *sufficient* is a variable that needs to be determined for each individual, and we will address that issue in several more places throughout the book.

Within limits, the more often and the longer you can subject these muscle fibers to a mostly aerobic stress, the more mitochondrial mass will be produced (Harms and Hickson, 1983). In one study researchers found a near-linear relationship (up to a point) between the duration of work and the aerobic adaptation of the muscles. Provided that a certain minimal intensity is maintained, a doubling of exercise time resulted in performance improvements of between 40 percent and 100 percent (Harms and Hickson, 1983).

Aerobic Enzymes as a Determinant of ATP Production

Recall that the mitochondria are full of enzymes, which aid in the aerobic metabolism. The more of these critical enzymes that are present, the speedier the Krebs cycle will proceed. These enzymes react to aerobic training stress by increasing in quantity (Harms and Hickson, 1983). This enzymatic adaptation *occurs within minutes* but begins to diminish after even a short break of a few days off from training. Hence, aerobic adaptation requires frequent stimulus to maintain and enhance. It is important to understand that enzymatic adaptations also respond to the duration of the exercise.

Because these enzymes respond immediately to a training stimulus, for many years one of the best ways that researchers have had of testing for an aerobic adaptation to certain types of training has been to measure the level of one of these enzymes known as cytochrome-c (Hickson, 1981). Higher cyctochrome-c levels indicated that the test subject was increasing his or her aerobic capacity.

The intensity of the training mainly determines which muscle fibers get selected for the training effect. We'll discuss this concept in depth

Cytochrome-C Level's Response to Training

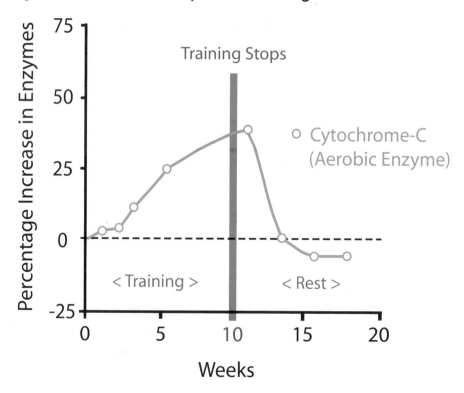

The level of cytochrome-c (an aerobic enzyme) drops quickly upon cessation of training, returning to their initial levels after only three weeks. Source: Hickson, 1981.

in the next section. Training extensively beyond a certain intensity results in a decrease of the aerobic enzymes in the slow-twitch muscle fibers. This can result in a decrease in aerobic capacity.

Capillary Density as a Determinant of ATP Production

Capillaries are the tiny blood vessels that perfuse the body. Capillaries are so tiny that their walls are only one cell thick, which allows these vessels to deliver oxygen to muscle cells and remove metabolic by-products. The closer the capillaries are to the working cells, the less distance the oxygen needs to diffuse to get to the mitochondria. **We grow new capillaries in the working muscles as a response to training.** (Billat et al., 2003) The more capillaries and the denser their networks, the faster oxygen can be delivered to muscle cells. Increasing these capillary beds' density serves a vital function in speeding the transfer of oxygen to the mitochondria and, in the end, increasing the speed of the Krebs cycle's production of ATP. Capillary growth involves growing new structures and takes from weeks to months of consistent training. Anecdotal evidence indicates that the capillary density can continue to increase for many years.

Training the Heart

Our discussion would not be complete without considering the role the heart plays in all of this. Why has the term *cardio* become a mainstay of the current fitness lexicon? Aren't heart rates a great way to monitor aerobic training? The heart is the pump that delivers the oxygen, via the blood, to the working muscles wherein the above three processes help the Krebs cycle crank out more ATP. But the heart is also a slave to the brain and the skeletal muscles. It increases its output of blood and oxygen at the command of the brain, which is getting messages from the muscles that they require more O_2 in order to produce more power. So the cardiac muscle gets trained whenever the demand is greater due to the muscles' requirements.

The heart's response to this increased demand is to increase its output, called the *cardiac output,* which you can think of as the amount of blood pumped in a minute. It does this in two ways: First, by increasing the rate at which it beats (your heart rate), and second, by an increase in its stroke volume, the amount of blood moved with each beat. The stroke volume is a very trainable quality.

Extended periods of elevated heart rate have the training effect on the cardiac muscle of increasing the pumping capacity of the heart. This occurs primarily as a result of an increase in the size of the heart chambers and the contractile qualities of the cardiac muscle itself. The noticeable effect of this cardiac adaptation will be a lowering of both the resting heart rate and a lowering of all sub-maximal workload heart rates. As your aerobic fitness improves, you will notice a drop in your perceived effort for all sub-max work levels. You'll breathe easier and your HR will be lower.

The best training stimulus to increase the heart's stroke volume varies depending on several factors, including age, gender, and fitness level. Fitness is the most important factor for our discussion. For the less well trained, there is very strong evidence that the stroke volume reaches its maximum level at much lower intensities. This means that for many aspiring athletes, even moderate training intensities will have a very beneficial cardiac training effect.

The fitter you are, the greater the intensity needed to elicit a training response from the cardiac muscle. For well-trained to elite-level athletes, the most effective stimulus to improve stroke volume is to

A climber with a high level of cardiac fitness will have a lower heart rate during demanding leads. Here Steve House climbs Colorado's Ames Ice Hose in thin conditions.
Photo: Richard Durnan

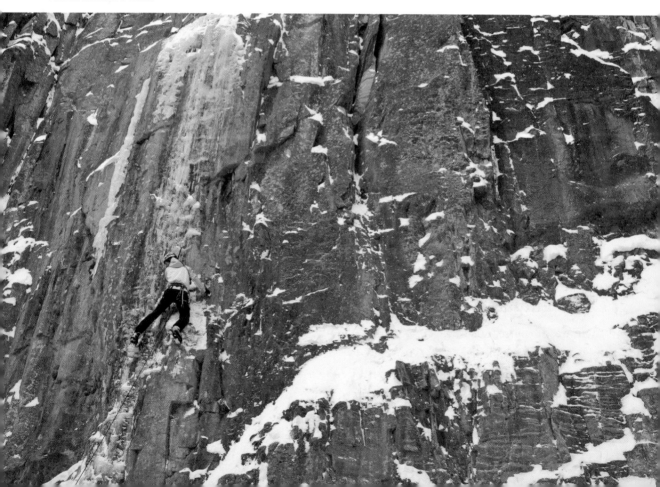

raise the heart rate to near-maximal levels for periods of several minutes (Helgerud et al., 2011, Costill and Trappe, 2002).

During exercise, the best way to raise the heart rate to near max (90–95 percent of the individual's maximum heart rate) in a healthy person is for the brain to call upon a large percentage of your big muscles and maintain that effort for at least several minutes. Through this recruitment of a large muscle mass, the heart has to respond by supplying more blood and oxygen. It does this by upping the cardiac output through an increase in the heart rate and the stroke volume.

This creates a conflict with the training stimuli of the other three determinants of ATP production (mitochondria, capillaries, and enzymes) discussed above that rely on prolonged low- to medium-intensity exercise. While beneficial for training the heart muscle, if sustained for too long and too often, this level of intensity has some undesirable effects down at the skeletal muscle level that can actually lower your aerobic fitness as well as lead to exhaustion and overtraining. We'll delve deeper into this later in the chapter. As a result, there needs to be a careful balance in the application of these two distinct training stimuli.

Endurance Performance Limits

Among coaches and researchers, there is no clear consensus about which of these two systems places the greatest limitation on aerobic power: the central system (cardiac and pulmonary) or the peripheral (skeletal muscles). For less-well-trained and younger athletes, it is thought that the central system may provide much of the limitations to aerobic endurance. It seems that as the athlete becomes more fit, the limitations shift toward the peripheral system. For the fittest athletes, this implies the need for a carefully balanced approach to training. While much debate in current exercise science centers on the question of which system is dominant, there is consensus that the two systems are closely linked and exist in a state of interdependence (Costill and Trappe, 2002).

Other Limitations

There are, of course, other determinants of aerobic power, and we'll only mention a couple here that respond well to training. The first is blood volume and the second is the amount of myoglobin in the muscle cells.

Hemoglobin (Hgb) is the protein in red blood cells that binds with oxygen and carries it to the working muscles. An increase in overall blood volume implies an increase in the amount of Hgb in the blood. The more Hgb, the more O_2-carrying capacity. This increase in the supply of O_2 can allow the aerobic process to proceed faster. Blood volume can increase by 10 percent over several months of endurance training (Helgerud et al., 2011). The blood volume and Hgb issues will be discussed in more depth in chapter 12.

Myoglobin is a protein in the muscle cells that binds with oxygen and acts as a temporary storage for the oxygen. Myoglobin responds rapidly to aerobic training by increasing in quantity and aids in the O_2 transport needed in working muscles.

SUMMARY: AEROBIC CAPACITY ENHANCEMENT

You can greatly enhance the aerobic energy production pathway through correct training that affects:

- The muscles' mitochondria content

- The aerobic enzymes that speed up the aerobic metabolism

- The capillary density in the working muscles

- The pump volume of the heart

- The oxygen-carrying capacity of the blood

- The oxygen-storage capacity of muscle cells

It is necessary to monitor and control the intensity of training to create the conditions necessary for these aerobic adaptations to occur.

MORE PIECES OF THE AEROBIC FITNESS PUZZLE

There exist several competing and overlapping theories about what limits the ultimate work output of the human body. While the details are primarily of interest to physiologists (Davis et al., 1981), and we will not engage in physiological hair splitting, these can offer insights and guidance to coaches and athletes as to the "why" of training. In the following sections we'll take a look at some areas of interest to us as aerobic athletes.

The Nervous System

The central, or supply side, of your body's propulsion systems consists of your lungs for extracting oxygen from the air you breathe and your heart and blood vessels for pumping that oxygen to the muscles. The muscle cells and the energy-conversion processes inside them make up the demand, or peripheral side, of the system. These systems exist in a delicately balanced feedback and feed-forward loop controlled by the central nervous system (this includes the brain and motor nerves), which regulates the amount of muscle mass engaged at any particular moment. The nervous, peripheral, and central systems all respond to training and together are responsible for important improvements in endurance.

The ability to extract useful work from your body ultimately rests with your ability of your central nervous system (CNS) to innervate the muscles. In effect, the CNS seems to be the ultimate driver and limiter of human performance. It does this through the motor nerves that control the muscles, and are responsible for propelling you up the mountain. Another less obvious system of nerves exists, called the autonomic nervous system.

The Autonomic Nervous System (ANS)

This insensible system controls the myriad unconscious activities that go on in our bodies such as heart rate, respiration, digestion, and the release of hormones. It also offers a critical feedback system to let the brain know what is going on throughout the body. In many ways the ANS controls your response and adaptation to training. This creates one aspect of your body's amazing feedback loops that constantly tries to maintain your body's homeostasis or biological equilibrium.

Fight or Flight

The ANS is divided into the sympathetic and the parasympathetic nervous systems (SNS and PNS). A simplified explanation of these is that the SNS is the system responsible for speeding up the body's processes, such as increased heart rate and respiration and the shutting down of digestion. It can be thought of as the evolutionary adaptation of the fight or flight reflex. It brings your body to a higher state of readiness for action.

The PNS does the opposite and can be thought of being responsible for the rest and digest response. It slows many body processes in preparation for rest.

These two systems exist in a delicate give-and-take relationship that, ideally, will result in a balance. Chronic overstimulation of either can result in a fatigue effect and a dysfunction of that system so that the balance is thrown off. We wrote more about this in the overtraining section of chapter 2.

Muscle Fibers

The approach we take throughout this book is one that exercise physiologists term *The Muscle Power Model*. This model assumes that the main limiting factor of aerobic athletic performance occurs at the muscular level. As stated above, the heart and lungs are slaves to the demands of the working muscles. Therefore focusing on training the specific muscles used in climbing is the best way to adapt the many systems involved in making you fitter.

Our muscle cells are joined together into fibers. All the fibers that are *innervated* by a motor nerve are called motor units (MU). To illustrate this concept we'll discuss a couple of examples.

The big muscle in the calf, the gastrocnemius, contains about 1.5 million muscle fibers and about 500 motor units, meaning that one motor nerve controls roughly 3,000 fibers. Because of this rather crude electrical wiring hook-up between brain and muscle, we do not have much fine motor control over this powerful muscle used for propulsion. In big muscles where many fibers must move together to make large movements, precision is sacrificed for power. In contrast, the muscles in our eyelids, over which we do exert a lot of fine motor control, have about 50,000 fibers divided into 500 motor units. Each motor nerve controls only 100 fibers, allowing very minute control over one of our principle means of facial expression.

Fiber Types

Muscle fibers can be divided into three basic types: slow twitch (ST) (also known as type 1), fatigue-resistant fast twitch (also known as type 2a or FTa), and fast twitch (also known as type 2b or FTb). The ST fibers are the predominant fibers used in endurance sports. They are highly fatigue resistant because they contain a high density of capillaries and mitochondria with their attendant aerobic enzymes. These assets allow them to make many thousands of contractions without

Central Nervous System/Muscle Connections

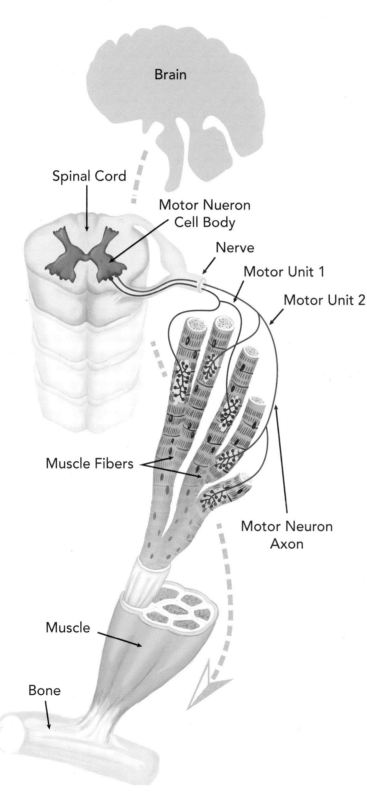

This diagram shows the connection from the brain to the bone that results in movement at your joints and thereby gives rise to locomotion. The brain, spinal cord, and nerves are all part of the central nervous system. A motor unit is composed of a group of muscle fibers and the nerve(s) that innervate them when a signal comes from the central command. Motor units are called into action on an "as needed" basis with the number recruited corresponding to the force you are trying to overcome to accomplish the task at hand. A scheme known as the size principle is responsible for the order of recruitment: In general, the slower/weaker motor units are engaged first with larger and stronger being recruited as the effort required increases.

Ultra-Training

By Krissy Moehl

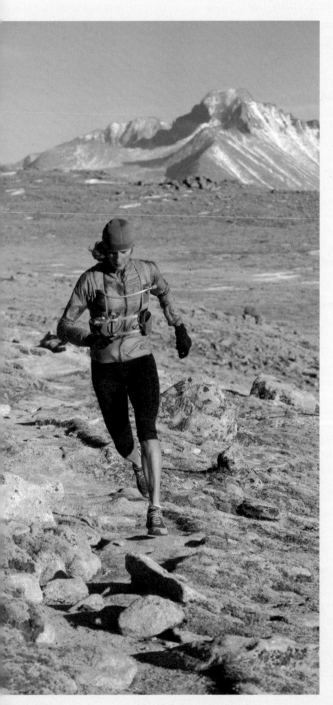

Endurance training is hard work. Pursuing goals that put me out in the elements and pushing my limits is challenging. Training for big goals gives me ample opportunity to focus, visualize, and grow. If I pay attention, I learn not only about training but also about myself.

Endurance training is a cumulative effort. I did not gain all of my fitness in one workout or even one season. From year to year my muscles, tendons, and ligaments are strengthening in response to the workload. My lungs, heart, and brain adapt. I am fine-tuning my senses to know what I need emotionally, nutritionally, and physically. Discovering my limits, and ability to push them, to become more aware and comfortable in my own body is grounding and affirming. These experiences create memories and become the cornerstones that mold my life.

On high alpine ridges and pounding pavement through cities, I have learned commitment, focus, play, and patience. I have reaped the rewards of focused intention and experienced regret when I lost touch with this path. In twelve years of ultra-distance trail running, I know I am the person I am because of the miles I have run, the experiences I have shared, and the lessons each mile has taught me.

Krissy Moehl is an ultra-runner, race director, and coach. She's twice won the Ultra-Trail du Mont-Blanc ('03 and '09), as well as the Hardrock 100 ('07), Wasatch 100 ('04), Ultra-Trail Mount Fuji ('13), and numerous other ultra-marathons. She is the race director of the Chuckanut 50K.

Krissy Moehl runs the Ute Trail in Rocky Mountain National Park. Longs Peak (14,259', 4,346m) is in the background. *Photo: Fredrik Marmsater*

fatigue. Trained endurance athletes have a much higher concentration of ST fibers than the general population. These fibers have a low
electrical threshold for activation. This means that the electrical nerve
impulse needed to contract the fibers of the motor unit is low, so they
are usually the first to be called upon by the brain to begin a movement.

The caveat is that muscle fiber types exist more along a continuum
rather than as discrete types. The classification of a fiber as either more
slow twitch or more fast twitch is based on the protein makeup of the
various parts of the fiber. Many variations are possible, for simplicity
they are usually divided into basic sub-groups.

Slow Twitch Fibers Are Your Endurance Machines

The ST fibers are known as slow twitch because their rate of firing is
about one-third to one-half as fast as that of the FT fibers, and they
generate lower forces than the FT fibers. Because of this they are not
able to produce as much power as the same mass of FT fibers. However,
these ST fibers have a higher density of mitochondria, a smaller
diameter, and greater capillarization, as well as high levels of aerobic
enzymes. These characteristics allow them to process oxygen more
quickly than their FT fiber neighbors and thereby aerobically produce
greater amounts of ATP via the Krebs cycle. Through long duration
and low- to medium-intensity training, these ST muscle cells can be

Mitochondrial Density in Different Muscle Fibers

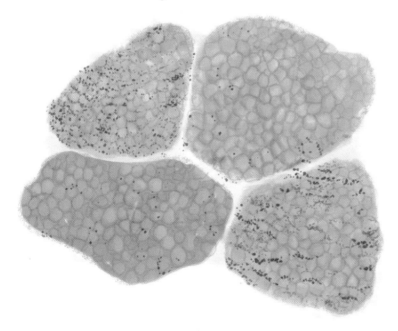

This diagram shows the cross
section through some muscle
fibers. Notice that two of the
fibers have a much higher density
of mitochondria as depicted by
the small blue specs. As you've
learned, mitochondria density
endow these smaller slow twitch
fibers with higher aerobic capacity
than their fast twitch neighbors.
You can also see that these ST
fibers are a little smaller in the
cross-sectional area, which means
that oxygen does not have as far
to travel as it diffuses from the
capillaries to the mitochondria.
These qualities help to give them
greater endurance than their FT
neighbors.

trained to utilize fat as their primary fuel while only sipping at the glycogen supply.

This glycogen conservation is important for endurance athletes who do long-duration activities, typically defined by physiologists as exercise lasting more than two hours. In long-duration activities such as alpine climbing where fat supplies the bulk of the energy for ATP synthesis, glycogen and the by-products of the glycolytic metabolism remain crucial for the function of the Krebs cycle. Even the most fit athletes will be reduced to a near walk if they completely exhaust their glycogen reserves. The common term for this is bonking. Because the brain requires glycogen for fuel, bonking will result in a loss of muscle coordination and slowed cognitive function. An athlete in this state will often be off balance and a little confused or slow witted.

Long-term, effective endurance training will result in quite high power production being sustained for long periods using mainly ST fibers. World-class marathon runners are able to run twenty-six back to back 4:45 miles, all the while deriving 95 percent of the required energy aerobically from their ST fibers using a blend of fat and sugar for fuel in a mix that relies on the abundant energy supplied by aerobic fat metabolism. In contrast, less-fit runners cannot produce the power required to run even one mile at a sub five minute pace without having to utilize a much higher percentage of the energy required from the more wasteful glycolytic metabolism. As a result they cannot sustain this pace. This is because their ST fibers are not powerful enough (well trained enough) to propel them at this speed without resorting to higher contributions from glycolysis with its concurrent lactic acid production and some assistance from their FT fiber neighbors.

Due to the limited glycogen fuel storage in the body, this higher power output cannot be maintained for longer than about one to two hours, depending on the individual. This makes balancing the energy output to complete longer-duration outings somewhat of a challenge. Push the pace a bit too much too early and you will likely bonk and be forced to slow dramatically as your very limited glycogen reserves run low. Eating early on during a climb and continuing to eat often is the best method to avoid bonking. This will be discussed in more detail in chapter 11.

Balancing Your Training

The intensity of training determines which muscle fibers are recruited by your brain and this in turn determines both the main fuel source and training effect on the muscle fibers. Go at an easy to moderate pace and the ST fibers are the predominant ones used with fat as their primary fuel. Speed up a bit and the ST fibers will need to start using more glycogen. Go faster still and the FT fibers will be added to the pool of fibers and the increased glycogen will be used exclusively to power them. These facts reinforce the importance of emphasizing training at a slow to moderate pace with carefully controlled doses of higher-intensity training.

Detraining ST Fibers with High Intensity

Coaches have long known that if they kept the intensity meter turned up too high for too long, especially without maintaining a lot of low-intensity training, their athletes' performance would flatten and fall off. Much of this was put down to the reduction of aerobic enzymes present in ST fibers when those fibers were exposed to prolonged high-intensity training. With the recent advances in genetics, new research has shed fascinating light on why this happens.

Researchers found that increased acidity in muscle cells (as described earlier in the chapter) leads to an inhibition of a certain gene's expression (Lin et al., 2002). This particular gene, known by the catchy name PGC-lalpha mRNA, is responsible for mitochondrial biogenesis. When this gene is inhibited, a host of effects occur that result in a lowering of aerobic capacity. As is often the case, the coaches figure stuff out and then it takes a while for the scientists to find out why it happens that way. The lesson from both the coaches and scientists: **Train too much at too high of an intensity for too long and your aerobic fitness will drop.**

Fast Twitch Fibers' Contribution to Endurance

Fatigue-resistant fast twitch (FTa) fibers tend to be larger in diameter than the ST fibers and have a lower mitochondrial density. They rely mostly on glycolytic metabolism. Recall that glycolytic metabolism can occur as an anaerobic process that takes place outside the mitochondria and allows these fibers to produce ATP at a rate as much as two to three times that of ST fibers. As a result of the glycolytic process and the increased contractility of these fibers, they are about five times more powerful than ST fibers (Widrick et al., 1996). The threshold of electrical stimulation required to activate these FTa fibers is higher than ST fibers. This means that the brain must be more active in engaging them through the motor nerves. In other words it takes more effort to engage and hence train these fibers. FTa fibers appear to be very trainable for endurance and with training can develop endurance properties more like ST, if not actually converting completely to ST fibers.

Muscle Fiber Conversion

Numerous studies have shown that fiber type conversion (such as FTa fibers taking on characteristics of ST fibers) is possible in laboratory animals (Wang et al., 2004; Lin et al., 2002; Pette and Vrbova, 1999). But very few controlled studies have been conducted on humans due to the length of time needed to observe changes. The conversion process seems to take years of sustained training at a high volume, which results in chronic low-grade microscopic muscle damage and subsequent repair (Rusko, 1992). It also seems to be reversible when training ceases. This conversion process is the best explanation for why endurance athletes tend to have a higher percentage of ST fibers than the general population.

Not only is this phenomenon possible (Dudley et al., 1984), it is essential for top-level athletes to effectively train these powerful fibers to become more fatigue resistant. The same basic mechanisms of training stimuli occur for the fast twitch fibers (both FTa and FTb) types as explained for the ST above. Duration of the exercise is key, and the muscle fibers need to be stressed by repeatedly contracting and relaxing for long durations in order to stimulate mitochondrial biogenesis along with the other aerobic adaptations, like increases in enzymes. Bear in mind that long duration for an FT motor unit may be only 20 seconds due to their lack of fatigue resistance. Because they quickly fatigue, an interval method (see chapter 2 for a more detailed discussion of interval training) will need to be used in order to accumulate a high volume of time at this higher intensity.

While these FT fibers respond to the duration of the training stimulus the primary stimulus is intensity because it takes high intensity just to engage these fibers. These FT fibers are harder to engage because they have a higher electrical threshold than the ST fibers, and the muscle has to be called upon by the brain to contract with a

Justin Merle chucks a lap near Ouray, Colorado. *Photo: Steve House*

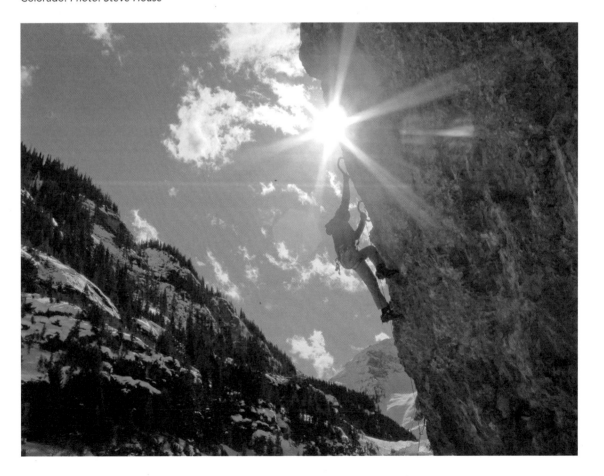

substantially greater force in order to get these fibers into action, giving them a training effect. Producing the force necessary to engage FT motor units requires real mental effort and concentration. At the same time that we are trying to encourage these FT fibers to shift toward a more aerobic metabolism, they will also be receiving a strong stimulus to develop their anaerobic capacity to new levels due to the intensity of the exercise required just to get them into the act.

While these adaptations are essential for an 800-meter runner or in the forearms and shoulders of a sport climber seeking to climb at his limit, this adaptation in the legs of an alpinist is of much less importance as it represents a miniscule part of his or her total energy budget. This, again, is due to the duration of the event (or climb) being in excess of two hours in almost every case. For shorter duration events this type of training is much more important in terms of the energy it can contribute to the total. This is not to say that it has no place in your training but you need to recognize why we recommend only a small percentage. We'll talk about how to balance this training in the Planning Section.

It is important to remember that whenever these FTa fibers are working they are consuming primarily glycogen, as opposed to the fat that is the preferred fuel for the ST fibers. Also recall that glycolysis requires nineteen times as much fuel input to produce the same amount of ATP, which is the energy source for propelling you up the mountain. Given this radically wasteful use of your energy stores, it behooves any climber to concentrate on developing the maximal amount of aerobic capacity of the ST fibers and their hyper-efficient metabolism, and only supplement with training of the FT fibers.

Muscle Fiber Specificity

Only the motor units of the muscles responsible for the movements being trained will show the effects of the training they have been subjected to. **This means you must use the muscles in your training in very similar ways that you hope to use them in the mountains.** This concept is defined as specificity of training.

Fiber Recruitment

In general, as exercise begins, the first motor units called into action by the brain are the ST because they have the lowest electrical threshold for activation. This is known as the size principle and it holds mostly— but not always. When more force is required, more ST motor units

Asynchronous Motor Unit Recruitment

Research shows that ST fibers within a motor unit can be activated asynchronously, so that some can be resting while others are working. It is thought that this quality is part of what adds to ST fibers' endurance. This ability to asynchronously engage a small number of fibers in a motor unit is also what allows us to perform tasks requiring a great deal of dexterity, like playing a piano or writing. Our brain can exert fine motor control of the few slow twitch fibers needed to perform these low force movements.

As opposed to ST fibers, when the requirements for force are high enough to recruit FT motor units, the brain tends to activate them synchronously. In other words all the fibers in an FT motor unit are either activated or not, depending on the signal from the brain. Thus the high forces required to perform powerful movements are not as susceptible to fine motor control. This is why newcomers to a sport have jerky, uncoordinated movements. It can make it very difficult to learn complex athletic movements that involve both strength and grace; this is one of the reasons why we admire demonstrations of high athleticism. Through proper training the pool of high-powered FT motor units is increased so that they too can be cycled in and out of action resulting in increased endurance at high power levels.

Muscle Fiber Recruitment

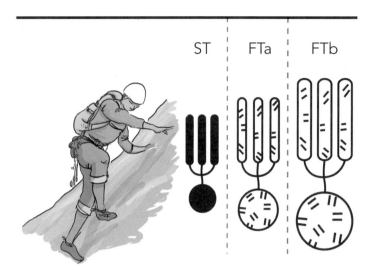

On easy terrain with a light load the climber will be mostly engaging the Slow Twitch Motor Units which can supply the low forces needed for this easy activity. These fibers have high endurance so this activity can go on for an extended duration.

As the climb becomes steeper and/or the pack gets heavier the climber must begin to use some of the intermediate fibers called Type 2a or Fast Twitch a. These can provide much higher forces than the ST fibers can. FTa fibers are also very trainable for increased endurance so they can become a major contributor to sustained difficult climbing.

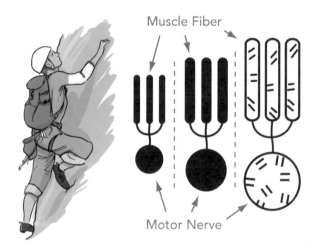

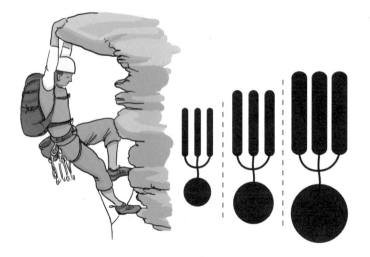

When the climb gets steep or the pack gets very heavy the climber will be forced to recruit a significant portion of his available pool of motor units to get up the pitch. The most powerful of these motor units are composed of FTb fibers which by definition will not be so well trained for endurance and will fatigue quickly. This puts a time limit on how long this climber can sustain these difficult movements.

are called in to join the effort. As the power requirements continue to climb the pool of ST motor units will get fully tapped and the brain will be forced to recruit FT motor units to add to the total motor unit tally contributing to doing the job at hand.

As an example of the difference between slow twitch activation and fast twitch fiber activation, imagine the following two scenarios:

1) First, you are out for a casual jog on a flat trail at a relaxed and easy pace. From what you know now it should be obvious that this predominately requires the slow twitch fibers and probably not even all of them since you are running well within your capacity. You can let your mind wander to any sort of thoughts without disturbing the level of power the muscles are making. In fact, you can become distracted enough to carry on an involved conversation while your trusty ST motor units that are responsible for driving your legs through the running cycle keep right on as if on autopilot, seemingly with no real conscious effort. A very small amount of your brain's motor cortex is needed for a simple and familiar movement like running slowly.

2) Next, imagine that you are standing below an overhang that is going to require a powerful lunge at the lip. From your knowledge of muscle fiber types, it should be pretty obvious that even Alex Huber is going to need to focus on these powerful movements in order to call upon his fast twitch fibers to have any chance of pulling this move. Think you could be doing mental long division or chatting away to your belayer while pulling that move? Not likely. Ever notice how you stop talking when you get to the crux of a pitch? Most of us would have to be supremely focused and have every one of the needed FT motor units firing in the exact right sequence in order to complete such a high strength, very complex movement. Your brain's motor cortex is in a hyperactive state to accomplish this task.

Certainly this is an extreme example, but it illustrates that in order for the brain to engage the FT fibers (even the FTa ones), you must make a concerted effort. In a running analogy you would have to force yourself to run harder.

At the Limit

There will, of course, be an ultimate limit to both the force that any muscle is capable of and the endurance of these crucial FT fibers. At some point the brain just can't call any more FT motor units into

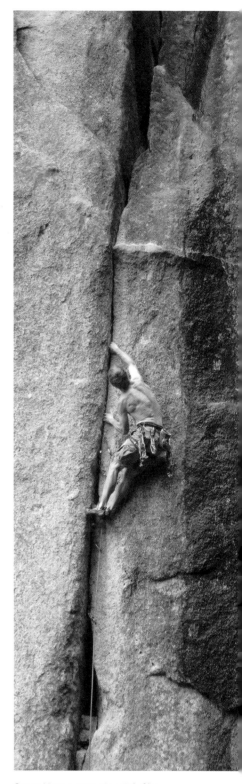

Steve House engaging FTb fibers to climb a steep granite crack in Mizugaki, Japan. *Photo: Eva House*

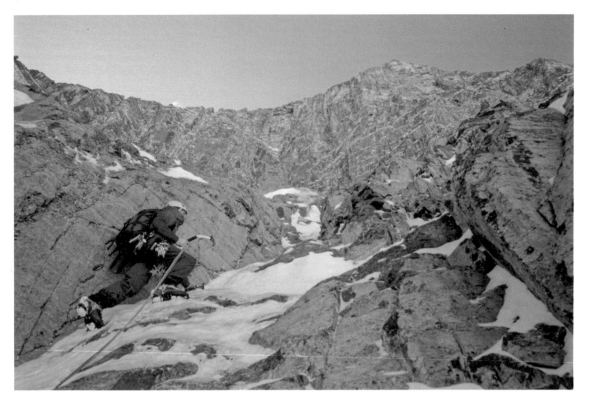

Marko Prezelj uses his slow-twitch fibers to efficiently ascend a moderate mixed pitch on the north face of North Twin (12,241', 3,371m). *Photo: Steve House*

action. This limits the amount of force the muscle can produce. Next you'll be limited by the ability of those FT fibers to maintain that level of force over time. As stated in the previous section, the brain has a nifty way of helping improve endurance: By cycling motor units in and out of action. It replaces the fatigued ones with fresh or fresher ones. If there is a large pool of available motor units within the muscle that are available to pitch in and help out, then this cycling technique can enhance the endurance of these FT fibers significantly. However, if the force required is close to the maximum that the muscle is capable of producing and most of the pool of available motor units is already called into play then, there will be far fewer motor units available to cycle in as replacements when the working motor units become fatigued. Training increases both the size of the available motor unit pool and the endurance of those fibers.

SUMMARY: MUSCLE FIBERS

- Fibers can be classified according to their characteristics as either slow twitch (ST) or fast twitch (FT).

- ST fibers are the main fibers used for long endurance activities like alpine climbing. They rely mainly on the aerobic energy production of the Krebs cycle to power them.

- While all fibers exist somewhere along a continuum from slow to fast twitch, conventionally FT fibers are further divided into FTa and FTb fibers. FTa fibers have some of the endurance characteristics of ST fibers but can contract more forcefully. These can be trained to become even more endurance oriented. They rely on glycolysis for ATP production.

- FTb fibers are the most powerful, but they fatigue very quickly and so are useful only for maximal efforts lasting only a few seconds.

- Fibers can convert from one type to another if they are exposed to many hundreds of hours of consistent training stimuli.

- Only the actual fibers or groups of fibers called motor units (MU) that are being trained receive the training adaptations, so specificity in exercise is important in training effectively.

- Motor units tend to consist of one type of muscle fiber. These MUs are recruited as needed by the central nervous system. For movements requiring low force, the brain recruits ST motor units. As more force is required the brain calls for more ST fibers. For still higher force generation, the brain begins to recruit FT fibers until the task is completed or the maximum strength of the muscle is reached.

- The different fiber types get the maximum training stimuli at different intensities of training. What causes the best adaptation in ST fibers probably won't even give a training effect to FT fibers. What is the best training for FT fibers is too short in duration to give a boost to the ST fibers.

PUTTING ALL THE PIECES TOGETHER

We understand that this chapter has required some heavy lifting on the reader's part and it was not without a great deal of thought and labor that we included such a detailed and complex discussion in this book. In the end we felt that to best serve our readers we needed to delve a little into the physiological depths to give you the basis for understanding why we are so adamant about our approach to training. Let's take the next few pages to bring all this chapter's information together into a coherent theory of endurance training.

Acidosis, a Primary Cause of Muscle Fatigue

If FT fibers can produce more power, why don't our bodies just recruit them more often? And, as a result, we could climb faster. The answer lies first in the fact that these FT fibers fatigue more quickly than the ST fibers and that their fuel supplies (glycogen only) are much more limited. As discussed earlier in the chapter this fatigue is brought on due to the anaerobically synthesized ATP (using glycolysis outside the mitochondria) having the undesirable side effect of increasing the acidity in the working muscle fibers. The increase in acidity is the result of an increase in hydrogen ion (H+) production. It is this H+ that causes a problem for us by lowering the muscle cells' pH (increasing its acidity) as these hydrogen ions begin to accumulate. This increased acidosis has a cascade of negative effects (Mainwood and Renaud, 1985).

Complex Feedback Loop

Our muscle cells have a natural pH balance of 7.1. When the intramuscular pH drops (increasing in acidity) to 6.9, the process of glycolysis (used for the synthesis of the all-important ATP) in the muscles begins to decrease. At a pH of 6.4, muscle cell glycolysis ceases (Spriet et al., 1987; Hargreaves and Spriet, 2006). It is important to remember that glycolysis is the metabolic process used to produce ATP when your power requirements outstrip the capacity of the slower fat-based metabolism. Also recall that glycolysis is the primary source of energy that powers the fast twitch fibers. As you now know, these FT fibers are the ones responsible for high power athletic movements.

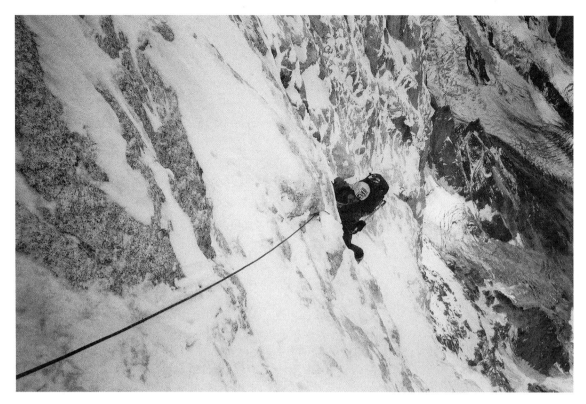

Steve House following a difficult mixed pitch at 23,000' (7,000m) during an attempt of Kunyang Chish East (24,278', 7,400m). *Photo: Vince Anderson*

It should be easy to see from this explanation that producing too much power for too long will raise the muscles' acidity, resulting in a virtual shutdown of those very muscle fibers that are providing the power. Most of us have experienced this feeling of absolute, temporary exhaustion when, say, we sprinted uphill too hard for too long and were forced to slow way down for several minutes before continuing. Or perhaps you have had a nasty forearm pump when your grip completely failed and you were spit off that route you were working. That is the sensation of your muscle pH dropping to below 6.4, producing complete muscular failure.

Slow Twitch Fibers Limit High-Intensity Power

The limitation imposed on high-intensity work by the low-intensity aerobic system is a salient point not understood by some popular exercise trends (such as CrossFit) that emphasize high-intensity training all the time. This is a very common misunderstanding, so let us look in more detail to the mechanisms involved.

Training for Alpine Climbing in the Former USSR

By Alexander Odintsov

In the USSR, alpinism was considered an official sport by the state. For this reason, the training process always included elements of competition. The greater the skill of the climber, the more frequently he found himself participating in various competitions.

The pluses of the Soviet system, in my view, include the fact that we developed and applied a methodology of athletic training. The Federation of Alpinism developed training requirements for athletes involved in climbs of varying levels of difficulty. These were contained in a 200-page book, which spelled out the expertise required of climbers at various skill levels; the exams they needed to take; the lectures they needed to attend. There were both practical and theoretical tests. Here are some of their titles: "Group Movement on Rocky (Icy, Mixed, Snowy) Terrain," "Pair Movement on Complex Rocky

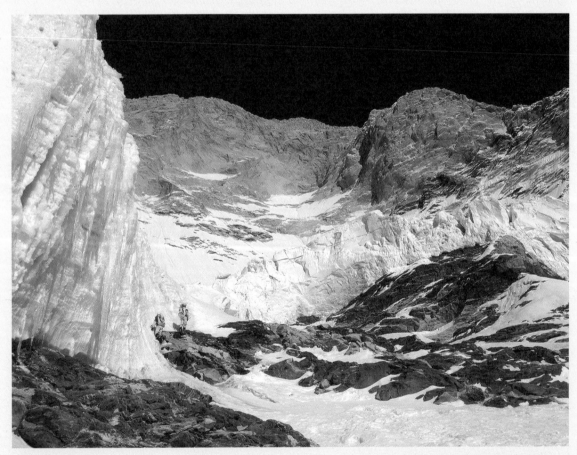

Steve House and Vince Anderson approaching the west face of Makalu (27,825', 8,481m) for an alpine-style attempt in 2008. In 1997 a Russian expedition led by Sergey Efimov ascended the huge, right-hand buttress visible in the right side of this photo. *Photo: Marko Prezelj*

Terrain," "Establishing Belays on Rocky (Icy, Snowy) Terrain," "Providing First Aid," "Transporting Victims on Rocky (Icy, Snowy) Terrain," "History of World Alpinism," "History of Soviet Alpinism," and "Survey of Mountain Regions of the World."

A trainer of young climbers bore serious responsibility for the students' level of preparedness, and therefore before attempting an advanced-level ascent, an alpinist would have completed from forty to one hundred simpler climbs. Accidents were rare, and each one was subject to careful analysis. Every year, an analysis of all events in the mountains was published and was required study material at alpine base camps.

I was exceptionally lucky with my trainer. I ended up in the hands of a person who began as my trainer, continued as a rope-mate, and finally ended up as my friend. He was Aleksey Rusyayev, known colloquially as Russo. I am indebted to him for everything I know, everything I am capable of in alpinism.

Rusyayev was brilliantly athletic in nature. He feared no challenge. He made optimal use of the competitive element in training. His imagination was boundless. Even when working on climbing knots, we competed against one another. Training was mainly aerobic in nature. Russo knew how to vary the exercises such that the classes were never monotonous. In climbing, the emphasis was on the amount of work completed. It was considered normal for a person to climb 1,000 meters (3,281 feet) on a wall during a training day. The most attention was paid to rope work. Each element—Dulfersitz abseil, pendulum, the setting of belay points—became automatic. Each exercise was completed against a stopwatch. Our trainer also paid attention to physical stamina. We practiced racing cross-country in the mountains, and in the winter the entire group skied. Even despite the fact that in the winter we spent one month in the mountains, we managed to Nordic ski as much as 1,000 kilometers (621 miles) in a winter.

At that time we practiced competitions known as alpine marathons. Participants in the competitions would receive a list of sixty to eighty routes located at the site of the championship, in the Caucasus or the Pamirs. Each route was given points rating the difficulty. Over the course of twenty days, the athletes could climb whatever routes they chose. The victor was the one who had accumulated the highest number of points. All that was required was physical training, the ability to allocate one's strength over twenty days, the ability to make expert choices in logistics, and the ability to endure. Participation in these competitions required daily training during the off-season; and second, a special relationship to the mountains. The mountains become a place of regular habitation rather than the hostile environment to humans that they are.

Many people use the mountains as a test site for self-validation: This virus afflicts the majority of young people who come to alpinism to some degree. I won't claim that this is a bad thing, but for me that state was, thanks to Russo, unfamiliar. He forced us to understand that in giving your soul, strength, time, and money to the mountains, you must not demand anything in return; that a relationship of equals with the mountains is impossible; that a person is only a grain of sand in the ocean of existence; that the most important thing in the mountains is the people, your friends, and your relationships; and that not a single mountain is worth a single frostbitten and amputated little toe. Further, he taught us to act equally kindly toward people of a fanatical inclination (those who dedicated themselves body and soul to the mountains) as toward those people for whom this love was not the most important thing in their lives (those who loved the process of mountain climbing but were not prepared to dedicate their entire being to it).

Aleksey Rusyayev was unfortunately one of the forty-five people buried on Friday, July 13, 1990, by an avalanche that fell on a camp at 17,390 feet (5,300 meters) on the slope of Lenin Peak. After his death, I skipped the 1991 summer season, the only time I did so in my thirty-seven-year climbing history.

Russian mountaineer and master of sport Alexander Odintsov began climbing in 1975. He is the head of the Russian Big Wall Project, which aims to climb the ten highest walls in the world's mountains.

Lactate Shuttle

A 1985 study by Davis et al. described a process now known as the lactate shuttle, whereby the lactate produced by gylcolysis is shuttled to adjacent ST fibers. This lactate, which used to be considered a waste product, is now known to be a ready and important source of fuel for the Krebs cycle of the ST endurance fibers. The better aerobically trained the athlete's muscles are, the better the shuttle works, the less the requirement for ATP from glycolysis in FT fibers, and hence, the better the blood's acidity is kept in check as the intensity of exercise increases (Brooks, 1986).

To re-state: The better the aerobic capacity of the ST fibers, the more lactate they are able to utilize as fuel.

The athlete can then produce a higher power output for a longer time with less fatigue: These athletes have better endurance.

From this comes the following understanding: **Even though the FT fibers are the ones largely responsible for the higher muscle power outputs that give you the faster pace, the length of time that you can sustain this fast pace is almost completely dependent on the aerobic capacity of the ST fibers.** This is the seemingly contradictory and counterintuitive reason why the aerobic base is so important to high exertion levels.

Climb Your Fastest

This is where we pull together these many seemingly disparate concepts and relate them to how you can climb faster.

- The enhanced aerobic capacity of trained slow twitch fibers is manifested as an elevation of the individual's aerobic threshold.

- Raising the aerobic threshold to its highest level puts you in the best position to raise your anaerobic threshold.

Recall from chapter 2 that the aerobic threshold is defined as the point during a graded (slowly increasing) exercise test where the blood lactate level begins to rise above the base level. This rise indicates that the metabolism fueling the muscles is shifting to one made up of slightly more glycolysis (sugar). It is reflected as an increase in breathing rate and depth. For those without a lab or lactate monitor there is a handy way to evaluate your own aerobic threshold: We have observed a close correlation between the measured blood lactate level and the point where breathing through your nose becomes noisy and labored.

Also recall from chapter 2: The highest intensity that one can maintain for an extended time (30 minutes to one hour) is determined by the anaerobic threshold. This is the point where the lactate shuttle mechanism we've been talking about has reached its shuttling capacity. At any higher intensity the shuttle can't keep up and the lactate levels begin to rise rapidly. This lactate rise is accompanied by a rise in muscle acidity, which will result in the onset of fatigue and subsequent drop in power output.

Referring again to chapter 2 you may recall that your anaerobic threshold is the point at which your fractional utilization of VO_2 max is maximized and is one of the best predictors of endurance performance. This point is highly individual and it is also highly trainable. By training near the intensity of the anaerobic threshold you can improve the power output you are capable of sustaining for extended periods.

Recall the concept of maximum lactate steady state. Now is when that concept ties into the reality of performance: **The higher the muscle's maximum sustainable lactate level and the power produced at that level (the anaerobic threshold), the faster you can climb.**

A high aerobic threshold power is the best support for a high anaerobic threshold. This potent combination means you can get up and down the route with a bigger safety margin.

Training to improve these thresholds is the primary goal of any successful program for any endurance sport.

THE BASE IS CRUCIAL

Hopefully you now understand that what gave Steve the ability to function at a high level of exertion during the North Twin climb at the beginning of this chapter (despite the significant setback of losing a boot) was his very high aerobic capacity or base. This gave him an endurance reserve that helped him survive a dangerous situation. When the situation on a climb where you are already near your limit turns nasty, will you have that same reserve to allow you to get down safely?

We cannot overemphasize that the aerobic base building period is the most essential phase of training, as it plays a critical role in the development of aerobic power. Base is an appropriate term because it forms the foundation upon which rests the harder, more specific

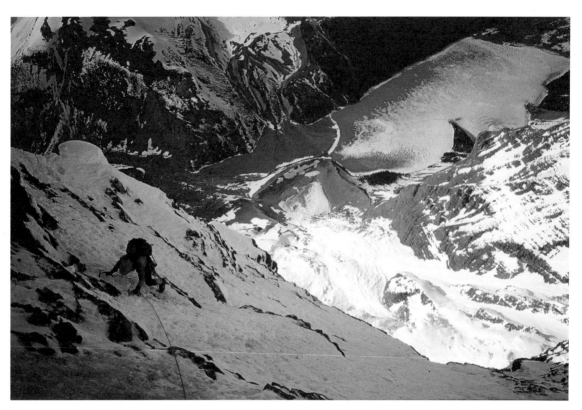

Colin Haley climbing the Emperor
Face of Mount Robson during the
first ascent of the Haley-House route.
Photo: Steve House

training to follow. We can use the building of a house as an analogy for training. A solid foundation will allow the rest of the structure to be built higher. While the roof is an essential element of the house, you would not try to put the roof on until all the supporting structure was in place. For that same reason, you do not want to apply the finishing touches, such as higher intensity aerobic/anaerobic training, to your training until you are sure that the base can support it. If you shortcut this base phase or mix in too many hard aerobic/anaerobic efforts, the specific training phase later on will be much less effective.

This is the foundation of all training for any endurance sport lasting longer than about two minutes. Omit it at your peril.

SUMMARY: PATHWAYS TO IMPROVE THE AEROBIC AND ANAEROBIC THRESHOLDS

What follows is the basis for what we lay out in the Planning section of the book.

Number One: Improve the ultimate aerobic power of the ST fibers. This is done by a high volume of training done at low intensity at or below your aerobic threshold. This is what increases a person's aerobic qualities and establishes a metabolic base of support for improving the lactate shuttle process. This improvement of the aerobic threshold (AeT) manifests as an increase of the pace that is sustainable at lower intensities for hours on end. Over years of correct training this increase can be profound. It is what allows elite male marathoners to run twenty-six consecutive sub-five-minute miles.

Number Two: Progressively increase the relative volume of training (time or distance) spent at moderate intensities to accomplish several goals: Improve the lactate shuttle's effectiveness, increase the power of the ST fibers, and improve the aerobic capacities of the FT fibers needed to produce higher power levels. These will jointly have the effect of improving your pace at the anaerobic threshold.

Having number one is essential in order to maximize the improvement in number two. In other words: The improved shuttling capabilities brought about by the higher aerobic threshold and increased aerobic power of the ST fibers is what allows the most effective endurance training of the higher power FT fibers.

We owe much of our natural endurance to our mitochondria and the aerobic enzymes contained therein. With the proper training stimulus, you can maximize the adaptations (increased mitochondrial mass, aerobic enzyme production, and capillary growth) that improve your ability to generate aerobic power many times over the untrained state. This increase in aerobic endurance is what allows the top athletes in all endurance sports to perform seemingly superhuman feats. With a correct progression of training, these adaptations will increase from year to year.

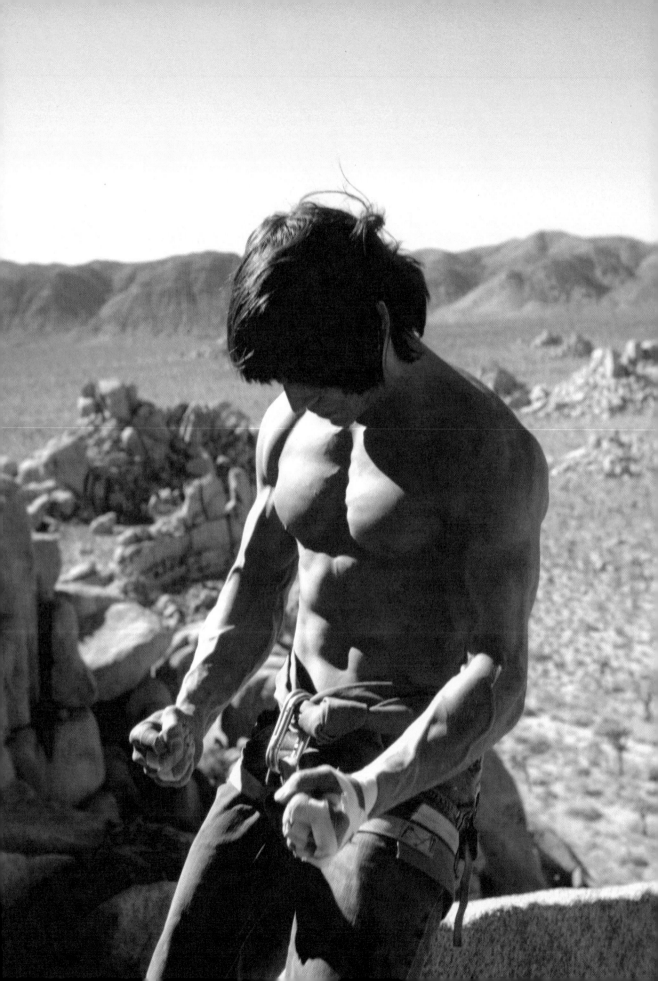

Chapter 4

The Theory of Strength Training

"If you don't have the strength to pull a single move . . . there is nothing to endure."

— TONY YANIRO, legendary rock climber and climbing strength coach

STRENGTH: EVEN FOR ENDURANCE ATHLETES?

Despite the popularity of strength training there exists a lot of misinformation among athletes about this very effective tool.

Not many years ago strength training for endurance athletes was considered a no-no. The thinking went something like this: Conventional endurance sports—like running, cycling, rowing, and swimming—rely on relatively low strength movements repeated for many minutes or even hours. These forces are well below the maximal force capacity of the muscles even in untrained individuals. If the forces required are so far below maximal then why spend precious training time to increase the maximal strength? This made intuitive sense to many coaches, and thus one of the cardinal rules for endurance sports was born: No strength training.

Opposite: Tony Yaniro after making the first free ascent of Equinox, 5.12c, in 1981 in Joshua Tree National Park, California. *Photo: Randy Leavitt*

It was also assumed (wrongly) that increasing maximum strength would likely result in an increase in body weight. Because of these two ideas a decades-long anti-strength bias prevailed and most endurance coaches had a poor understanding of correct strength training methods. This bias still remains in some quarters even today.

New Evidence

These arguments sounded so reasonable that they went generally unchallenged for many decades despite a handful of coaches using various forms of strength training very successfully for their endurance athletes. Then, in the 1990s Norwegian exercise physiologist Jan Helgerud completed a couple of studies in which he had high-level cross-country skiers train to improve their maximum strength. The outcome of these studies was that the skiers radically improved their time to exhaustion (just as it sounds, this is a very good measure of endurance) of an exercise simulating the specific cross-country ski movement of double poling. In the most dramatic case involving elite women cross-country skiers, their time to exhaustion in the double-pole motion improved by 100 percent after adding only nine weeks of thirty minutes per week of maximum strength training to their regular training routine. This staggering improvement in endurance for the minimal time investment put to rest any notion that endurance athletes could not benefit from strength training.

The phenomenon of developing strength to improve endurance, alluded to in Yaniro's quote on the previous page, has come to be termed *strength reserve*. It refers to the difference between your absolute strength and the strength needed to complete a given task specific to your need. Let's look at a couple of climbing-specific examples:

1) You are headed off to climb Denali's West Buttress.

You've been reading up and found out that most people are carrying a sixty-pound pack when they move from 14,200 feet (4,328 meters) to the 17,200-foot (5,243-meter) camp. Just for fun you load up a pack with sixty pounds and put on your double boots, harness, ascenders, and camera, along with the other incidental stuff you'll wear, and then do a little box step-up test. What you find is disturbing: Wearing all this gear, if the step you need to take is more than twelve inches, you can't make it. You just can't step up with that much weight attached on your body.

You've read that some of the steps going up the headwall from about 14,300 feet (4,359 meter) to 16,000 feet (4,877 meters) can be at least knee high. How are you going to make 1,700 feet (518 meters) of these kinds of steps (at altitude and after a week of hard work) if you can't even make one of them in your own basement? Suddenly, Yaniro's words hit home. He wasn't just talking about 5.12 rock climbers when he made that observation. He was talking about you, in your basement, who can just barely squeak out the move of stepping up twelve inches once.

So what do you do about this? Do you just step up and down a smaller box a million times or do you just use a lighter pack for training? Hell no! You need to get stronger first and build up your strength reserve. This will give you a base of strength from which you can develop endurance. At this point you are operating in excess of your strength reserve (SR). You must increase your SR to have any hope of pulling off this move for 1,700 feet (518 meters).

2) Before any of you tough-guy alpinists scoff at this exercise in vertical backpacking, here is an example you can sink your teeth into:

Steve coaches a young climber who takes part in ice and mixed competitions. Steve noticed that this guy often fell off the routes because he could not hold on to his tools during critical crux moves despite not feeling pumped. It was pretty clear after talking to this climber that his SR was too small. He had been operating close to his maximum strength for too long on the route; when he came to the crux he no longer had the strength reserve needed to grip the shafts tightly for one powerful move. To overcome this problem he'd been training to improve his muscular endurance, thinking that was his limitation.

Steve and Scott advised that he change his training to improve his maximum grip strength. Steve devised some very demanding workouts of hanging one-handed from his ice tools while carrying weight hung from his waist. Within a few weeks of this training his endurance on the steep cruxes had improved dramatically. He'd boosted his strength reserve, and voila! More endurance.

How it Works

How does being stronger improve endurance? While there is still some debate about the underlying adaptations that result in improved endurance among those who improve their maximum strength, there is a hypothesis that seems to explain it well. Scientists propose that by engaging in maximal strength training the athlete increases the pool of motor units that become neurologically hardwired so that these motor units can be easily accessed by the brain when needed and thus readily available for use during exercise. **A common maxim is: Muscles that wire together, fire together.**

This training is more of a neurological adaptation than it is purely building strength in the muscle and results in smoother, more coordinated movements. Much of what passes for sport climbing training involves doing laps on climbs that are just above your current ability. Recall the last time you went sport climbing consistently; say in the spring, after a long layoff from rock climbing. Your endurance probably improved dramatically in the first few weeks, right? That was your strength reserve improving and giving you increased endurance.

The training effect at work here is exactly what Helgerud did in his study on the skiers. This is not at all dissimilar to gymnastics training where individual tricks are trained and then linked into full routines by this delicate interplay of the nervous system and muscle. In a complex, highly technical sport like gymnastics, or climbing, coordination and fluidity play a huge role in success. There is nothing wrong with gaining endurance in this way, but it can be maximized by doing focused strength training at the right time in your training plan.

Training for maximum strength has a large neurologic effect by improving the brain's ability to recruit more fibers. Once these new motor units become more readily accessible via the improved neurological connections, they can be recruited on a rotating basis as needed for lower-force contractions like climbing or hiking uphill. As individual fibers and even entire motor units become fatigued they are rested when new fibers are brought into the act. With a larger pool of fibers available, there are more fibers to share in the workload on this rotating basis. Thus higher power outputs can be sustained for longer times, and improved endurance is the result.

Strength as the Foundation for Endurance

As we hope you can see by now, strength is the basis of endurance.

The idea that endurance depends on strength may seem counterintuitive because your real-life experiences probably tell you that the most powerful athletes do not exhibit the greatest endurance. Otherwise Olympic weightlifters would be winning the marathons. So what gives? Well, there are certain metabolic restrictions that eliminate power athletes, like Olympic lifters, from running fast marathons.

Allow us to share an analogy that Tony Yaniro has used in his strength coaching for rock climbers that does a good job demonstrating the system your body uses to develop strength and athletic ability.

The Piano Movers

Louie formed a piano moving company with a few guys (the motor units). At first these guys were not very good at moving pianos because they were not very strong, nor could they all lift and pull in coordination. With practice however they became pretty darn good at piano moving and began to get requests to do more jobs with bigger pianos. Louie, being the brains in the group, realized that he could recruit some more guys and get more work done. He'd have to serve them all lunch and he'd have to take them to all the jobs but hey, it seemed like a no-brainer because he'd make more money in the end.

Well, these new guys turned out to be really lazy and bumbly. So much so that they got in each other's way and dropped pianos. It was mess. So Louie decided he had to give them more supervision and train them to work as a team. Sure enough, after a few weeks even these new guys were really good at moving pianos. But jeez, could they pack away the lunch. They were eating him out of house and home. But the jobs kept coming in and now Louie was making real money.

Then the bottom dropped out of the piano moving market. Louie was still obliged to transport all these, now kind of useless, workers around to the few jobs he could find, just in case new work came in. To make matters worse, he still had to feed them. It became obvious pretty fast to Louie that this was no way to run a business, and he needed to reduce his crew to just the number of guys needed to get the immediate job done.

The Olympic-style weight lifter can afford to carry a lot of guys around in his truck and he can afford to feed them as much as they want to eat. When he needs them for that big moving job he needs every single one of them and they need to be sharp and ready to pull together as a team. The marathoner or the alpinist can afford neither the cost of the lunch nor the cost of carrying all these guys around that he may never need to put to work. The alpinist must have his minimalist crew so well trained that they can handle any moving job that comes their way.

Typically, athletic activities have limited budgets, so the goal is to get the most efficiency from our bodies. We need enough muscle strength and mass, but not too much. Then we must tune what we have to perfection.

From Tony's analogy we can understand why the Olympic lifter won't be the best marathoner. However, if you look at a group of marathon runners, or any other uniform grouping of endurance athletes, the individuals who produce the most power will be the fastest in their respective endurance events. Surprisingly, there is a very strong correlation between short-term power and endurance. For most of us, improvements in strength and power will also result in improved endurance.

As we learned in the previous chapters, training technical climbing skills, power, and endurance need to be carefully and correctly balanced to optimize your preparedness. For any big-mountain objective your

Specific Qualities Required for Different Sports

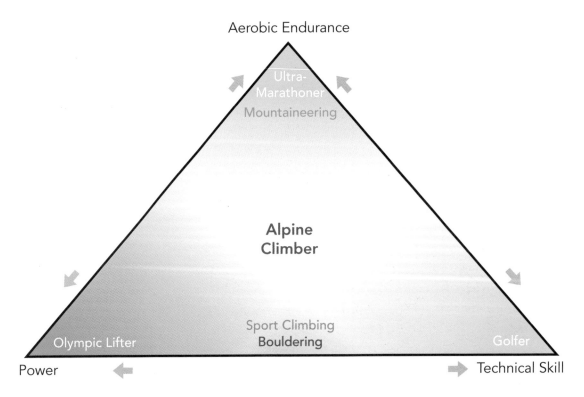

We have chosen three conventional sports to represent the extremes of aerobic endurance, power, and technical skill. To give some perspective we have fit the extremes of climbing activities into the same model, which is based on the most important sport-specific qualities needed to perform at the top level in each. The mountaineer is best served by a very high level of aerobic fitness. Both the boulderer and sport climber need a good balance of technique and power. The sport climber tends to need more muscular endurance than a boulderer due to the length of routes. Of course none of these aspects of climbing exist in isolation but it is apparent that the alpinist above all needs to be the most well rounded in training specific qualities. Keep in mind that there will always be a trade-off between power and endurance. Maximal development of one will always mean drop in the other.

training will be a balance of strength and endurance. The figure on the facing page illustrates how tradeoffs between technical skills, power, and endurance relate to the type of climbing you might train for.

Clearly bouldering requires lots of power, and classic mountaineering endless endurance. This book is concerned with training for climbing in the mountains, so we'll ignore training for bouldering. We've included it to illustrate that the more difficult the individual moves are on a route, the more power you need to incorporate, but the less endurance you will have. The reason no one will ever climb 5.13 at 8,000 meters is that the energy systems required for those two circumstances (altitude and difficulty) are mutually exclusive. Just as in the figure on the left that illustrates that the most powerful athletes, Olympic-style weight lifters, are never going to run the best marathon.

Basic Physics

For the purpose of our discussion we'll use the words *force* and *strength* interchangeably. It might help to review a couple of simple formulas from high school physics to get reacquainted with the relationships of force, work, and power.

Work = Force x Distance (Work is the mechanical energy to move.) This means that when a force acts on an object in such a way as to move that object some distance, work has been done to the object. Carrying a 30-pound pack 1,000 feet (305 meters) uphill does 30,000 foot-pounds of work to the pack. This is a gross simplification of course because you have also done work by moving your own body up the hill. Not only that, most of the energy of moving the climber and the pack went into heat that the body had to dissipate. The human body is not a very efficient organism in terms of transferring the chemical energy in the food you eat into the mechanical energy of moving you and the pack up the hill. In terms of efficiency we are about on a par with the internal combustion engine in your car; only about 20 percent of the available chemical energy in the fuel (food for us, gasoline for your car) ends up being converted into useful mechanical work. In both the car's engine and your body most of the rest gets wasted as heat.

This seeming gross inefficiency is an example of the Second Law of Thermodynamics. While very small changes in efficiency are possible—some cars can convert 21 percent of their fuel energy into movement, and training on rough footing will make you a little more efficient—in general this transfer from chemical to mechanical energy by whatever means is depressingly inefficient.

The Difference Between Power and Work

By Tony Yaniro

When I was eighteen, I was invited to compete in a really horrendous made-for-television competition called "Survival of the Fittest."

It was a test of all-around outdoor skill and strength, involving racing up mountains, swimming class-V whitewater rivers, climbing rope courses, and other crazy events. Accomplished athletes from different sports were invited: triathletes, World Cup cross-country skiers, mountaineers, rock climbers, Navy Seals, and the like.

The idea was to put the best-conditioned athletes head-to-head in events designed to be grueling tests of all-around fitness that none of the athletes had specially trained for in their respective sports. It seemed like the usual winners were cross-country skiers and climbers.

I decided I needed to train my cardiovascular system and leg strength to keep up with those pesky cross-country skiers, who seemed to be able to prance up the steep hills without effort. Having no experience with training, I did what I thought was the logical thing. I put on a big pack and started hiking up hills.

I worked hard. By the next event I was really strong. I could slog up thousands of feet with a 150-pound pack.

On race day (many of you will be able to predict what happened) I attacked the hills right behind the XC skiers. And that is where I stayed: behind. At the top of each hill, I could hear everyone else breathing so hard that it sounded like they would pop a blood vessel in their head. I, on the other hand, felt great . . . but slow. As hard as I tried, despite my lack of fatigue and easy breathing pace, I could not get my legs to move fast enough to keep up with the other guys who were killing themselves. Why?

You guessed it. I used too much weight in the pack so that my leg speed during the training was slow. I got really strong, slow legs, but could not generate much power.

Even muscle speed during training will respond specifically. What you do exactly is what you get better at. I got good at carrying big packs up hills slowly. While my speed would probably be fast compared to other pack-toting competitors, in the race, nobody had a pack.

Virtually all athletic endeavors are dependent on power. The more power you can produce, the better will be the athletic outcome. Power has a place in endurance sports too and not just in events like sprinting and jumping. Athletes need to understand that endurance is strength utilized over a long duration.

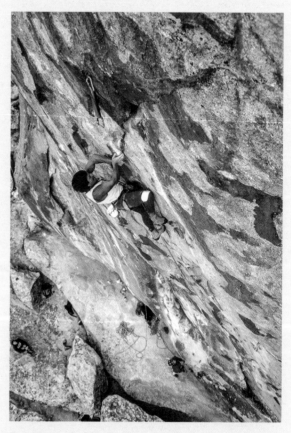

Tony Yaniro climbing Calypso, 5.13d, at the City of Rocks, Idaho, sometime in the 1980s. *Photo: Greg Epperson*

Tony Yaniro is known in climbing circles for his early difficult first ascents and for his work coaching climbers to be stronger.

Power = Work / Time (Power is how fast the work is done.) This simple mathematical expression is the embodiment of many athletic pursuits. Power is the measure of how much work you can get done in how short of a time. It is probably intuitive to most people that the climber who can carry that 30-pound pack 1,000 feet (305 meters) uphill in 30 minutes did the same amount of *work* as the person who took an hour to climb the same 1,000 feet. The pack still moved uphill 1,000 feet. But the 30-minute climber produced twice the *power* of the one-hour climber because he did the same work in half the time. Power is simply the rate at which the work gets done.

We make the point often in this book that speed in the mountains is one of your biggest safety features. The amount of time it takes you to complete that 1,000-foot (305-meter) climb can be the difference between safety and danger. All other things being equal, it should be obvious that the more powerful climber will have a better chance at success and have a bigger safety margin than the less powerful.

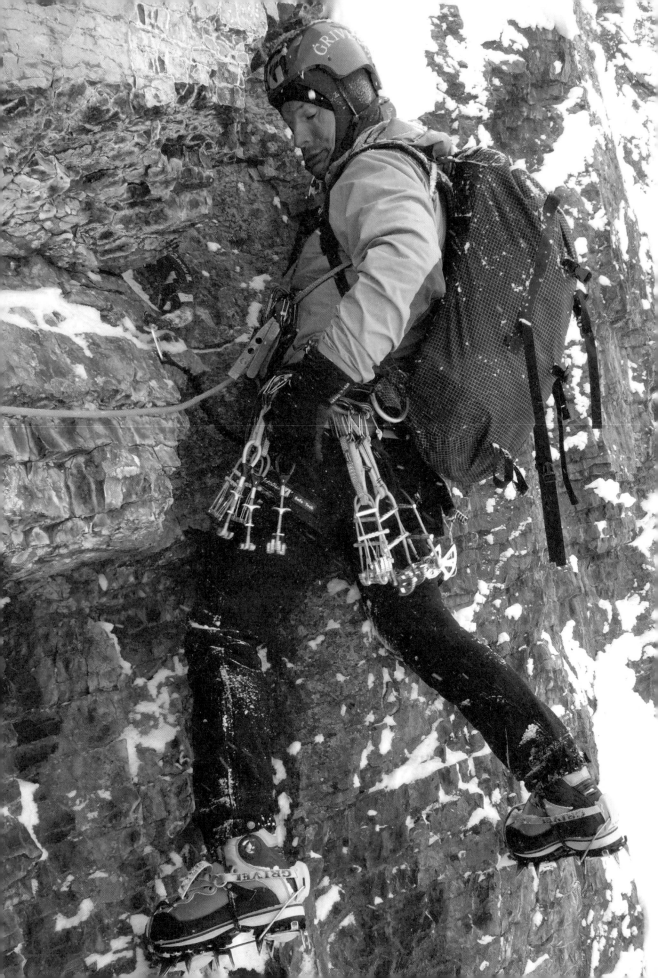

Strength on Mount Alberta

By Steve House

Fragments of snowflakes float upward as the wind gently blows against the steep black rock of Mount Alberta's North Face. Grunting, I grab the top of a flake with a gloved hand and pull up, eye-level, to its top edge. I press up and stand on the two-inch-wide fin of rock. Both my hands touch the wall for balance. As I catch my breath, I start pawing the wall, feeling for holds above me.

Vince Anderson and I are nearing the end of the first day of an attempt on a new route on Mount Alberta's North Face. The sun of late winter is drawing out the shadows of the countless wilderness summits behind us. Thirty feet (nine meters) above me, and fifteen feet (four and a half meters) left, a couloir of snow snakes toward a dramatic 200-foot (61-meter) long icicle hanging high in the face. That icicle has never been climbed. Linking our route to the icicle and then up some as-yet-unknown way through the upper headwall is the line that we came to climb.

The dark limestone before me is smooth and solid. The pitches to here have ascended square-cut edges alongside one- and two-inch-wide cracks. I kneel delicately and tie slings around the flake I'm on to rig some kind of protection. Standing, I see a good-looking pocket up and left, just out of reach. I place the front points of one foot precisely on edges the width of two matchsticks, torque my right tool behind a flake at head-height, and press up gently, tightly balanced. I reach my other tool to the pocket and find a shallow but positive hook. I contract my body, my core pulled in, keeping my points of contact motionless and secure. With quick, tight breaths I scrape dirt out of the pocket with the pick and place my smallest cam. It's shallow, but the rock is solid. My breath feels like it's burning, I reverse the moves to the ledge to catch my breath. A minute later I climb up again, scrape another crack clean and place another small cam and clip it to the rope. Smoothly I reverse the moves to my perch on the narrow flake.

Over the next forty minutes I climb up and down these first several moves—thin tool placements with long lock offs requiring lots of core tension—until the moves become more familiar, easier. I discover two small, but solid, nut placements. Above my highpoint is several body-lengths of climbing, finishing with a long reach far to the left, with no footholds, to a wider, fist-size, crack; a move I doubt I'll be able to reverse. But the protection there, if I make it, looks good. Then I have to traverse six or eight protectionless feet to the couloir, and the crux of the route is behind us, the way to the ice-dagger is open.

I breathe, swinging my arms, noticing that the narrow edge no longer feels so desperate. I breathe into my focused place, tip my pick into the now-familiar hold, lift one foot up on the wall, exhale sharply, and begin to climb.

Opposite: Steve House on Mount Alberta (11,873', 3,629m) starting the pitch described in this story; the crux section came 100 feet higher. *Photo: Vince Anderson*

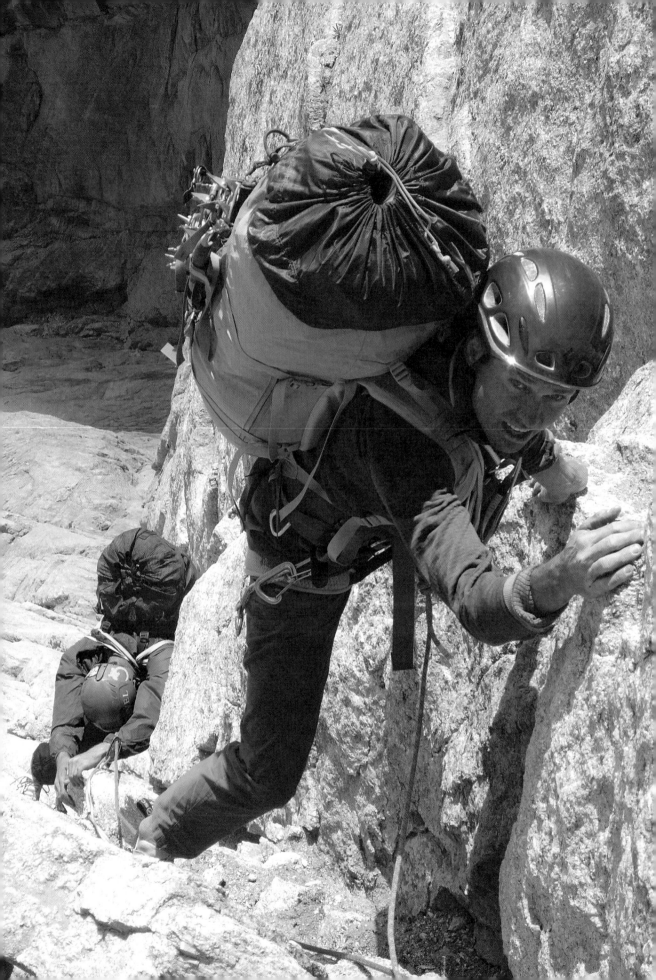

Chapter 5

The Methodology of Strength Training

"Let me state that simply going climbing is *not* the best method of strength training for climbers."

– ERIC HÖRST writing in *Training for Climbing*

WHAT IS STRENGTH?

Strength is the force generated by the contraction of muscles. This muscle force exerted across a joint is thereby translated into the movement that propels an athlete. All movement takes some level of strength. But what did the strength required by Steve while working out the crux moves on Mount Alberta have to do with being able to do twenty pull-ups or squat 300 pounds? The answer to this question lies in the maxim we proposed in the beginning of chapter 2.

There are two types of training:

- **Training that prepares you in a general way for the event-specific training.** This is general conditioning with a mix of both strength and endurance training and may not be climbing specific.

Opposite: Marko Prezelj and Vince Anderson arrive at the top of a 5.10 pitch climbed at 16,600 feet during day one of the first ascent of K7 West (22,500', 6,858m).
Photo: Steve House

■ **Training that prepares you in a specific way for the event you are doing.** This consists primarily of climbing or workouts that model directly the specific demands of climbing.

It is important to understand that the nonspecific training is not necessarily intended to be of direct benefit to your climbing, though for all but the most fit, it will. Its purpose, instead, is to provide a base of support that enhances the specific workouts and climbing. In the case of Steve on Mount Alberta, he had spent many training sessions raising his maximum strength by using the same kinds of workouts prescribed later in this book. Knowing that one of the main qualities needed for technically demanding alpine climbing is the ability to hang on for a long time, he then converted that raw strength into more climbing-specific muscular endurance again using a strategy we'll detail later in the book.

There is no way you can anticipate the exact combination of movements and muscles you'll need to power safely through the crux moves on your next climb. So the best way to prepare is by building a broad base of general strength and then honing that base to be more climbing specific.

As you read the next pages, remember that this chapter focuses on teaching you the reasons, theories, and methods behind training strength so that in the subsequent chapters (in the Planning Section) we can go right into planning strength workouts.

WHAT IS STRENGTH TRAINING?

The term *strength training* is a catch-all for several different methods of resistance training. Any training that improves the contractile qualities—either the force, the power, the endurance, or the coordination of contraction—of the muscles can be grouped in the general category of strength training.

In the popular lexicon, strength training is most often associated with heavily muscled men and women laboring away in gyms lifting massive weights and posing in front of mirrors. While this type of strength training is popular around the world, it is the least applicable to most athletes. It represents only one of several methods, taken together, that make up the continuum of strength training. Unfortunately, body building (an aesthetic pursuit, not an athletic one) and power lifting have gained so much traction in gyms everywhere that people sometimes follow the precepts of body building in a misguided attempt to become better athletes.

In light of the misconceptions it is ironic that strength training in its various forms is the most studied and best understood of all athletic training methods. Prescriptions for achieving improvement in any aspect of muscle contractility are readily available. In this book we use tried-and-tested methods specifically developed for preparing athletes. This method starts with a general strength and conditioning period followed by a period that emphasizes maximum strength in a few large muscle groups in a semi-sport-specific way. The base of strength thus built will provide you with the ability to handle more climbing-specific training, which in the end is the training that will make you a better climber. The bigger that base of conditioning, the more of the hard, specific work you will be able to handle and hence the better climber you will become.

As with any athlete, climbers do not view strength gains as an end in themselves. We don't get stronger just to be stronger. We gain strength so that we can climb longer, harder routes.

WHY SHOULD CLIMBERS TRAIN STRENGTH?

More so than any other conventional sport, gymnastics has much in common with hard, technical climbing because of the reliance on the mix of strength and technique for competency. Check out what a standard gymnastic coaching manual for USA Gymnastics (USAgym.org) has to say about conditioning training:

> *Without doubt, technical ability and preparation is paramount in gymnastics training. However, technique can only be applied within the boundaries of physical fitness—be it strength, power, or anaerobic capacity. By developing a sport-specific base of strength, power, and flexibility proper technique can be coached and acquired more easily.*
>
> *Performing more gymnastics [we could substitute climbing here] does not guarantee even a minimum level of strength to perform the skill correctly. Instead, conditioning is required so that the athlete can learn the skill correctly.*

So even gymnasts, with the highly technical requirements of their sport, spend a considerable amount of time on nonspecific conditioning. Does it not make sense that climbers can benefit from developing a base of more general strength and conditioning?

Why Get Stronger?

Athletes get stronger so they can do their sport better. What this means is that they use strength to help them become faster, more powerful, or have better endurance in their sport. Unlike a weight lifter, who gets strong to be able to do something like bench press more weight, an athlete has a highly sport-specific goal to his or her strength training.

Another important benefit of strength training is protecting yourself from injury. Being stronger is one of the best ways to avoid injury in the rough-and-tumble alpine environment, where you carry a heavy pack and put yourself in awkward positions that can place very high stress loads on your joints.

Of course the higher the standard of skill needed, the more climbing specific the strength training must be. For instance, almost any strength training will benefit a 5.7 rock climber where as a 5.13 climber will need to spend more training time using more sport-specific conditioning exercises.

HOW STRENGTH TRAINING WORKS

Without going into much detail, there are essentially two ways in which a muscle can increase its strength. The first, *hypertrophy*, is the result of an increase in the size and number of the elements within the muscle that allow it to contract with more force. The second, which we've already touched on in our discussion of strength reserve, is known as Max Strength, which relies to a large extent on the motor-neural adaptations that allow the central nervous system (CNS) to contract the muscle more effectively and hence produce more force.

It is this second method that holds the key for the best results for endurance athletes, especially those who must bear their own body weight. Studies have found that even well-trained athletes are able

Ueli Steck soloing the Colton-MacIntyre route on the north face of the Grand Jorasses (13,806', 4,208m) near Chamonix, France.
Photo: Jonathan Griffith

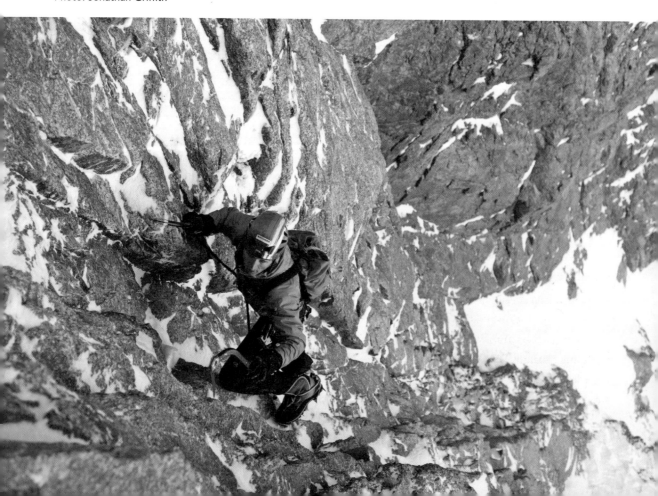

to recruit only about 30 percent of any muscle's total fibers during a maximal voluntary contraction. Untrained individuals may be able to access only 15 to 20 percent of the muscle's total fiber pool. Thus we can see that there is a lot of upside potential for any athlete to increase the total volume of muscle mass that can be accessed by the CNS. Much of the increase in strength, especially early on in a training program, comes about from the nervous system wiring making better connections so that the firing of the muscles becomes more effective.

Double-digit percentage gains in strength are possible from just the neuromuscular adaptations that come during a Max Strength training program of six to eight weeks with no increase in muscle size or weight. We advocate this approach to increase your strength and will explain it in detail shortly.

WOMEN AND STRENGTH

It can be very difficult for most women to gain appreciable muscle mass, especially in the upper body, even with specialized training. This being said, it will benefit women with high athletic goals to spend some of their precious training time and energy focusing on a Max Strength plan, because it will help with injury prevention as well as making them stronger climbers.

We have observed large gains in strength in women athletes using only a well-crafted eight-week maximum strength program that we will describe later in the book. They did this without gaining weight or increasing muscle bulk. Much of a woman's strength increases will come about due to the neurological adaptations mentioned above.

The cruel fact remains that a female alpinist's pack is going to weigh just as much as her male counterpart's. This makes it all the more imperative for her to improve her strength-to-weight ratio.

LIFTING WEIGHTS

Most of us think of weight lifting in a gym when we think of strength training. While this is perhaps the most common way to increase strength it is certainly not the only way. Weight lifting has gained its popularity as a means of gaining strength due to the control it allows in the progressive overloading of the muscles. It is an expedient, safe form of adding resistance loads especially when those loads need to be high in order to achieve the desired effect, such as in building maximum strength in the legs.

After Injury:
The Long, Long Road Back

By Tony Yaniro

Sadly the load that any tissue can handle post-injury, and which it needs to achieve a stimulation that requires it to adapt via the training effect, is many, many, many times less than was needed to induce a training effect before the injury. Athletes need to avoid injury at all costs. It is the surest way to derail your plans.

The training effect is the model that explains the recovery from an injury—rest and reinforcement, then re-stimulation—but now the training or stimulation must be conducted at an exaggeratedly low effort. A very minor tear in a tendon will require many weeks to heal. You cannot train it at the previous levels during this time. After healing, it must be rehabilitated with light progressive loading in order to reinforce itself and be ready for a normal training load—this can take at least many weeks. In total, such an injury needs several months to heal, *if* the injury was recognized immediately and was not irritated by more stress.

Injuries will be bathed in inflammatory cells and fluids. These must be gone before significant stress is applied to the tissues. If they remain, chronic tendonitis, scarring (meaning that the tissues may never fully heal properly), and calcification will occur. Some of these changes can take years to remedy, if not longer.

The gradual progression of your training that is advocated throughout this book is the best long-term method of ensuring continued success and avoiding injury. Taking that extra easy day, or more, of recovery as needed is a much better and faster way for genuine long-term fitness gains. There is no secret and quick method of improving fitness. It takes hard work—and time.

Train hard, rest hard.

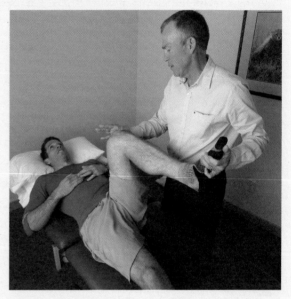

Overuse injuries usually lead to missed training time. Don't let this be you. *Photo: Scott Johnston*

Tony Yaniro is a doctor of naturopathy who has never suffered an injury from climbing or training for climbing despite his infamously brutal finger-strength workouts.

Many athletes will use weight lifting in a gym setting for only the periods required to develop maximum strength as described in the periodization section of this chapter. We discuss methods and programs both within and without a weight room.

Machines versus Free Weights

Weight lifting machines like you find in most gyms today are of limited use for climbers. Machines were developed for, and are excellent at isolating, certain muscles or muscle groups. This isolation has advantages when one is trying to rehabilitate an injury or correct a muscular imbalance. Machines allow body builders to target certain muscle groups in order to perfect their physique. Another advantage is that machines are much safer than free weights. They avoid the potential for injury both in using the machine and in handling heavy weights. Gym owners like this from the liability aspect and the fact that they allow people to move through exercise stations more quickly.

For climbers, free weights offer one distinct advantage over machines: the ability to coordinate many muscles into powerful movements that involve the precise firing in exactly the right sequence of many thousands of motor units. Any real-world movement, such as front pointing up an alpine couloir, requires that some of the active muscles act as stabilizers of the joints so that the big, prime-mover muscles can do their job effectively. The roles of the myriad muscles involved in a simple action like walking are constantly shifting from stabilizer to prime mover in an incredibly complex web of neuro-muscular interconnections controlled by the central nervous system usually without our conscious thought.

Because your ultimate goal is an improvement in athletic abilities, you will make much more progress toward that end by foregoing machines except when they offer their unique advantage of isolation.

STRENGTH TRAINING TERMS AND CONCEPTS

1) Body weight: The resistance to movement is provided only by your own body weight such as in a normal pull-up.

2) Repetition or Rep: One complete movement cycle. One pull-up movement would be one rep.

3) Set: A grouping of repetitions. A set might include as few as one or two reps when building maximal strength and as many as a hundred reps when building muscular endurance. Sets allow a way to control the end result of the strength training because they are separated by a rest interval.

4) Recovery Time: This is a rest interval between sets of the same exercise or between different exercises when using a circuit. During this time, critical energy sources in the muscle are restored. As we will show, by adjusting this time you can target which metabolic system will predominate in supplying the energy for the muscle contractions.

5) Strength Reserve: The difference between your maximum strength and the normal level of strength needed to do the movements of an activity. The greater this reserve, the lower the percentage of your maximum strength needed to perform your sport. Example: Say that your maximum twelve-inch box step is eighty pounds on top of your body weight. You'll be carrying a thirty-pound pack on your attempt on the Cassin Route on Denali in June. You have a fifty-pound strength reserve. The bigger this reserve is, the less of your capacity you need to use to perform a task, and hence, the more endurance you will have for that task.

6) Circuit: A strength workout done by completing one set each of several exercises in quick succession before returning to the first exercise and repeating the circuit. Can be repeated multiple times with various rest periods as needed for different training effects.

CORE STRENGTH

All movement originates with the body's core or torso. Even the simple act of lifting a fork to your mouth requires many stabilizing muscles along the spine, shoulders, and hips to go into isometric contractions. This happens because your arm weighs, perhaps, twenty pounds and lifting it would otherwise cause your spine to bend and you would likely fall over if not for the core becoming more rigid to counter this imbalance.

The Weak Link in the Chain

The core is of particular interest to climbers because when the terrain steepens, humans, normally bipedal, revert to using all four limbs (quadrupedal) for locomotion. The core figures heavily into even third-class scrambling but becomes increasingly important as the climbing becomes steeper. Climbers often engage in what are called diagonal movements. These are actions where you are in balance on only two points of contact: the opposite arm and leg while the climber repositions one or both other limbs. The core serves the vital function of connecting the shoulders to the hips in a stabilizing action so that the limbs can exert useable forces to the terrain you are moving over. Having very strong arms and legs connected to their respective anchor points of shoulders and hips is great, but if the connection through the core is weak you will not be able to transmit the needed force though the core to propel yourself upward efficiently. Whether you are hiking to the base of a route using poles or climbing M8, you are still acting as a quadraped and need that vital core strength.

Most of the exercises we'll describe using either weights or your body will involve the core directly as part of the movements. This is exactly why we prefer the exercises we've chosen, but supplemental core training can be very beneficial. Core training will be part of each period even if only for strength maintenance, and we'll detail our prescription in terms of the exercises and the periodization of them in chapter 5. In that same chapter we'll provide you with some ideas on building your own strength program.

PERIODIZATION FOR STRENGTH TRAINING

One of the most common questions we get from climbers is how to manage all this training around their climbing. Clearly something has to give. Spend all day pulling down and it's unlikely you are going to feel inclined toward a hard gym strength session, nor would you get much out of it. You have only so much energy. And, as you well know by now, it takes time to recover from an activity, whether you call it training or recreation. Trying to do everything all the time is a recipe for exhaustion.

This is why the concept of periodizing training is the most successful model of training for sport. Every athlete is faced with the dilemma of how to fit it all in. The solution that conventional sports have devised is to use different periods for different purposes. For instance, the Base Period is not intended as an end in itself. It is meant to be a building period where you are trying to increase your capacity for absorbing more and more hard work. You are setting yourself up to be able to handle more hard climbing-specific training in the Specific Period.

What we commonly hear from climbers who do not understand the benefits gained from following a periodized plan is that they want to climb hard all the time, and they want to be at the top of their game all the time. That is just not possible. Sure, you can climb pretty well all the time but you are not going to do your best climbing without a more structured approach. Look at it another way: If your climbing level has been the same for a long time, now you know why. Keep reading!

Just as Usain Bolt can't knock off a sub-twenty-second 200-meter run whenever he wants, climbers need to understand that they must prepare diligently for months and months in order to have a performance that breaks a personal record. A talented, lucky few sometimes keep on a roll for weeks at a time before needing to return to basic training again. The simple fact that top climbing performances have often come at random times and with a random approach should hint at how far climbing is from realizing its potential.

The reason the climbers we speak to have trouble fitting hard climbing and hard training into the same time frame is that they don't want to back off the hard climbing during the base-building period. When we tell them that their absolute climbing ability will suffer if they don't, it's a hard pill for them to swallow.

For the same reasons we apply periodization to the aerobic training we use, we apply the periodization principle to strength training. Each period is necessary to prepare your body for the subsequent periods. And just as with endurance, the final period is the one that develops the sport-specific qualities to their maximum level.

The model we will utilize incorporates the following periods:

- Transition Period

- Max Strength Period

- Conversion to Muscular Endurance Period

We'll come back to specific guidelines for each of these periods again in the Planning Section, which will help you create a strength training plan.

Transition Period for Strength Training

For those with little or no strength training background, or returning from a long break, six to eight weeks is necessary for this period. An injury from strength training is the last thing we want to induce, especially since one of the primary goals of strength training should be to buffer you against injury. This general period can be as short as four weeks for those who already have a long history of strength training and are returning to if after only a short break of less than a couple of months.

We are going to recommend exercises that are varied and general in nature with many muscles targeted, which aligns with the knowledge that general training must occur first to support climbing-specific training later. The overall volume of work done during these workouts will be high but there is not a high concentration of any particular exercises. By avoiding doing many sets of a single exercise you can avoid some of the stiffness and soreness normally associated with starting a strength program and minimize the risk of overuse injuries. To these ends we will recommend using a circuit style of workout involving about eight to ten different exercises and running through the circuit two to three times. None of the exercises should be done to exhaustion or muscular failure during this period.

Max Strength Period

This period is intended to build as high a strength reserve as possible while remembering Tony Yaniro's piano mover analogy. A sizable strength reserve will make for greater gains during the next period of conversion to sport specificity, which in the alpinist's case entails specific muscular endurance. During the Max Strength Period we will pare down the number of exercises to three to four at the most. This is where more climbing-specific exercises enter the program. You'll have to decide which ones to include based on your personal strengths, and more importantly weaknesses, along with your goals.

Choose a resistance that allows you to do between two and four reps without reaching muscular exhaustion. A resistance of about 85–90 percent of what you are able to do for one repetition will be about the right amount. You'll do three to five sets with rests of three minutes between sets. It has been our experience that when done properly these workouts leave the athlete feeling invigorated and have a restorative effect. We often insert them after other more exhaustive workouts to both aid recovery and act as maintenance of strength during later periods. If these leave you feeling drained you are doing them too hard and not getting the most benefit.

Hypertrophy Training

Normally a high-level strength building periodization plan would place a phase between the Transition Period and this Max Strength Period.

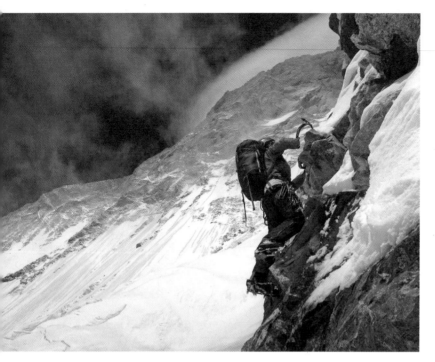

Marko Prezelj during the first day of a 2011 attempt on the west face of Makalu (27,825', 8,481m).
Photo: Steve House

This is called the *Hypertrophy Period* and its purpose is to actually add muscle mass. There are very sound reasons for a Hypertrophy Period in many sports and in cases involving young or very lightly muscled individuals it is a hugely beneficial to include it, even for climbers. However, its very name reveals why we are not recommending it for most alpine climbers. It is usually undesirable for an otherwise lean and fit person to gain muscle mass that he has to haul up the climb with him.

Recall Tony Yaniro's piano mover analogy again: Do you really want to have to feed and transport all those hungry mouths that you may only need occasionally? Hypertrophy training differs in one essential feature from what we are proposing in the Max Strength Period: You continue each exercise to complete failure repeatedly with multiple sets. Your body's response to such exhaustive training is to build more muscle tissue. If you are especially weak or an adolescent, then you might do well to consider adding a Hypertrophy Period; strength training books abound that will help guide you through this. Most adult alpine climbers we know are obsessed with weight and are too busy cutting labels off of long underwear and removing the mosquito netting from their tents to consider adding bulk to their body.

Using Isometrics for Rapid Maximum Strength Gains

The word *isometric* is Greek in origin and means equal length. In an isometric exercise the muscle remains at a constant length. The joint the muscle crosses does not change angle. Think of being locked off on your ice tools and you'll get the picture. An exercise done isometrically involves a static muscle contraction. This is a very effective way of increasing the maximal contractile force in a muscle. The problem with it is that the strength is trained at the specific joint angle used and provides limited benefits at other joint angles.

However, isometrics provide a clever way to help you bust through a strength barrier. Say you are struggling with a one-arm lock off on steep ice. Hook your tools over a pull-up bar and do three to five five-second holds at various elbow angles followed by at least three minutes of rest using your current maximum pull-up weight. This will almost always help you break through that strength plateau. We've used this numerous times with everyone from teenage girls to crusty sixty-year-old rock climbers still chasing 5.12.

The Conversion to Muscular Endurance Period

As we explained earlier in this chapter, athletes do not gain strength simply for strength's sake. They gain strength in order to become better athletes. Nonspecific strength gains have to be converted into real improvements in athletic performance or they are not useful. Hence the name for this period. In it you convert the general strength you have built into the climbing-specific qualities that you choose.

For alpine climbing we believe that the specific quality best enhanced in this conversion period is long-term muscular endurance, especially in the big muscles used to get you to and up the climb. If you are mostly concerned with short, hard single-pitch routes then this conversion period will focus on building power and short-term power endurance. There are numerous excellent books available to help you improve these qualities as they directly relate to rock climbing. The series of training books by Eric Hörst are packed with good information.

Here is where alpinists-in-training get down to business. This period takes the raw and somewhat unspecific strength you have built up and turns it into a resistance to fatigue that you have never known before. You'll do it via very sport-specific movements in workouts using up to hundreds of repetitions.

This is exhausting work. It is the stuff that has direct application to alpinism, and like the specific training described in the Endurance section, it is the sexy stuff. So, why not just go immediately to this phase of strength training and avoid wasting precious time and energy on the preceding two periods? Just like the aerobic endurance base is critical in order to maximize aerobic endurance, the two previous periods of strength conditioning are necessary to provide the strength base needed to be able to handle this demanding work. And this period is the one that will provide you the key to attaining your top level of performance in the mountains.

It is worth noting that the higher your level of aerobic endurance, the better the support is for Muscular Endurance (ME) training by virtue of the lactate shuttle discussed in chapter 3. A large aerobic base is critically important in realizing your ultimate potential with this training because it will allow you to do more and do it harder, and thus reap bigger gains. Specific Muscular Endurance training is critically important if you have high altitude alpine climbing goals.

The Ability You Are Training

What you are trying to accomplish with this muscular endurance routine is to improve the ability of the muscles to contract at a higher force for a longer time than they currently can. From what you learned about muscle fiber type recruitment you can understand how it is possible to target different types of fibers by selecting the load you use and the number of repetitions used in a set.

Here is a simple example: It should come as no surprise that if you use fifty pounds and do five sets of one hundred repetitions of half squats you will be focusing more on the endurance of different fibers and motor units than if you use 150 pounds and do five sets of fifteen reps.

Higher resistance will necessitate more motor units being recruited into the task. The ones that fatigue the fastest will be the ones that are less endurance trained, the faster twitch fibers. They'll be the ones complaining to you as you near that fifteenth rep. Of course there will be different ones complaining when you use the fifty pounds and do one hundred reps. When their complaints finally get loud enough you'll be forced to stop and take a break. That will be one set.

If you are using a higher load and lower reps, like in our example of fifteen reps, you'll need to give those fibers that complained the loudest a long break. Those FT fibers do not have much endurance capacity and will need two to five minutes, depending on the resistance, to (mostly) recover before you subject them to the next set. This kind of Muscular Endurance training can be applied to any major muscle group that has the right base training and can be very useful in preparing for short, hard climbs near your limit.

On the other end of the scale if you are using the one hundred rep example you won't need such a long recovery. With the lower resistance you are using, you will be affecting mostly the slower twitch fibers, which have better endurance properties and recover much faster than their fast twitch neighbors. Thirty seconds to one minute can be used to separate these longer, lower-intensity sets. This kind of Muscular

Endurance training is mostly useful for the legs, and possibly the pulling (down) and grip-strength groups for technical climbing, to greatly extend your existing absolute endurance.

So how do you choose which end of the scale to use? Do you go with a heavy weight and a killer burn in twelve to fifteen reps? Or do you go for the slow bake that comes with one hundred reps and a light weight?

As with most things, it depends. If you are relatively new to this training method it will benefit you most to enhance the power of the slow twitch fibers that comes from many reps using a lighter weight. This will help maximize the fatigue resistance of those slow twitch fibers you'll be relying on for long days in the mountains. If you are a more advanced climber with many years of carrying a pack up and down mountains, you can use a heavier load and fewer reps to help enhance the fatigue resistance of the faster twitch fibers. This can be a big asset when it comes to speed and can give you another gear. These two methods can be combined into one progression to provide the ultimate benefits.

It is critical that you develop progression and gradualness in order to get the most benefit from this training method. We'll devote considerable time laying out various workouts and progressions in the Planning Your Training Section.

Muscular endurance workouts can take many forms limited only by your imagination. These can range from simple two- to four-station circuits in a gym to elaborate outdoor circuits with several stations. You can do an interval-style workout by including a hike up a steep incline with a heavy pack. Steve has used a long, easy alpine route and done several fast laps on it to add variety to his ME workouts. Designing your own ME circuit can be a fun challenge and you can customize it to suit your individual needs. We'll give you some planning suggestions in chapter 8. Just keep in mind the principles of continuity and a gradual progression.

The Value of Specific Strength Training

By Tony Yaniro

As a high school kid I came across a boulder problem at Joshua Tree National Monument that had only a few ascents. I tried this mantel problem and could hardly start the move. I realized that it took a very specific group of muscles that was rarely used in combination. I tried doing push-ups, presses, and the like. I got better at the presses, but still came no closer to doing the problem. I finally thought: I need to either move to Joshua Tree and train directly on the climb, or find a way to replicate the move at home.

One day I noticed on the roof of my house that the dormer roof lip and wall below was very similar in orientation to the move on the boulder problem I could not do. I decided to use this as a specific training apparatus. I put a wood block under the eave and placed a toe on it. I then replicated the movement with a little help from my toe. Over the next month, I would go up there and do sets of reps in the typically prescribed method for building strength. I felt the strength come as it had done before with the push-ups and presses.

When I returned to the boulder problem, I found that the dormer was actually a bit more difficult. The boulder problem was disappointingly easy—but I was hooked on specific training.

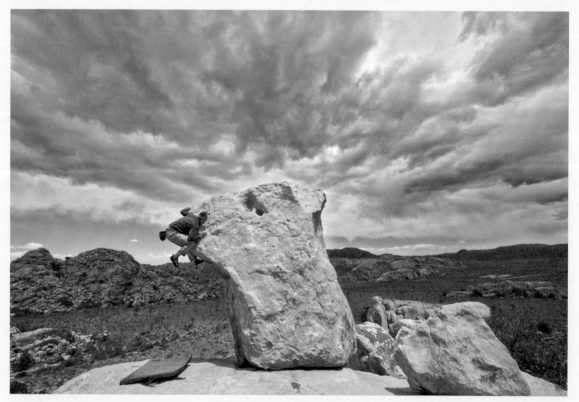

Vic Zeilman pressing out the exit mantle on the North Arete, Bullwinkle Boulder, in Joshua Tree National Park, California.
Photo: Greg Epperson

SUMMARY: SOME REAL-WORLD ADVICE

The correct progression is absolutely fundamental to improving all of the various qualities that each period seeks to impart. Due to its quantified nature, strength training lends itself to monitoring your progress pretty easily.

- The Transition Period can be a bit of a shock to your body if strength training is new to you. It is likely to leave you stiff and sore after the first few workouts. By doing these workouts in a circuit style we hope to minimize this unpleasant stiffness. By all means don't spend your first day in the gym doing multiple sets of any exercise unless you like being stiff and sore for a week and missing training time because of it.

- During much of the alpine climbing activities you participate in there is not much pushing of your strength reserve. In other words, in your preparation you will actually train at a higher degree of strength than you encounter during most of your climbing activity. This gives you the needed buffer above and beyond. But if you do not regularly include some maintenance stimulation of this Max Strength during this Muscular Endurance Period, and even into the climbing season, you are relying on your activities alone to keep up your strength and you will eventually lose the buffer you have built up through your training. This can reduce the effects of the Muscular Endurance work as well as set you up for potential injury. It can pay big dividends to include an occasional Max Strength session even as a warm-up for another strength workout.

- If you notice a stagnation in improvement, or even a drop off, and you have been consistent in your workouts, the most likely reasons are (a) you are not recovering from the training. Perhaps the other training you are doing is carrying over some fatigue into the strength workouts or vice versa. Or (b) you are progressing too fast. If you are in a heavy strength period it has been our experience that a reduction in the volume of strength training will remedy any short-term stagnation. Try cutting back on the number of sets for a workout or two and see if that helps.

- If you experience a plateau in strength gains during the Max Strength Period, this can be overcome by utilizing isometric contractions for one or two workouts.

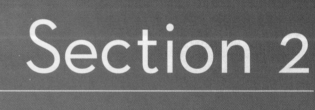

Section 2

Planning Your Training

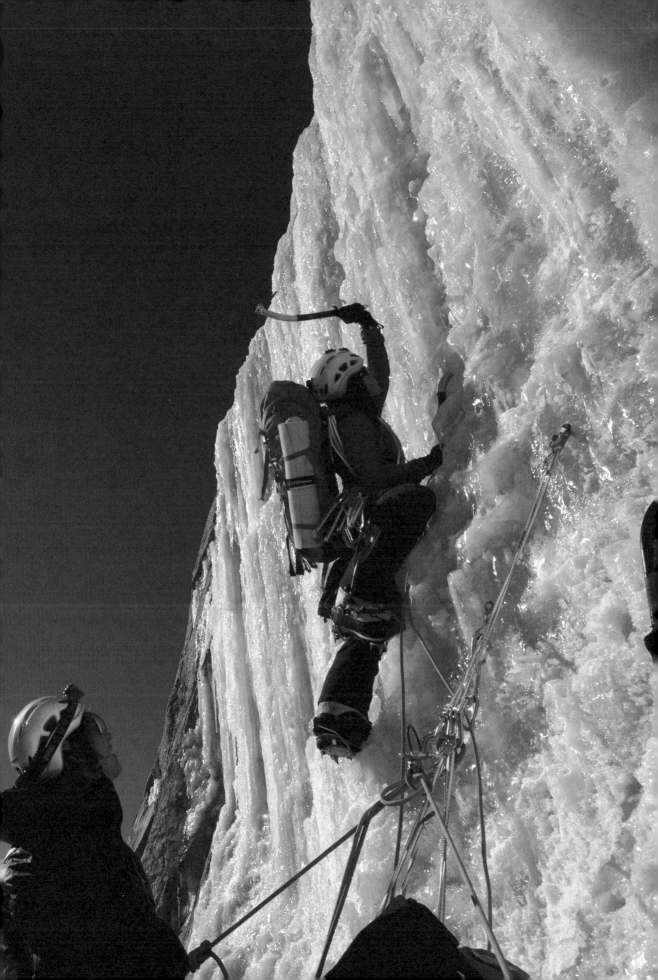

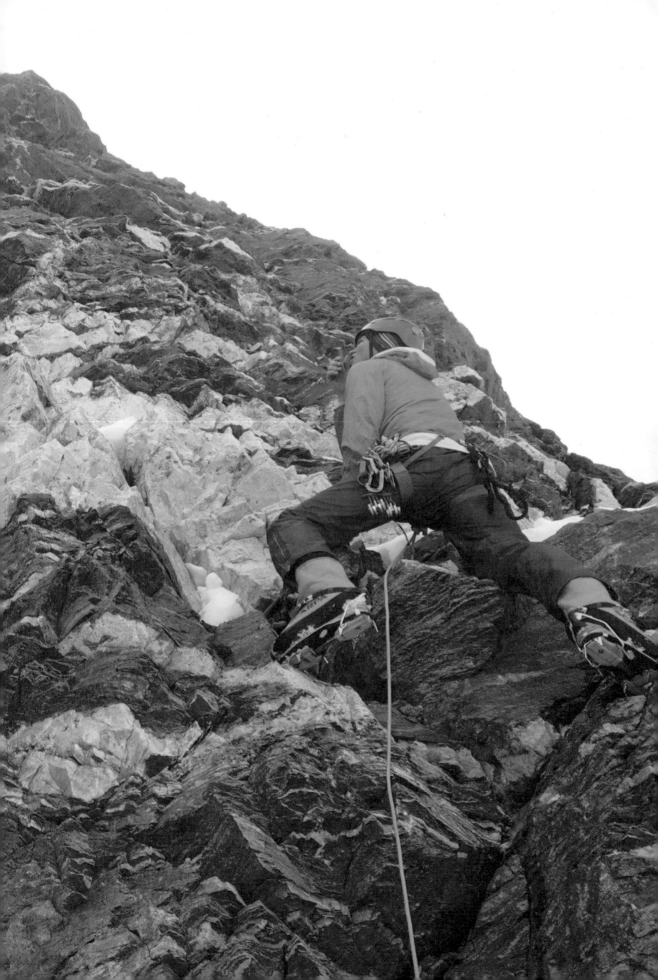

Chapter 6

Assessing
Your Fitness

"Ambition, to me, has always seemed preferable
to memories."

– GASTON RÉBUFFAT, pioneering French alpinist and writer

MAXIMIZING YOUR FITNESS

The first step in planning a training program is to map your course.
You must know where you are, where you want to go, and when you
want to arrive. This chapter gives you a simple, reproducible general
fitness test. By a general test we mean that the test will measure some
basic fitness qualities rather than measuring directly how fast you can
climb a particular alpine route, even though that is the ultimate goal
of your training.

Aside from the obvious difficulty of developing and prescribing a
universally meaningful test, we want to assess fitness and not your
technical proficiency. The purpose of this book is to help you train
your strength and endurance in the mountains. It is this foundation
that will support your climbing, and we have found that measuring
some basic fitness qualities that relate well to real climbing can give you
a very good idea of where you stand.

Opposite: Marko Prezelj tackles the
first difficult pitch during an alpine-
style attempt on the west face of
Makalu in 2011. *Photo: Steve House*

Previous spread: Ines Papert leading
on Kyzyl-Asker (19,170', 5,842m),
Kyrgystan. *Photo: Thomas Senf*

Twelve Hundred Feet

By Caroline George

My accident was not the result of coincidence. We were skiing a steep southerly face in the middle of the afternoon on a hot spring day. We were tired. We had little experience. The snow had softened to make skiing this steep slope a pure delight. I wanted more and decided to indulge in a few more slushy turns before taking a sharp left to avoid the 1,200-foot (366-meter) drop below.

One turn. Two turns. And suddenly, something hit me softly, throwing me off balance. The soft slide that released from above spun me around. I had little control over my gear. It all happened in slow motion. Yet, I was so close to the edge that it all unraveled quickly. While falling down the 1,200-foot (366-meter) face, I kept thinking to myself, "*I need to stop. I am going to die.*" I tried to stop myself, yet there aren't many ways to self-arrest while free falling. I hit twice, on two separate ledges, before landing in the soft afternoon snow on the glacier below.

A helicopter scooped me up and delivered me to the Swiss hospital: twenty-five fractures in my ankle, a broken and displaced sacrum, broken ribs. During the two months spent lying flat on my back in the hospital, I realized that I didn't have the appropriate skills that were required to climb big mountains. I wanted to learn those skills, but I would need partners to take me and show me. Since I didn't know the right people, I grabbed a friend who had never really been in the mountains before and took her climbing. We started with a mellow snow climb, then an easy ridge, and eventually up bigger and harder climbs.

Our first big alpine route was on the Aiguille du Chardonnet in Chamonix. We hiked through wildflowers and spent the night in the damp Albert Premier hut. The route, the Forbes Arête, is not a hard climb, though it offers a bit of everything: a treacherous approach on a glacier; exposure to a serac at the start; a long, steep snow climb to reach the ridge proper; and a technical and sometimes knife-edge ridge with many gendarmes to climb and contour, requiring efficient rope management.

As I climbed, I watched what other parties were doing. I tried to remember what I had read in books and listened to my gut feeling. I not only had my life to watch out for, but also that of my friend. I felt a deep sense of responsibility to keep us both alive. We climbed—neither quickly nor efficiently. An exposed and complicated descent brought us down from the summit. We missed the last chairlift, forcing a long walk back to the valley floor.

We successfully climbed a mountain, and I had gotten us up and down. Safely? Well, safely enough. The greatest lesson was that I had so much to learn. But I also learned that I could do it—I could climb a mountain by my own means with a weaker partner.

This ascent gave me the confidence to keep climbing mountains, and I decided I wanted to become a mountain guide. Over the following years, I acquired the skills to make this decision a reality: I climbed a lot, in all sorts of terrain, weather, and conditions. I kept taking my friend to the mountains as my guinea pig. I learned rope management, rock and ice climbing techniques, how to move efficiently on ridges, how to read terrain, how to navigate in whiteout conditions, and how to assess and manage objective hazards.

I realized that although accidents can happen, the risk can usually be identified and mitigated, and the accident avoided. This is one aspect of alpine climbing that I still work on, by going into the mountains with people weaker and stronger than me, by learning from my mistakes, by acknowledging my limits, and learning how to push them safely. I try to be a proactive and solid partner, a good climber, and the best guide I can be.

Caroline George is an AMGA-IFMGA certified mountain guide and lives in Chamonix, France, with her husband and daughter.

Opposite: Caroline George belays on the 1938 Route on the Eiger North Face, Switzerland. Griffith. *Photo: Jonathan Griffith*

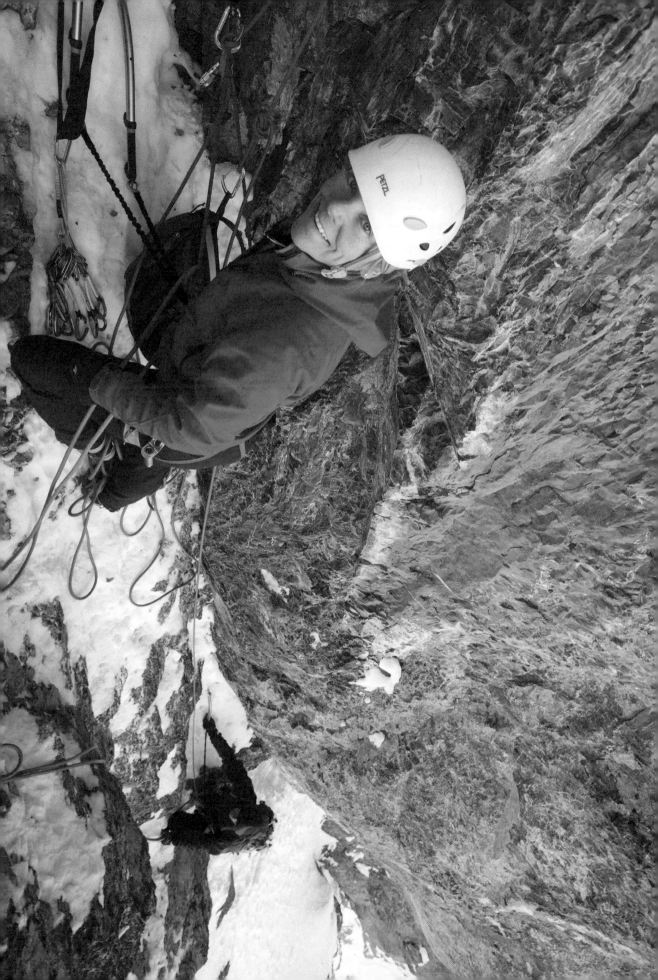

Testing the Components of Fitness

Why do we want to test the component parts of your fitness? How do general qualities relate to climbing-specific ones? These are good questions, and to answer them, let's use an analogy from the National Football League. The NFL uses a series of tests called the NFL Combine, administered in late February every year. Coaches, scouts, and team executives along with every aspiring NFL draftee show up in Indianapolis for the Combine. The athletes are run through a battery of physical and mental tests. Each test measures some basic quality of the athlete. Some are more closely related to the sport of football than others, but none of them actually involve having the aspirants play football.

There are millions of dollars and many reputations riding on this selection process, so why would the NFL not want to see these guys play football? Simple: The tests can compare athletes easily, and they know that without a certain level of proficiency in these basic skills the chance of a player having what it takes to play in the NFL is about zilch. If a guy can't break five seconds for the forty-yard dash he does not have enough speed to be a decent running back no matter his ball-handling skills. If a player does not have a thirty-inch vertical leap he is lacking in the kind of explosive power the sport demands.

Many other sports organizations use a similar process. The former Eastern Bloc countries were the first in making early selection of very young athletes by measuring basic predispositions in sporting aptitudes. Because of the money involved, the NFL is probably the most structured example of this method of testing. As mentioned earlier in this book, other sports have a lot to teach alpine climbers.

The test we will propose will address basic qualities of physical strength and endurance that, when taken together, we believe you need to have in order to be successful in alpine climbing. Sure, you can be a good climber if you can only do ten pull-ups. Yes, you can still get up the big routes if you can't climb at 3,000 feet (915 meters) per hour with a twenty-pound pack. But we're not talking about being merely good. We wrote this book to help you break boundaries.

Alex Lowe was one of the most forward-thinking and smartest guys in alpine climbing and he recognized the value of maximizing his basic fitness as a foundation for improving his climbing. There was a good reason why Alex trained like a fiend and was known to routinely train these very basic qualities we are proposing.

JUDGING YOUR CURRENT STRENGTHS

To help assess your fitness it is important to first look at your goals and what specific fitness will be required for those goals. Your end goal may be a one-day ascent of the north face of the Eiger or a climb of the west buttress of Denali. They are very different objectives, but the basic aerobic fitness required for these climbs is really no different. It is in the climbing skills area where the big differences lie. The skill requirements for the Denali climb will be fairly low technically with glacier travel and moderate-angle snow climbing and cramponing on ice being the most important. The Eiger, on the other hand, will require technical prowess on steep ice and rock while wearing crampons, the ability to simul-climb or solo confidently, and the ability to transition at belays quickly to climb the route safely. In both cases aerobic endurance will factor heavily into your success and as such, needs to factor into the test you undertake as well as the subsequent training you do in preparation. We will show you one test that we use that measures whole-body strength and aerobic fitness, but you can design your own test. Just bear in mind when you do so that you want to break down climbing into some simpler component parts so you can see where you need to improve.

Testing Basic Fitness

So how do you get this climbing-specific fitness that applies to your climbing goal?

Start with general fitness. To assess this we've developed the Alpine Combine. The beauty of this test is that it is simple, reproducible, and universal, but you are going to have to do some math.

- Timed 1,000-foot (305-meter) vertical ascent on steep second- to third-class terrain carrying a pack weighing 20 percent of your body weight (BW). Ideally this will be somewhere local that you can come back to for regular re-test. If you do not have easy access to this, then use the next method. Timed box step with a pack weighing 20 percent of BW to reach 1,000 vertical feet (305 meters). The box height should be approximately 75 percent of the height of your tibia (from the floor to three-quarters of the way to your knee), usually eight to twelve inches high. Wear boots.

- Number of dips in sixty seconds

- Number of sit-ups in sixty seconds

- Number of pull-ups in sixty seconds

- Number of box jumps in sixty seconds

- Number of push-ups in sixty seconds

Basic Fitness Test

	Poor	Good	Excellent
Box step, 1,000' with 20% of BW pack	40–60+ min	20–40 min	<20 min
Dips in 60 sec	<10	10–30	>30
Sit-ups in 60 sec	<30	30–50	>50
Pull-ups in 60 sec	<15	15–25	>25
Box step ups in 60 sec	<30	30–45	>45
Push-ups in 60 sec	<15	15–40	>40

Why these exercises? They don't really seem to have anything to do with climbing. The aim here is to measure a general, overall foundation of fitness. Without a good foundation, the specific training of climbing will not yield as good of results as it will with a higher level of basic conditioning.

Once you have results from this or a similarly simple, reproducible test you can come back to it later to assess your progress.

Don't feel constrained by our Alpine Combine. You can invent your own test—let your imagination run wild.

SETTING GOALS

We encourage you to plan your climbing goals around one-year cycles. While it is possible to achieve near-peak fitness two, even three times a year—with excellent coaching—it is difficult to hold that form for more than a few weeks. Achieving one's highest fitness levels multiple times, or for an extended period, in a year is beyond the scope of most athletes. A self-coached or nonprofessional climber will achieve a higher and longer single peak, lasting four to eight weeks, by following the steps presented in this book.

We understand that this full process will not be practical for everyone. If you are training for a climbing trip less than twelve weeks away, you will have to abbreviate the whole training cycle, and will not see the optimal gains.

Some of you may want to plot five- or ten-year plans, which we encourage. In 1990 Steve set a goal to someday ascend Nanga Parbat's Rupal Face, which took him fifteen years to accomplish. Long-term goals can be very powerful motivators. While it is great if you can see that far into your future, don't worry if you can't. Training has a way of being transformative in many ways. By the time you've repeated this process for yourself every year for several years, you'll be in a much different place than you are now. Keep in mind that as you age you'll be more physiologically predisposed to attempt endurance-focused objectives since it takes years to maximally develop your endurance capacity.

The Box Step Test: An Unpleasant, But Useful Tool

Box steps are a bit like drinking castor oil: effective but unpleasant.

For this test you'll get decked out in mountain boots and put on a pack that's equal in weight to the one you use on your goal climb or a minimum typical alpine pack of twenty pounds. This weight represents a light kit for a day's alpine climbing, and the kit will weigh roughly the same regardless of age, sex, or body weight.

You will probably want to conduct this test in the privacy of your own home lest you fall victim to the guffaws of any witnesses.

You'll need a sturdy box or stair to step up and down on. We'd suggest something in the range of eight to twelve inches in height.

Now comes the tricky bit (wink, wink). You got it! Step up and down off this box as fast as you can until you've tallied 1,000 feet (305 meters) of vertical gain. To count one full step, you must have *both feet* on the top of the box before you step off.

Keep track of your steps by using one of those gate-keeper clickers that counts attendees at high school basketball games. One click for each step on to the box. Before you start, calculate the number of steps you'll need to make to gain 1,000 feet (305 meters), based on the height of your box.

We don't recommend using a Stairmaster device because on that sort of machine the step is actually falling away beneath you and you do not have to raise your body weight with each step as you do in real uphill or on the box.

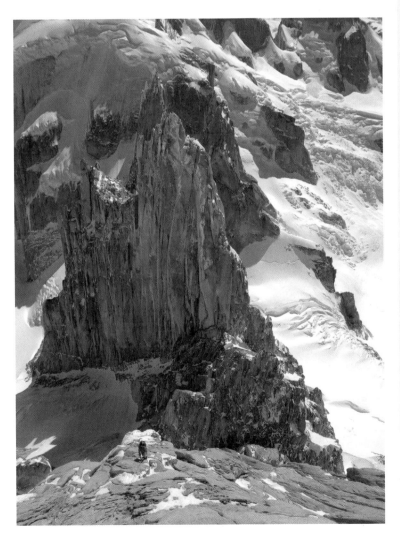

Alessandro Beltrami climbing Festerville on Aguja Standhardt, with Aguja Bífida in the background, Patagonia. *Photo: Rolando Garibotti*

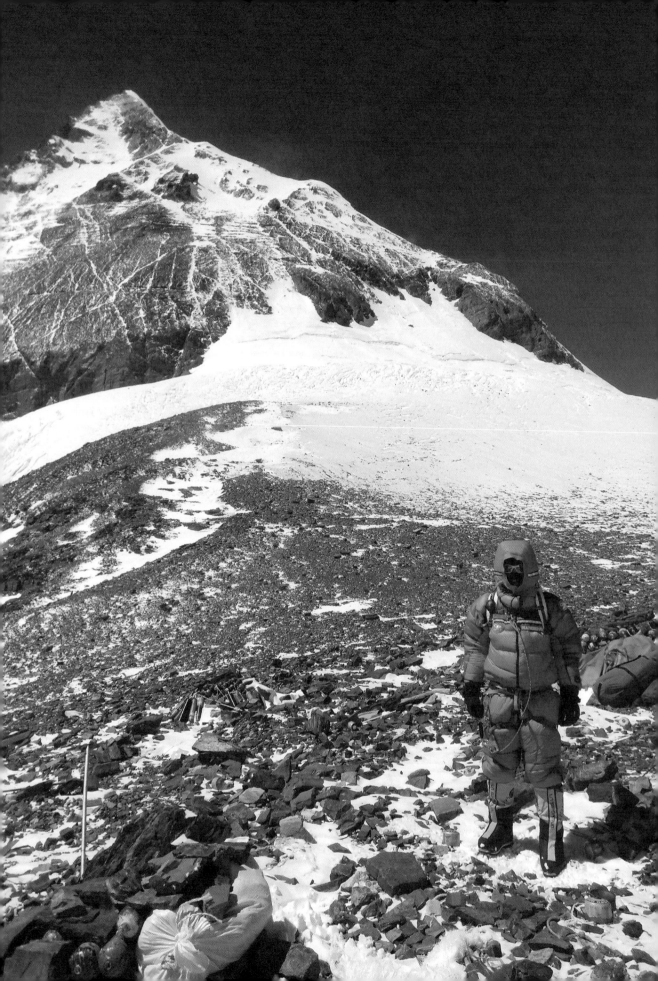

The Quest to
Climb Everest in a Day

By Chad Kellogg

When you begin training for an alpine objective you must give the problem a thorough analysis: How much vertical gain must you ascend, what are the difficulties, how long will it take? Your task then is to become the physical and mental solution to the problem. The problem of speed climbing Everest is to go from base camp to the summit and back to base camp within a single thirty-hour period. The main objectives to overcome are the extreme altitude and having the endurance to push for that long.

Here is how I sized up the Everest speed objective: The starting elevation is 17,300 feet (5,273 meters) and the summit is 29,035 feet (8,850 meters). To get to the top via the Southeast Ridge is approximately twelve miles. The total vertical gain is about 11,700 feet (3,566 meters). The technical difficulties are minimal.

I began training in 2008 by hiking 3,600 vertical feet (1,097 meters) quickly using ski poles to harness my arms. After a couple of weeks I could run the same hill without poles much faster. Then I added a second lap at a walk/run pace. After a couple of months I could run three laps for over 11,500 feet (3,505 meters) of vertical gain. Then I began to do 10,000-foot (3,048-meter) climbs on Mount Rainier, then I doubled it and kept going until I could climb the mountain from the parking lot three times in succession in a thirty-three-hour period.

In 2009 I went to a trainer and told him I wanted to put on fifteen pounds of leg muscle for Everest. My logic was that the high altitude would eat my muscle mass away and I would lose twenty pounds of muscle and ten pounds of fat. Before I left for Everest in 2010 I weighed 185 pounds. This was not a good strategy. All that body mass slowed my acclimatization. When I went back to Everest in 2012 I weighed 31 pounds less than I had in 2010: 154 pounds.

In 2012, for a second time, I did not reach the summit of Everest. This time my issues were with my nutrition. Our bodies cannot digest food well above 17,000 feet (5,182 meters). At high altitudes, for me above 23,000 feet (7,010 meters), I find that my body can only break down the simplest foods. On my second attempt I was on track for the new record when I vomited all of my food and water at around 24,000 feet (7,315 meters). The resulting shortage of calories caused a major drop in my pace and I lost two hours between Camp 3 (23,300 feet/7,102 meters) and the South Col (26,000 feet/7,925 meters). I was able to keep down some gluten-free granola and continue to 28,350 feet (8,642 meters). Seven hundred feet (213 meters) below the summit I turned back.

What have I learned from my repeated attempts? I learned that going into a climb at fighting weight allows me to go faster because my body is light and requires less oxygen to operate. I also learned that the more time I spend at altitude the easier my body is able to adjust to the stress of adaptation. I learned to wait for the conditions to match the objective I had in mind (i.e., crowds, air temperature, route conditions, time of year). I discovered that I had to experiment with nutrition to find the right types of food for optimum endurance and recovery. You need to know how many calories your body needs to function and not be in deficit. But most of all I found out that I needed to sacrifice whatever is standing in the way of my dream.

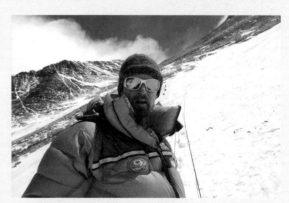

Chad Kellogg. *Photo: Rory Stark*

Chad Kellogg is a Pacific Northwest native and holder of the speed record to the summit of Denali (14:26). He has also climbed several impressive technical routes, including a difficult new route on Pangbuk Ri (21,736'/6,625m) with Dave Gottlieb in a fifty-hour push.

Opposite: Chad Kellogg at Everest's South Col (25,938', 7,906m); all dressed up and ready to sprint to the summit. *Photo: Rory Stark*

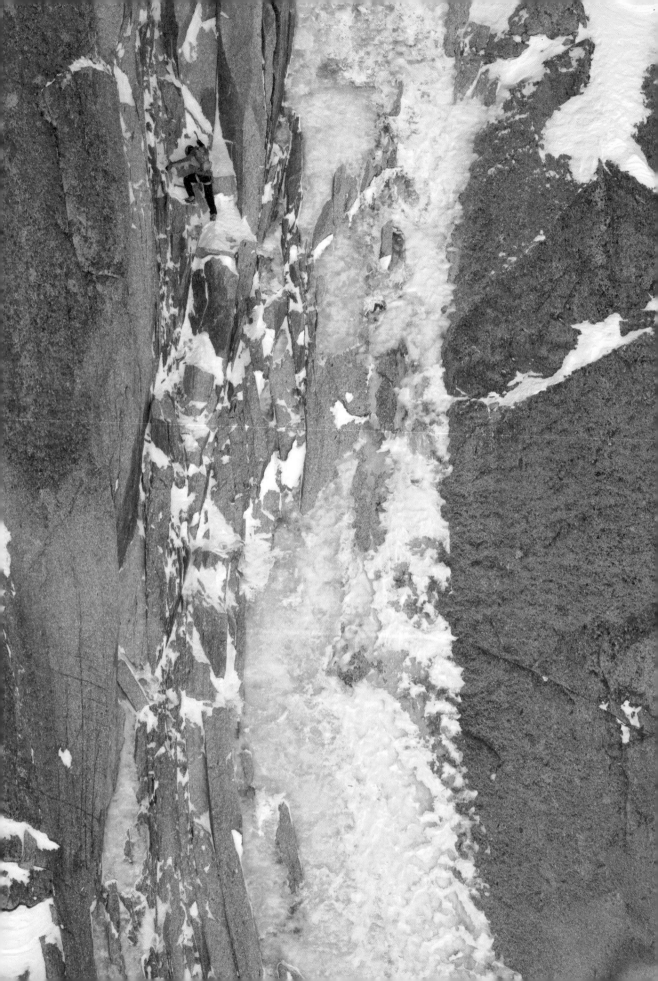

Chapter 7

Transitioning into Training

"If people knew how hard I had to work, they wouldn't think I was such a genius."

– MICHELANGELO

LISTEN TO YOUR BODY

It is impossible for us to tell you what an appropriate training load would be. By explaining the theory and the methods, by giving you real-world examples, and by equipping you with self-assessment and monitoring tools, you are now able to create and regulate your own training with the guidance of these next chapters.

No matter your climbing goal, your life, family, co-workers, and your body will all need to adjust to regular training. Training is not the same as exercising; training requires discipline, attention, and consistency. The challenge is to adhere to a schedule and gently coax your body into a regime, not bludgeon it into submission.

Continuity. Gradualness. Modulation. Those are our watchwords. Continuity is listed first for a reason. Without continuity, the other two will become moot.

Opposite: Ueli Steck climbing the Ginat Route on the north face of Les Droites (13,126', 4,001m) near Chamonix, France. *Photo: Jonathan Griffith*

Besides discipline and adherence, you need attention. We all have a lot to learn about our bodies. Part of the purpose of the Transition Period is to feel how you react to training. Be aware and attentive to the subtle signals your body communicates with. You'll learn how much volume you can handle. You'll learn whether morning or afternoon is the best time for high-quality training. You will learn to tell when fatigue is mounting and you need a break.

There will also be logistical aspects to this phase: finding the best local trails, getting your bike tuned up, buying new approach shoes.

THE TRAINING LOG

Attention includes recording. And recording means you need a training log to write down the training you've done, and more importantly record how it affected you and how you recovered. Grade each workout and be sure to record a few impressions about your daily training and climbing. These notes will often jog your memory when you review your training later and will help you remember specific workouts, or specific climbs and how they felt. In the future, these details will go a long ways toward helping you see the effectiveness of the training over time.

A good training log will come to act as a coach in the sense that it will provide you with feedback on how you are adapting. Your log will ultimately become the most important training book you have.

But don't become enamored of numbers in your log. Don't be a slave to the plan. Getting into a competition with yourself by posting impressive training results is a time-tested path to overtraining.

We find that a simple, durable notebook or calendar works well. Many people like to use their smartphone since it's always handy. Other people like to use spreadsheets or online- or smartphone-based training applications. We've included a couple of examples here that you can copy and use. You can also download the MS Excel files for these documents at www.stevehouse.net/downloads.html.

TRAINING PLANS: STEVE'S TRANSITION PERIOD BEFORE MAKALU 2009

Your training plan is meant to offer guidance in what you might do, not dictate what you will do. Things will come up, your body's response to the training, for any number of reasons, may not be what you expected. You will be forced to deviate from the intended plan, and that is OK.

Quarterly Training Log

Name:				Training Volume projection worksheet		
Year:			Goal:			
Week #	Period	Hours Zone 1	Hours Zone 3/4	Hours Strength	Weekly total	Cummulative
1						
2						
3						
4						
5						
6						
7						
8						
9						
10						
11						
12						
13						
14						
15						
16						
17						
18						
19						
20						
21						
22						
23						
24						
25						
26						
27						
28						
29						
30						
31						
32						
33						
34						
35						
36						
37						
38						
39						

Weekly Training Log

Date:

Name:

Week #:

Target Hours this week:

Actual Hours this week:

Someday I will climb:

Period:

Training goal this week:

Climbing goal this week:

A: I am Superhuman!

B: Good Workout

Partners this week:

C: I Felt Flat

Nutrition goals this week:

My zones:

55-75% 80-90% 90-95% D: Modified workout

F: Didn't complete workout

Date	Day	Activity by time				Altitude gained	Time in Intensity Zone				Workout Grade	Workout Notes
		Climb	Approach	Run	Ski	Strength		1	3	4		

Total time/activity

Total training time this week:

Routes, comments, observations, quote of the day, music of the day, inspirations, routes I want to climb:

Cummulative training time:

Total altitude gain this week:

Total altitude gain this year:

Weekly Evaluation:

Understand that the plan is an outline; your log is the actual story. The outline keeps you on track but offers some flexibility.

Let's review the first month of training for Steve's 2009 Makalu plan. Because he had been training consistently Steve didn't require much of a Transition Period to ramp back up into training form. We decided that six weeks would be sufficient to get him ready to start the Base Period of his training. This is as short a Transition Period as we'd ever recommend. Remember: Gradualness rules here.

Since Steve had trained close to 900 hours the previous years he could start with a simple formula: 900 hours/52 weeks = 17.3 hours per week on average. This allows us to see what level of work Steve's body is capable of handling. Jumping right back to that level would violate the cardinal rule of gradualness. So we need to pick a starting point.

If you have trained the previous year, you can use the rule of thumb that you can start at approximately 50 percent of your average weekly hours from the previous year. This means that Steve would start at 8.5 hours per week.

Considering Steve's long training history, and based on our experiences coaching, we decided it would be reasonable for him to make a 5 percent increase in hours each week during this period. Less-experienced climbers will need to make smaller incremental increases during the Transition Period.

The hours listed here are hours of training with his heart rate in Zones 1 and 2 (120<HR<160) and includes time for strength training.

First Six Weeks of Steve's 2009 Makalu Training Plan

Week number	Hours
1 (Begin strength training this week)	8.5
2	9
3	9.5
4	10
5	10.5
6	11

Even though his emphasis was on high-altitude mountaineering, he didn't emphasize climbing very much in this early stage. Priority was given to the aerobic system since it is the slowest to respond to training and so needs the longest period and the most stimulation. Time spent in the aerobic zone is what's important. Weight-bearing sports like running, hiking, and ski touring are best; though any modality will work. Remember, this is the period where specificity is least important.

PLANNING YOUR TRANSITION PERIOD

A dirty little secret of training is that the training plans during the Transition Period are very similar for everyone. The main difference will be the volume of training rather than what makes up the training. Those who do not have a history of structured training have to guess

Maxime Turgeon rappels after climbing the Bonatti Route, Grand Capucin (12,592', 3,838m) in the Mont Blanc Massif, France. *Photo: Steve House*

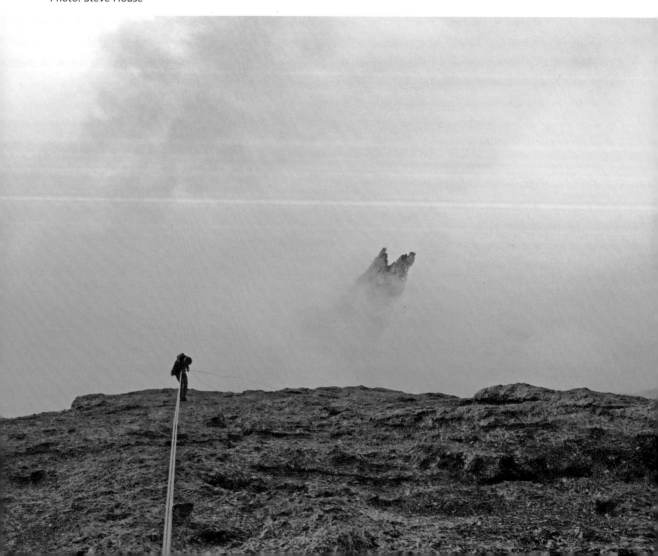

at a starting volume. Everyone else will use 50 percent of the previous year's average (as we did in the previous example). For all but the most experienced athletes this Transition Period will be eight weeks.

General Guidelines for Guestimating Your Annual Training Volume

Person	Hours
Active college student/climber	250
Working professional	200
Seasonal worker/climber	400
Working mountain guide	500

General Guidelines for Your Transition Period Planning

During these early weeks there is no difference in training for technical routes versus mountaineering. The principles of training dictate that we are best served building general strength and fitness first. This plan provides a gradual adaptation period: The training load is held constant for the first three weeks; after that an increase of 10 percent in volume is held constant for weeks 4 and 5. Then a 5 percent increase in volume is held constant for weeks 6 and 7. Week 8 is a reduced training load to give your body a chance to catch up before launching into the Base Period—the meat of the training.

General Progression of Transition Period Training Load

Weeks	Weekly volume
1–3	All three weeks the same at 50% of previous year's average weekly volume (or best guess)
4–5	Both weeks the same at 10% increase over week three
6–7	Both weeks the same at 5% increase over week five
8	Drop 50% of volume from week seven for consolidation

Returning to Training after a Layoff

A common trap for athletes is coming back from a layoff. Often people return to high levels of activity after they have left it for some reason other than injury. If there have been months, or years, of inactivity, there is a danger period in the initial stage of retraining.

Even though you have been out of shape for a while, when training restarts, the muscles and the neuromuscular interface will pop back into shape relatively fast. Actually, most people are amazed that within several weeks they begin to feel quite strong. This is a particularly dangerous time because during the layoff, not only did the muscles become weak, but the tendons and their attachment points to the bones also became weak. These connective tissues will need more time to reinforce than the muscles. If you add too much training load too soon (because it feels so good), you risk rupturing these other tissues.

Allow for a similar amount of time that it took to train the first time—at least for the first several months—so that the connective tissues have a chance to catch up. Don't become injured, it is not worth it.

The final take-away point is: Listen to your body. It will tell you when to back off or to forge ahead. Nobody else will train exactly like you. If you want to really improve, talk to someone experienced in your sport; learn from their mistakes and triumphs.

Remember the adage: Training makes you weaker, recovery is what gets you stronger.

Workouts for the Eight-Week Transition Period

Suggested workouts for each week are listed below. You'll need to slot these into the days that fit your schedule and plan for the required time based on your ability. For some people a one-hour hike may be long and for others a two-hour run may be more appropriate. No one can decide this for you.

Weeks 1, 2, 3 (for the active, but not trained individual) contain the following workouts:

- One long Zone 1 aerobic workout each week. Should leave you tired from the duration, not the intensity. This one workout should be 25 percent of the weekly aerobic training volume.

- Two General Strength sessions. Do Scott's Killer Core Workout as warm-up.

- One Zone 2 aerobic session at top of conversational pace. This should not last more than 10 percent of total aerobic training volume.

- Climb one day. Do a minimum of 5–6 pitches that are 1–2 number grades below your current top (redpointing) ability.

- Make up the rest of the volume with easy aerobic exercise at Zone 1, or recovery pace.

Example Training Schedule Weeks 1–3

	Monday	Tuesday	Wednesday	Thursday	Friday	Saturday	Sunday
AM	Zone 1	Zone 1	Zone 2	Off	Off	Climbing	Long Zone 1
PM	Strength	Off	Recovery	Strength	Off	Recovery	Off

Weeks 4 and 5, use the same workouts as weeks 1–3 but with 10 percent higher volume than week 3:

- One long Zone 1 aerobic workout each week. Should leave you tired from the duration not the intensity. This one workout should be 25 percent of the weekly aerobic training volume.

- Two General Strength sessions. Do Scott's Killer Core Routine as warm-up.

- One Zone 2 aerobic session at top of conversational pace. This should not last more than 10 percent of total aerobic training volume.

- Climb one day. Do a minimum of 5–6 pitches, 1–2 number grades below your current top (redpointing) ability.

- Make up the rest of the volume with easy aerobic exercise at Zone 1, or recovery pace.

Example Training Schedule Weeks 4–5

	Monday	Tuesday	Wednesday	Thursday	Friday	Saturday	Sunday
AM	Zone 1	Zone 1	Zone 2	Off	Off	Climbing	Long Zone 1
PM	Strength	Zone 1	Recovery	Strength	Off	Recovery	Off

Weeks 6 and 7, use the same workouts as weeks 1–3 but with 5 percent higher volume than week 5:

- One long Zone 1 aerobic workout each week. Should leave you tired from the duration not the intensity. This one workout should be 25 percent of the weekly aerobic training volume.

- Two General Strength sessions. Do Scott's Killer Core Routine as warm-up.

- One Zone 2 aerobic session at top of conversational pace. This should not last more than 15 percent of total aerobic training volume.

- Climb 1–2 days. Do a minimum of 6–8 pitches, 1–2 number grades below your current top (redpointing) ability.

- Make up the rest of the volume with easy aerobic exercise at Zone 1, or recovery pace.

Example Training Schedule Weeks 6–7

	Monday	Tuesday	Wednesday	Thursday	Friday	Saturday	Sunday
AM	Zone 1	Zone 1	Zone 2	Off	Off	Climbing	Long Zone 1
PM	Strength	Zone 1	Climbing	Strength	Off	Recovery	Off

Week 8 is at 50 percent of the total volume of week 7 and contains the following workouts:

- Two shorter Zone 1 aerobic workouts on hilly terrain.

- One General Strength session.

- One Zone 2 aerobic workout on hilly terrain.

- Climb one day, aiming to climb five pitches that are one number grade below your current redpointing ability.

- The rest of the aerobic volume is at recovery pace.

- This week is intended to act as a consolidation week to allow your body to catch up.

Example Training Schedule Week 8

	Monday	Tuesday	Wednesday	Thursday	Friday	Saturday	Sunday
AM	Zone 1	Zone 1	Off	Off	Off	Climbing	Long Zone 1
PM	Off	Off	Zone 2	Strength	Off	Recovery	Off

The last week should leave you refreshed, your legs bouncy, and your mind eager to launch into the Base Period with a high level of fitness and enthusiasm.

Strength versus Endurance

Hopefully by now you have gained a solid appreciation of the concepts of strength and endurance, and their differences. These two qualities exist in a complex yin and yang, a give and take, and your balance of these two factors will exist somewhere along a continuum. Only at the extremes of this strength-endurance spectrum will they exist in near isolation from one another. Everything in between will be a mixture where one quality will dominate while the other is supporting it.

STRENGTH TRAINING DURING THE TRANSITION PERIOD

Strength training is an integral part of every training plan because, as we've said before, strength forms the basis for endurance. By now you should understand that having a big aerobic base allows you to convert it into some impressive climbing-specific performances. Scott and Colin Haley's seven-hour round-trip on Denali's West Buttress (from chapter 3) and Steve's ability to make multiple attempts on the technically difficult new route on K7 can be attributed to their strong aerobic base and high strength reserve. With both aerobic endurance and strength you can build fitness for alpine climbing effectively by applying this proven, structured approach.

Goals of Transition Period Strength Training:

- General Strength. A wide variety of big, whole-body movements involving a lot of muscles forms a conditioning foundation for the next period.

- Flexibility. These movements require a full range of motion that require flexibility. Flexibility and strength are closely related. Often a deficit in strength is misdiagnosed as a deficit in flexibility.

- Coordination. Muscles that wire together, fire together. Make more and better neuromuscular connections.

CORE STRENGTH IN THE TRANSITION PERIOD

Core training does more than give you a nice six-pack. The importance of the core in climbing is that it connects the arms to the legs. Recall from our discussion about core strength in chapter 5 that climbing is a quadrapedal, as opposed to a bipedal, movement; especially the connection of the opposite limbs (for example, the right arm to the left foot). How often in climbing do you find yourself with your left foot hiked up high, and reaching for a hold with your right hand? This feels so intuitive that most of us scarcely give it a second thought. But the logic behind that movement is that a torque being resisted by your core musculature is what prevents you from barn-dooring off the wall. Furthermore, the steeper the climb, the more core strength it takes to

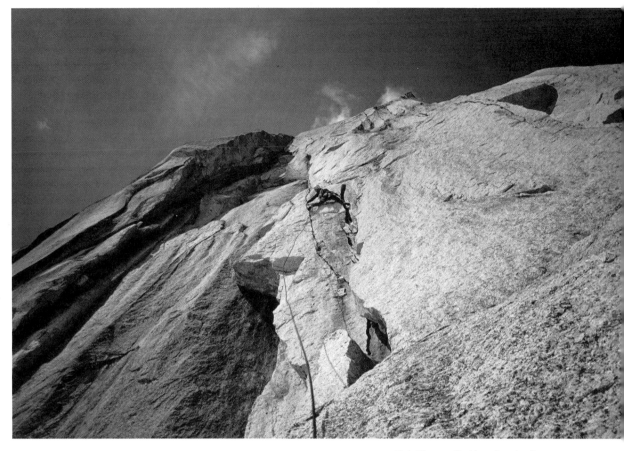

Rok Blagus climbing the classic
Cobra Pillar on Mount Barille (7,650',
2,325m) in the Alaska Range.
Photo: Marko Prezelj

keep your feet on. Steep climbs with small footholds require enormous core strength. Now imagine climbing with a backpack; functionally this is making the wall steeper in terms of the core strength required to keep pressure on your feet while reaching with your arms.

The core workout we have used for ourselves and many others, and recommend here, is not climbing specific. This is because training non-climbing-specific strength will provide the base of support for more activity-specific training to come. This explains why some climbers have success with circuit-style workouts (such as CrossFit): They are good general strength. But to do general strengthening workouts indefinitely results in a plateau because this typically ignores the principles of modulation and progression that we've discussed previously: Start generally and train more and more specifically throughout your training cycle.

The poorly understood secret about core strength is that our core musculature includes many deep and some superficial muscles. Some of them are composed mainly of fast twitch fibers and others are predominately slow twitch, both require some clever training methods

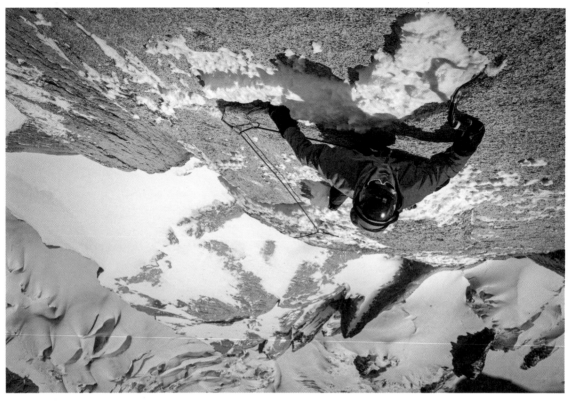

Stephan Siegrist climbing steep mixed ground near the summit of Cerro Standhardt (8,957'/2,730m) during a winter ascent of the peak. Patagonia. *Photo: Thomas Senf*

to engage. Sit-ups and crunches are not enough to fully engage the many other core stabilizers and often do not elicit an actual strength-building response. For instance, doing 500 sit-ups is great but it trains these muscles for endurance not strength.

Take a look at your abs of steel: Those six-pack muscles are the *rectus abdominus*. These are the guys that really work when doing spine-flexion movements like sit-ups and crunches. Because they are the most distant abdominal muscles from the spine they can exert the most force on the spine to effect a flexion of it. Repeatedly training crunches is strengthening the strongest link in the chain.

There is nothing wrong with a nice six-pack, but we want to train the weakest links in our athletic chain. A problem with athletic function arises when mono-directional training causes an imbalance in strength resulting in a lack of stability of the hips and shoulders. Reaching the deep spinal stabilizers can take some effort. It may surprise you to find that you are unable to engage some of these vital muscles. And if you can't engage them you will never train them.

Scott's Killer Core Routine

On the following pages is a core strength routine we have developed over the years to build good overall strength of virtually all the core muscles.

The idea for all these exercises is to hold the best, strictest form you can regardless of how few reps you can do, or how short a time you can hold a particular pose. When any of these things happen it indicates that the muscles have reached the point of failure and have received as much training stimulus as they can absorb. Do not allow poor form to take over. Unlike endurance training, quality is far more important than quantity.

Some of these exercises may be easy for you and some may be impossible. Try them all at first. If some are too hard, just keep trying them. If some become too easy you can add resistance by holding a weight or wearing a weight vest or changing them to increase the difficulty. Always be guided by the principle of maintaining maximum core tension. If some exercises are still too easy then leave them out of the routine and focus on your weaknesses. Do this once through as a warm-up for any strength training workout, or do it two or three times through as a stand-alone workout.

Let's review the five primary reasons for developing core strength for climbing:

- All athletic movements originate with the core musculature.

- Your core connects your arms to your legs.

- A weak core results in a less effective use of your arms and legs.

- A weak core exposes you to injury.

- Strength in the core will become the foundation for all your endurance.

The principles of Scott's Killer Core Routine are:

- Do this routine in a circuit fashion with thirty seconds between exercises.

- You're finished with the reps for each exercise when you can no longer hold the position, complete another perfect repetition, or if you begin to shake.

- Start with one circuit if you are a beginner or if you find the exercises are difficult for you.

- If you allow poor form to take over in order to get in more reps, you are defeating the purpose of this workout because you'll be compensating for weak core muscles by using some of your stronger ones.

- Don't hold your breath during the poses. Training yourself to breathe through this kind of core tension will transfer positively to your climbing.

Strict Sit-Ups

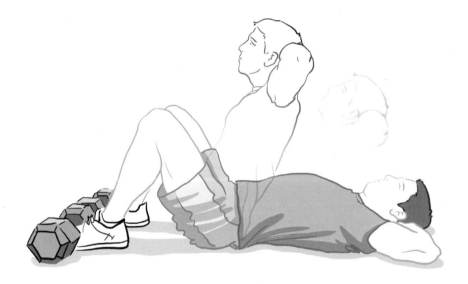

This version of the sit-up is meant to isolate the deep hip flexor muscles by eliminating flexion of the spine. Assume a normal sit up position: knees bent to about a 70 to 90 degree angle, back flat on the floor, toes hooked under something you can pull against. Link your fingers behind your head and keep your elbows as far back as you can. Do not allow your elbows to come forward as you sit up or you will be tempted to flex your spine. Now slowly, and in control, sit up by only flexing at your hips. Do not crunch by curling your spine. Keep your spine in a neutral (straight) position while coming up as high as you can. Return to the start position for one repetition.

Hitler's Dog

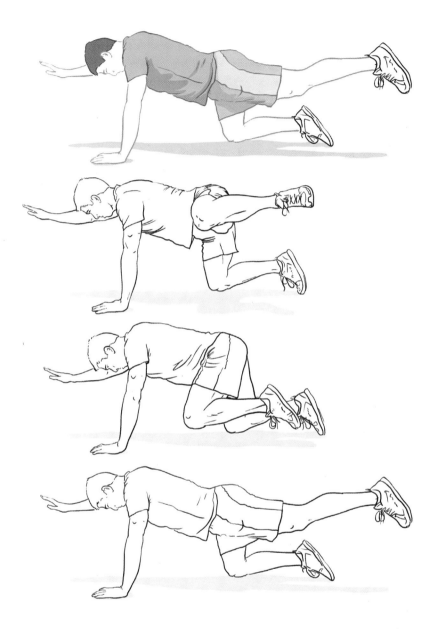

This oddly named exercise combines hip flexibility with transverse core strength. Get on all fours with knees directly below your hips and hands directly below your shoulders. From this decidedly doglike position pick up one leg and, while holding the knee bent at 90 degrees, move the hip joint through the full range of motion. This means drawing a big ellipse with your knee in the air. At the same time you are working hip strength and range of motion, pick up the opposite arm of the leg you are moving, and point it horizontally in front of your shoulder so that it is in line with your back. You may not feel this exercise is too tiring, but more than likely that is because you have poor hip mobility.

Windshield Wipers

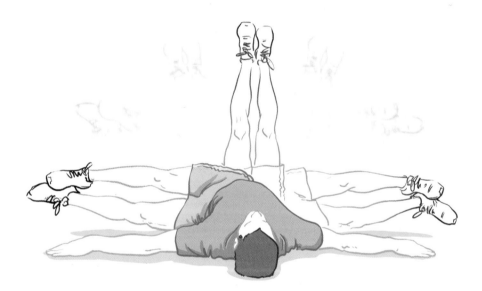

The name for this one suggests the action of your legs as they wipe across an imaginary windshield. Lie on your back with your arms outstretched from your shoulders with palms placed against the floor. Now flex your hips so that your feet are together with your legs pointed at the ceiling. Slowly rotate your hips so that your feet lower to the floor to one side; keep your feet locked together with knees straight. You'll want to resist the rotation of your shoulders by pushing down hard with your hand on the side you are rotating toward. Just lightly touch the floor with the side of the lower foot before raising both feet back to the 12 o'clock position, and on to the other side where the other foot will touch down. Return your feet to the 12 o'clock position to complete one repetition. Do this slowly and with control. If you cannot manage to keep your knees straight, or legs together, then bend your knees and do the same rotation while keeping your knees together and knees pointed at the ceiling when you are in the 12 o'clock position.

Three Point /Two Point

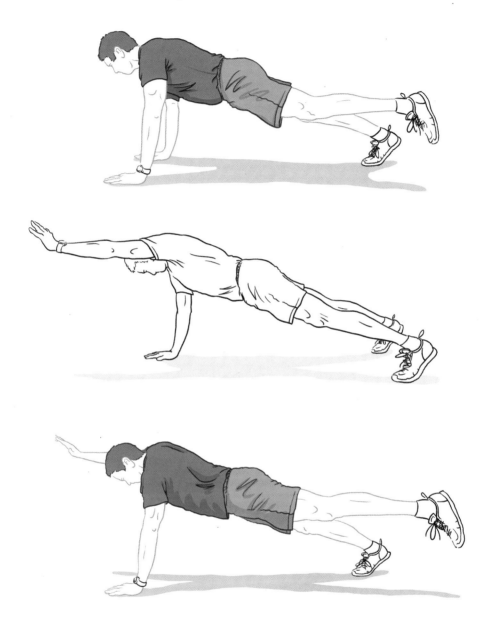

The intention of this exercise is to build a strong neural connection between opposing limbs. Assume a good push up position (a straight line running the length of your back and legs) with hands directly under you shoulders and feet spread about two feet apart. To start: Pick up one hand without rotating your shoulders or hip. Point that hand straight out in front and in line with your spine; hold till you feel your shoulders rotate, hips rotate, or your back sag—anything that gets you out of the straight line you were in when you started the push up position. In turn, pick up each limb and hold till failure. When this is no longer a challenge you can pick up the opposite hand and foot, and hold that position as long as possible. We have some athletes that do this exercise with as much as a sixty-pound weight vest.

Kayaker

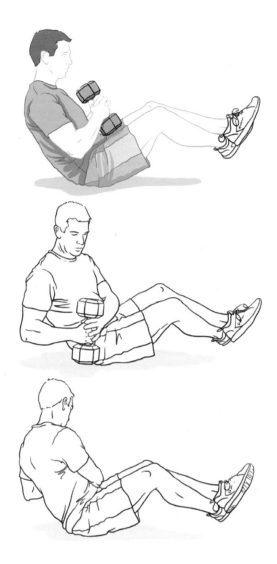

By mimicking the counter rotation of the hips and shoulders that a kayaker does we can target some of the deepest core muscles connecting the spine to the pelvis. Sit on the floor with legs stretched out in front of you. Bring your knees up to about a 90-degree bend and lift your feet a few inches off the floor. Clasp your hands together in front of you and rotate your shoulders so that you can touch your hands to the floor lightly just beside one hip. Rotate all the way to the other side and touch the floor again. Do this slowly and in control. Hold a dumbbell and touch it to the floor for added resistance.

Super Push-Ups

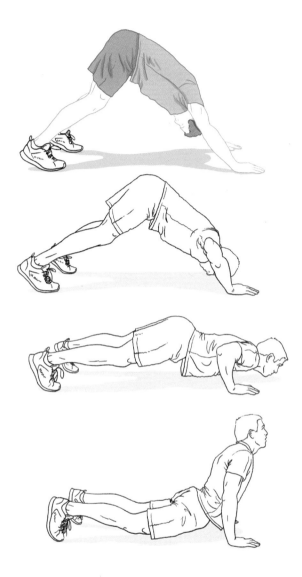

This exercise owes much to the yoga postures of downward dog and cobra. Start in a modified push-up position with hands and feet just wider than shoulder width. While keeping your arms and legs straight, walk your feet closer to your hands so that your hips rise up toward the ceiling. From this inverted V position bend your elbows to touch your nose to the ground between your hands. Then, without rising up, touch your chin, followed by your chest to the same spot. Brush the front of your body across this imaginary line drawn between your hands. As your rib cage reaches this line you begin to swing your head in an upward arc; at its apex your arms are straight again, your hips pressed near the floor, your shoulders pulled back and your spine hyperextended. Reverse this movement by slowly lowering first your ribs and then brush all the same body parts across the imaginary line between your hands until you are back in the inverted V starting position.

Bowls of Jell-O, Links of a Chain

By Scott Johnston

For a number of years I coached a junior cross-country ski team made up mostly of middle school–aged kids with the typical mixture of enthusiasm and lassitude. I was amazed at how weak the kids were. Cross-country skiing requires the ability to generate a lot of core tension to transmit the power developed in the arms pushing on the poles through the body via the core into the legs to make the skis glide on the snow. It is a long chain connecting the hand to the foot, and in the case of these kids not only were their arms and legs weak, their cores were more like bowls of Jell-O than links of chain.

I began a several-year process of remaking them athletically. One of the main things was to get them strong enough so that they could even be able to statically hold the body positions in the gym that are necessary in order to make powerful, dynamic movements while gliding on snow. A simple little circuit of core exercises with its lack of reliance on props helped several National Junior champions come out of this rag-tag group with one girl going on to place on the podium at a World Cup cross-country ski race.

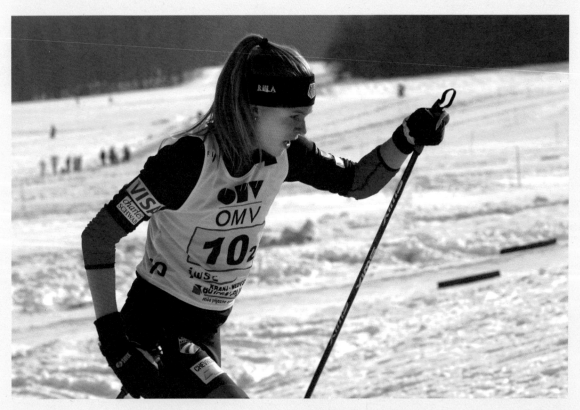

Sadie Bjornsen is one of the junior girls that Scott trained. When she started strength training with Scott at age fourteen she could not do a single pull-up. She did the same core routine outlined in this book. Here she is at fifteen, one of the youngest competitors at the World Junior Championships in Slovenia in 2006. She has since progressed to the World Cup where her best finish to date is a second place in 2011. Until recently top results by the United States at the world level have been rare as the sport has been dominated by the Scandinavians and Russians. *Photo: Scott Johnston*

Hanging Leg Raise (straight and bent arm)

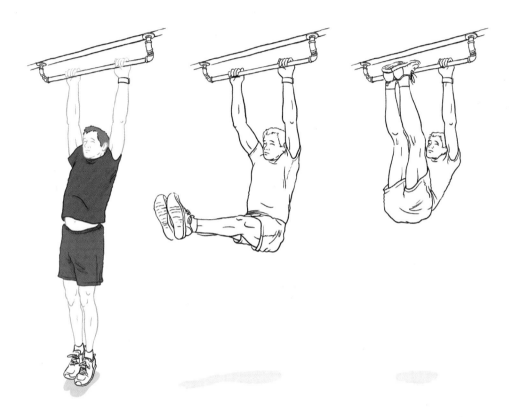

A great climbing-related exercise for steep routes. Hang from a bar with straight or bent arms (locked off at 90 degrees). While keeping your legs straight, raise your feet above the bar and slowly lower. This combines the climbing-specific shoulder position with core control. The more difficult variation is to hang straight armed from the bar and slowly raise your straight legs to touch the bar with your feet. Do not let your body swing from the bar with either variation.

If you cannot do this with straight legs then start by using bent knees in the locked off position and pull your knees to your chest. When you can complete ten reps of this, progress to straight legs by first holding the top leg position for five seconds and then lowering as slowly as you can with straight legs. Once you can do this for four or five reps then you are ready to start using straight legs.

If you have a partner, have them help lift your straight legs slowly up to the top and then, without assistance, slowly lower your straight legs to the bottom without swinging. If you have no partner then kick your legs to the top anyway you can and slowly lower them back to the bottom. Start with bare feet; we have known climbers who can do this with double boots on.

Bridge (w/leg extension for advanced)

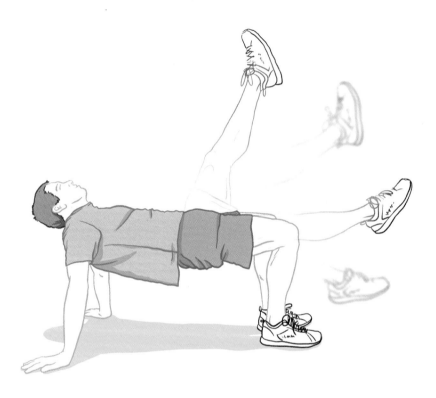

In this exercise you will form a bridge (or coffee table) by getting onto all fours with your belly facing the ceiling. Hands directly below shoulders, feet flat on the floor directly below your knees: All angles should be nice and square. The first step is to push your navel toward the ceiling as far and hard as you can. Hold that position for as long as you can. For many, this will be enough of a challenge. The next stage is to lift one foot off the floor by straightening that knee. Your straight leg will be in line with your torso. Hold this while pushing your navel up. If you can do this without dropping your hips, then you are ready for the last stage: flex the hip of that raised leg so that your toes point to the ceiling. Do this all while keeping your navel pressed high. Hold this end position as long as possible without your core sagging.

Gymnast L-Sit

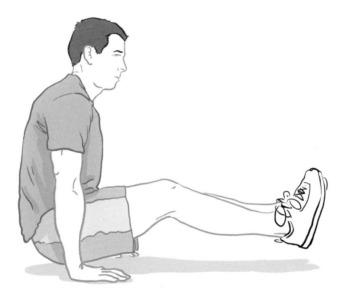

The gymnast L-sit teaches balance, hip flexibility, and tension from the fingers all the way through to the toes. Sit squarely on the floor, toes pointed, knees straight. Place your palms on the floor so that your fingers point toward your toes and the heel of your hand is about even with your crotch. Slowly rock your shoulders forward so that your shoulders come over your hands as your elbows straighten and your shoulders drop slightly. These two actions combined will lift your hips off the floor. Push down hard through your hands and lift your feet while keeping your knees straight. Don't be dismayed if you cannot get your feet off the floor at all, or if you can, it is only for a split second. Keep working at it no matter how short a time you can get your feet up. Eventually you'll be able to hold your feet outstretched for many seconds. Start with bare feet.

Side Plank

Make your body into a rigid plank, but do it while on your side with your shoulders supported by one hand and both feet on the floor. Keep your legs straight and in a straight line from your head, through shoulders and hips, to your feet. Raise the high arm and point the fingers to the ceiling. Slowly rotate about the weighted shoulder so that your high arm (while remaining straight) can come down and touch the floor next to the supporting hand. Raise the arm back to the top position for one repetition. When this is easy for you add a dumbbell in the high hand. It is important to maintain the plank-like straightness (both vertically and horizontally) along your back and legs. Don't sag or stick your butt in the air as you rotate about that shoulder.

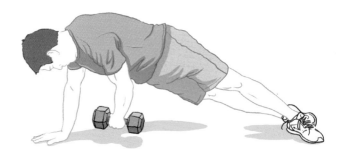

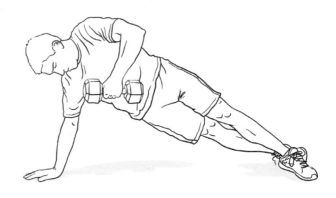

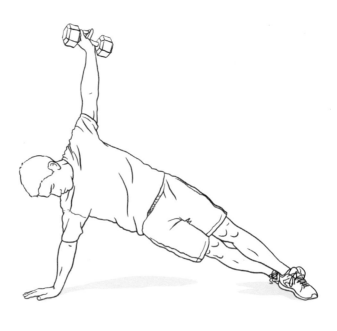

GENERAL STRENGTH TRAINING IN THE TRANSITION PERIOD

It is important to start a program of general strength training as soon as you start your Transition Period. There are two reasons for this that should now be familiar to you:

1. General strength will be an important basis for the more specific training to follow. The sooner you get a strength program underway, the better.

2. You will do the heaviest lifting, literally and figuratively, during the upcoming Base Period, and starting with general strength training now is needed to prepare your body for that.

First, let's review some terms that we presented previously:

- **Rep** is short for repetition. This is one complete movement cycle. For instance, one complete pull-up constitutes one rep.

- A **Set** is a group of reps. Reps in a set are completed continuously.

- **Rest** is the recovery time between sets. The length of period is used to allow at least partial restoration of the nutrients within the muscle cells so that the next set can be completed. In strength training this rest is usually done passively or with stretching.

- A **Circuit** is sequentially completing one set each of a group of different exercises, rather than completing all sets of one exercise before moving on to the next exercise.

Adding a couple of new terms will help as we move on.

- **Frequency** is the number of times each week that the routine is completed.

- **Load** is the amount of resistance used. For the Transition Period use 50–60 percent of your maximum. For the max period, use 85–90 percent of your maximum, or enough to allow only six reps.

Which Exercises to Do and Why?

In this book we recommend several workouts with groups of exercises. While these are the workouts we've used ourselves, there is nothing magical about them. There is solid, principle-based thinking behind the selection of exercises that make up each workout we've outlined here. However, there are other ways of accomplishing the goals of these workouts. We have explained the training principles behind each workout so that you will have the knowledge to be able to modify the workouts and vary or substitute the exercises based on what facilities and equipment are available to you. If you have any doubt, follow the recommended workouts.

The General Strength Routine

Notice that the exercises alternate between upper and lower body and need minimal props, which means that they can be completed almost anywhere. Start with one to two times through the circuit. Every two weeks add another lap through the circuit. Go one time through during the first two weeks, do two circuits during the third and fourth week, and so on up to four circuits in the eighth week. Move from one exercise immediately to the next. Take a three-minute break between circuit laps but try to move from one exercise to another within thirty seconds. Add more challenge whenever you can do more than ten repetitions of any one exercise. Repeat the same or slightly varied routine twice a week and feel free to create your own variations on the exercises. With this variety of exercises and with many of them being body weight, we have specified a recommended number of repetitions for each exercise rather than a more typical blanket prescription of four sets of ten to twelve reps. Do not push to failure. Look for details in the notes accompanying each exercise illustration and description. Don't expect it to be easy.

Turkish Get-Up

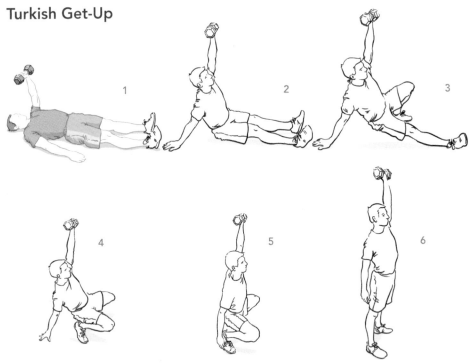

The difficulty is mainly due to shoulder and hip flexibility along with core, not leg, strength. Using a weight that is too light (a small dumbbell) will allow you to cheat the form and lose a lot of the benefit of this exercise. Once you learn the movement and develop the hip and shoulder flexibility, you need to increase the weight. Change dumbbell hands while you are supine. When you can do five reps of each hand, then increase the weight. For advanced users, try using a long barbell.

Split Bench Squat

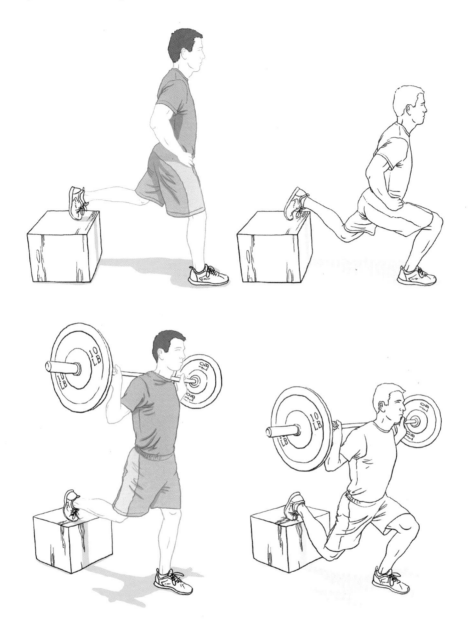

Similar to a lunge, this works the big muscles that propel you uphill and does it on one leg at a time, which requires balance and hip stability. Start by using a split stance with both feet on the floor and body weight only. Pull your hips up over the front leg, trying to use the back leg only for balance. Progress first by raising the rear leg on to a bench or even an exercise ball. Once balance is established add resistance via anything from a backpack or weight vest (easiest) to a barbell, which will be a big balance challenge. When you can do ten reps, start adding the variations to increase the challenge.

Push-Up

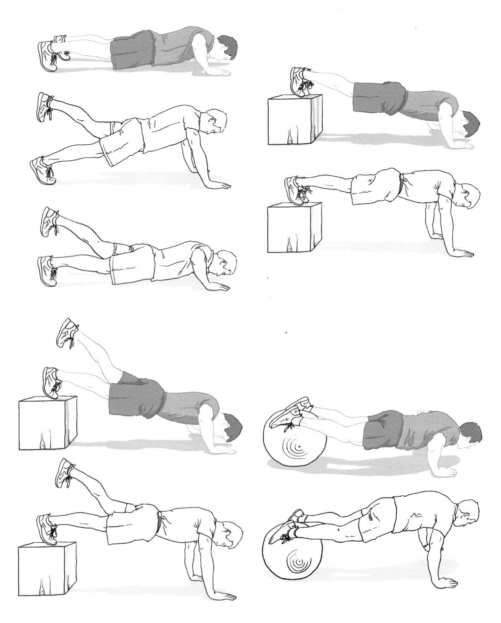

Great whole-body exercise that connects hands to feet. When you can execute ten reps progress to raising one foot off the ground while maintaining strict push-up form. When an elevated single foot gets easy, add a weight vest or place an exercise ball under your feet.

Box Step-Ups

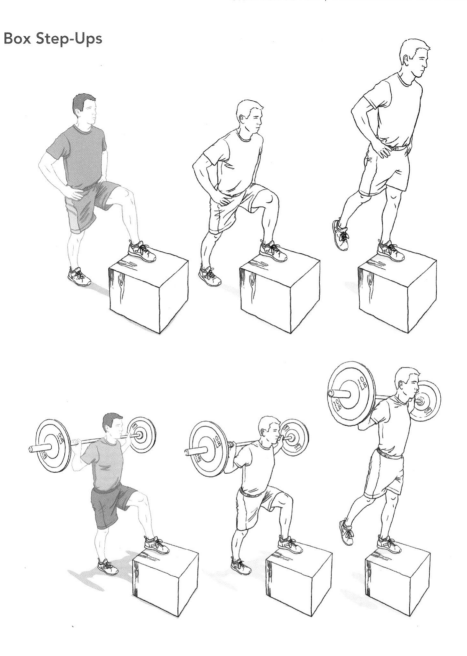

This is another exercise that effectively targets crucial uphill propulsion muscles. The higher the box, the harder it will be. The lifting of the foot onto the box is part of the exercise. Imagine punching steps up a steep snow slope. You know that feeling of stepping up two feet (0.6 meters) high and then standing up on that foot while it sinks as the snow compresses (but hopefully does not fully collapse). Now you get the feeling of what we are training here. This is mind-numbing work, but an essential strength for anyone spending serious time in the mountains. Step up and fully balance on the loaded leg before stepping back down. Repeat. When you can do ten reps increase either or both height (up to almost-crotch high) or weight. Use a pack, or for a real challenge use a barbell resting on your shoulders.

Pull-Ups

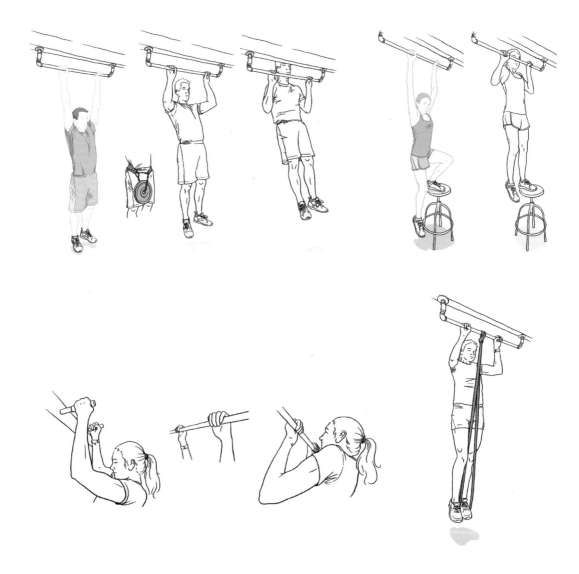

From the base of strength this exercise provides, you can come up with just about any sort of variation and progression you can dream of. Once you can do fifteen normal pull-up reps you are ready to mix it up a bit. You can do this either by doing one of the variations we list below or progressing the strength via the method laid out in the Max Strength section. Be aware that a high volume (many dozens in a day) of normal pull-ups from a bar can increase the likelihood of elbow tendonitis since the fixed handgrip forces your elbow into a restricted range of motion. Rather than go for volume with these, pick the one you see as building a more climbing-specific strength base. Here a few we have used over the years.

- Add weight to whatever variation you can do fifteen reps of.

- **Offset**—one hand higher than the other.

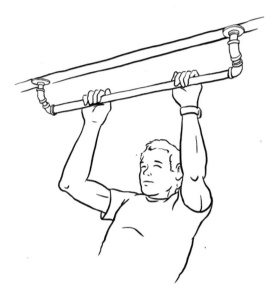

- **Lock off 90s to 120s**—Pull up, hold the full lock off for five seconds with your chin as far over the bar as possible, lower to 90 degrees, hold for five seconds, lower to 120 degrees, hold for five seconds. Vary the exact positions so you build lock-off strength in any arm position.

- **Frenchies**—This is an advanced pull-up technique that combines the maximum strength gains that come from isometric holds while taxing the muscular endurance of your fast twitch fibers. It's a great addition to the experienced climbers strength-training repertoire. Begin in the normal pull-up position with palms facing away. Pull up to the top position with chin above the bar. Hold that position for five seconds. Drop back to the bottom hanging start position and immediately pull back to the chin above bar position then immediately lower to the midpoint spot where your elbows are bent 90 degrees. Hold this position for five seconds and then lower to the bottom again. Once again pull all the way to the top, but this time lower to the point where your elbows are bent 120 degrees and hold for five seconds. This completes one full repetition. Weaker climbers should then take a break and drop off the bar and rest for three to five minutes before doing another repetition. Continue with that method until you can do five full repetitions. Stronger climbers can immediately begin the next repetition with no rest. If you are unable to complete three repetitions without stopping you make faster progress by taking a three to five minute rest break and doing more repetitions.

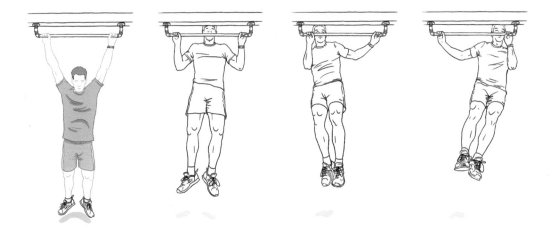

- **Typewriter**—with a wide grip, pull up on the right, traverse your chin along the bar, and lower on left. Make circles going in both directions.

- **Muscle-ups**—start with a pull-up then continue upward by pressing as in a mantel.

- **Deep pull-ups using ice tools**—lock off with your hand as far below your chin as you can. Really strong climbers can bring their hands down close to their waists.

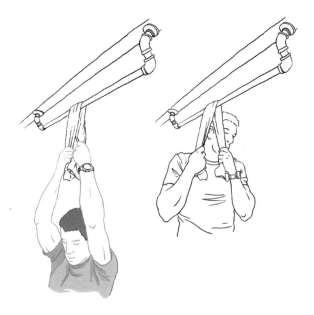

- **Towel pull-ups**—hang a towel over the bar and pull up while gripping each end of the towel.

Let your imagination take over. The possibilities are many.

Squat (with a Progression)

The squat is known as the king of lower-body exercises but needs to be learned and executed carefully. We prefer to start with a front squat and holding a light bar on the tops of your arms (1). Feet toed out a little and shoulder width. Do not let the bar roll forward. If it rolls you are leaning too far forward at the hips. Maintaining a neutral lumbar spine is essential in order to protect your back. A mirror or a knowledgeable partner will be helpful. Practice holding this neutral spine position through the full range of motion with light weight before adding any significant resistance. This engages almost the full core musculature and adds stability so your hips and legs can apply the lifting force. Many people are too stiff in their hips and legs to do this exercise properly. You can add a small lift under your heels to help tilt you forward. With time your flexibility will improve.

When competent you can progress to a conventional front squat holding the barbell on the front of your shoulders with the grip shown (2).

Once you are feeling solid with your technique you can progress to an overhead squat (3). For this, hold barbell with a wide grip. You will not be limited by leg strength in this exercise but by core and shoulder strength. In all forms progress to ten reps before adding more weight.

The back squat is the common form and allows the heaviest weight to be lifted, but we recommend mastering the above methods as a progression to heavy back squats as the potential for injury is greatest while doing heavy back squats.

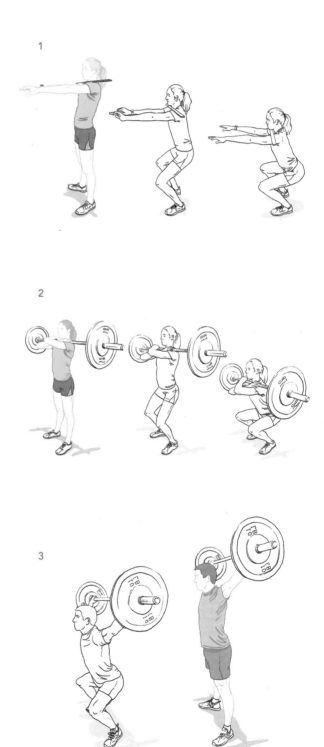

Dips

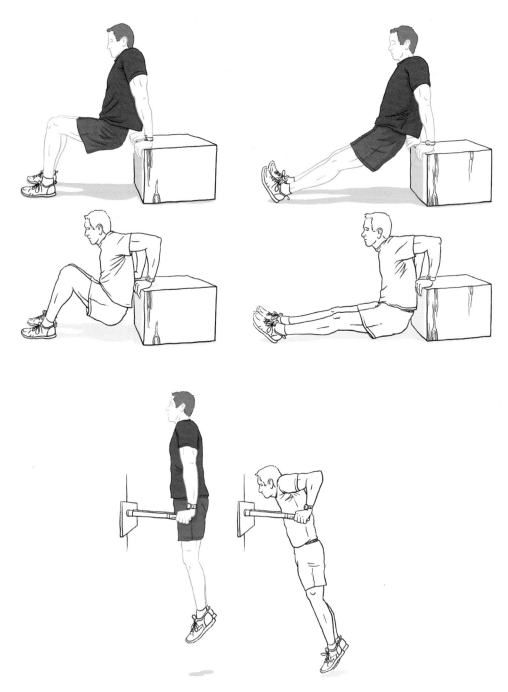

Great for general shoulder health and will help with those pesky mantels. Unless you have a shoulder injury, use a full range of shoulder motion: Drop so far down that you feel a good stretch in your pectoral (chest) muscles. You may need assistance on this one but still use full range of motion. When you can do ten reps, add more resistance.

Hanging Leg Raise (Progressing to Ice Tools)

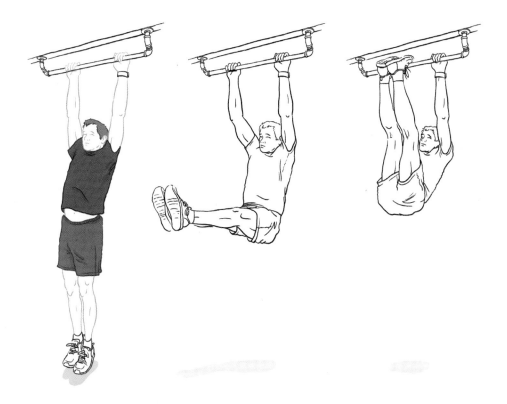

Hanging leg raises can be done with either straight arms or bent (as in a lock-off position). The main thing to remember is: Do not swing. You may need to start with bent knees and pull them to your chest before slowly lowering them. You may only be able to do one to two reps at first. This is a dramatic test of core strength. Work toward a straight leg raise and lower under complete control. Taking your shoes off for this will really help to start out. When you can do ten good reps with straight legs, add weight to your feet in the form of shoes and later boots. Can be progressed to a front lever by the most advanced.

Wall-Facing Squats

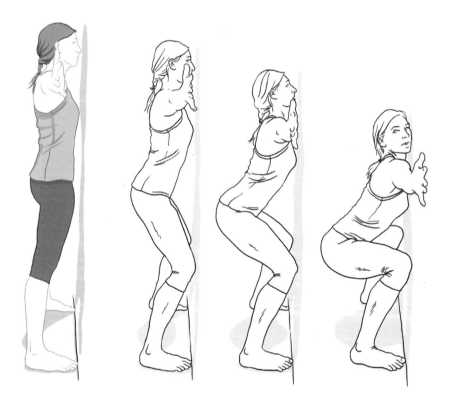

Start by facing the wall with chest and toes almost touching the wall, feet slightly wider than shoulder width. Squat down to a full squat depth, all the time keep upper chest in contact with the wall. Most people can't do this with their toes touching the wall the first time; find the point where you can have your toes as close as possible, but still do the full range of motion. This exercise takes balance and core strength; it is harder than it seems like it should be, but has incredible application to climbing. Start with three sets of five reps. Later you can add weight in the form of a weight vest for an extra challenge.

Isometric Hangs from Ice Tools

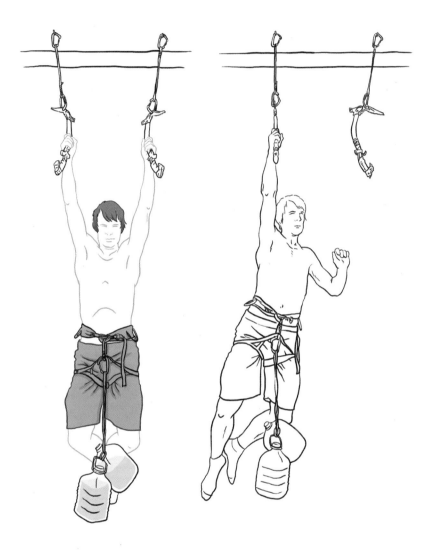

This works on grip strength specifically used with leashless tools. Just as weak crimp strength can limit your confidence in leading hard rock, having weak grip strength can undermine your leading ability on ice. Hang by one hand until grip failure. Then switch to the other (these two hangs constitute one set). You need to have a full recovery, so rest three to five minutes before the next set. When you can hang for more than thirty seconds, then add weight, usually two-and-a-half to five pounds of additional weight is enough. Once you master this you can make it considerably harder by gripping only the shaft of the tool without letting your hand weight the pommel.

Incline (horizontal) Pull-Up Progression

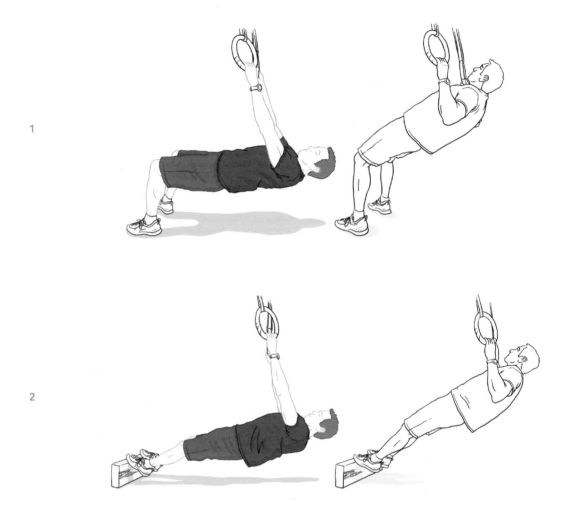

This is another good semi-climbing-specific exercise that combines core strength into a basic pulling motion. Using a squat rack, rings, or any bar that is between three and four feet off the ground, lie under the bar and grasp it in overhand grip or, using a higher bar, hook ice tools over the bar and grab your tools. Extend your legs with heels on the ground and pull your chest to the bar while maintaining your body in a straight line from your head to your feet. If you cannot do five perfect reps like this, then bend your knees till you can do five good reps while maintaining a straight line from head to knees (1). You can progress this exercise by elevating your feet (2), using one foot or one arm (3), placing your feet on an exercise ball (4), pulling with one arm, while twisting and reaching upward as high as possible with the other, pulling with one arm while gripping an ice ax or (harder) a towel and keeping the twisting/reaching component, and pulling with one arm while holding a weight in the opposite hand and still twisting and reaching as high as you can (5). Great crossover exercise for steep, dry-tooling routes.

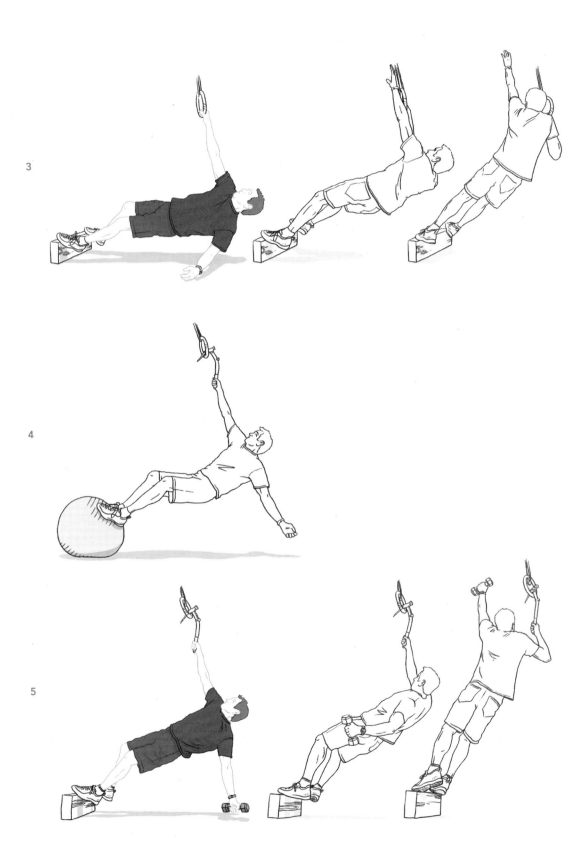

3

4

5

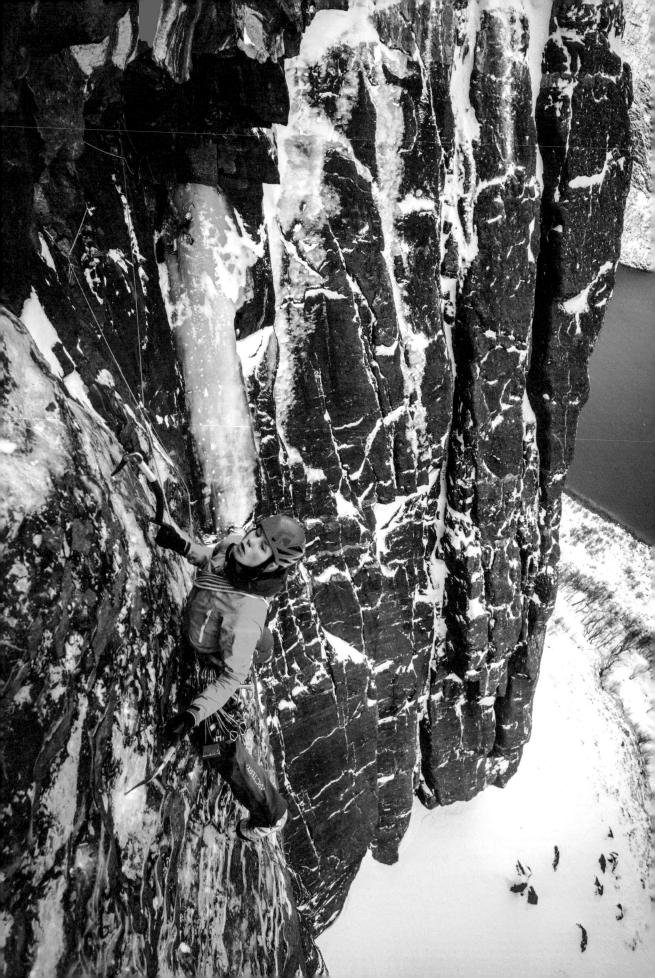

Chapter 8

Planning Your Base Period Training

"Training in rock and ice techniques must be accompanied by training for general fitness. The climber will need considerable stamina as well as being well acclimatized. He will be helped by long-distance training runs, especially cross-country, together with long sessions on crags—six to eight hours at a stretch."

– GASTON RÉBUFFAT, pioneering French alpinist and writer,
from *The Mont Blanc Massif: The Hundred Finest Routes*

THE IMPORTANCE OF THE BASE

The training that will help you to feel the strongest and most energized when you set off from high camp is a solid, structured Base Period. We've continually emphasized the necessity of building a solid endurance foundation before adding a high volume of specific training. Recall that the purpose of this Base Period is to toughen you up, to improve your fatigue resistance so that you can handle more hard climbing and hard climbing–specific training in the future. For most climbers this means many hours of basic conditioning as a supplement to regular climbing. And, as we have already emphasized: During

Opposite: Ines Papert makes the first ascent of Finnmannen (m9+, WI7, 400m) on Norway's Senja Island. *Photo: Thomas Senf*

Training Is Teamwork

By Roger Schaeli

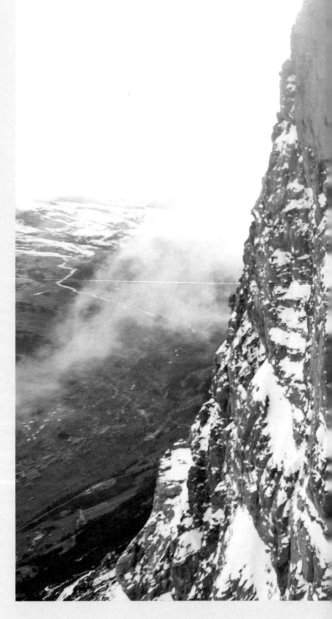

As a professional climber, training is an important part of my everyday life. Many different variables need to come together to realize my best performance on the big day—whether I am trying a hard sport climbing route or I'm on an expedition.

I start each day by going for an hour-long run and, depending on the training phase, my coach, Mäx Grossmann, adds maximum or endurance strength training. Depending on the current climbing project we then add either cardiovascular endurance or interval training. My plan is very strict and intense. But if I feel tired, I adjust the training schedule accordingly. Twice a year, after big projects, I take a recovery vacation of ten to fourteen days. As soon as I decide on my climbing projects for the coming year, I fix my training plan. If I'm training for a hard sport climbing route, my main focus is on going climbing. If I plan to go on an expedition I shift my focus to overall fitness and lung capacity with running and jumping. The fitter I am before an expedition, the less I get sick.

Resting is also a big part of training. My manager, Nik Ammann, has helped me to organize my time better in order to have time for my friends, my girlfriend, and myself. It's important to manage my time well so I get enough rest.

Another crucial part of my training is nutrition. Here again I consult an expert. I love to eat and to eat well. Giving up certain foods for my projects is not at all easy for me; I love pizza.

All the physical training in the world is useless if I am not able to apply it to the mountains. As a professional athlete I cannot ignore the importance of mental training. Mental training incorporates several elements: If I have trained my body well, my mental strength is improved. That's the first thing. Additionally, I practice progressive muscle relaxation daily. The third pillar of my mental training is my mental coach, Romana Feldmann. Every six weeks we meet and discuss my upcoming projects. We go through several scenarios like what happens if I fail, or we talk about conflicts, doubts, and fears. Fear can limit my physical performance. It's hard to know whether the mental or the physical preparation is more important since they go hand-in-hand.

The administrative part of being a professional climber is more challenging than training for me. We all have down days in our jobs. Then I recall how privileged I am to climb professionally. The down days are most common at the beginning of a training season when my routine is not clearly defined and I haven't gained momentum toward a goal. If I have a project, I am very motivated.

I enjoy climbing-training most of all. But since I'm so incredibly happy in the mountains, I also enjoy training for my expeditions. These are unforgettable experiences that shape me deeply. Every hour of training is worth it.

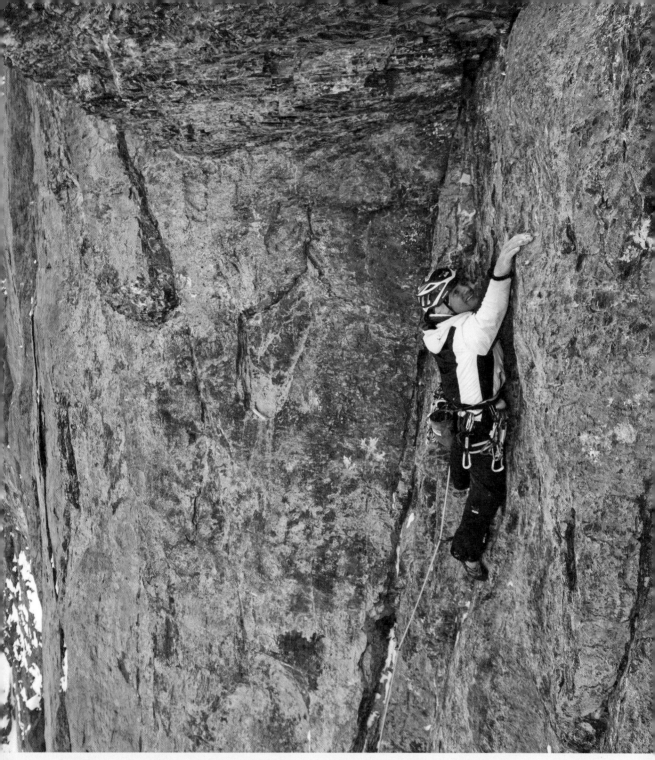

Roger Schaeli during the first free ascent of the Harlin Direct route (M8-, 5.11+) on the 5,900-foot (1,798m) high north face of the Eiger (13,024', 3,970m). *Photo: Günther Göberl*

Born in 1979, Swiss climber Roger Schaeli has ascended the Eiger's North Face thirty-five times by many different routes. Roger is adept on difficult rock as well as hard ice routes and he aspires to convey his utmost respect for the deeds of the pioneers of alpinism.

much of this period you will be too tired to climb your best and should not expect to. This gets back to the ideas Mark Twight discusses in his TINSTAAFL essay. There is no shortcut to doing this right.

Those who have many years of base training under their belts will need a higher volume of specific training to see improvement. Steve, with twenty years of accumulated base from climbing, guiding, and organized training, embarked on his program for Makalu in 2008, 2009, and 2011 with the goal of maximizing his specific training. This is what he and other top climbers need to put them in the best possible position on game day.

FITTING STRENGTH TRAINING INTO YOUR BASE PERIOD PLAN

In order to lay out a plan for yourself it will help if you understand what you will be doing for strength training as well as how and when you'll do it. In this next section we'll give you the details so you can integrate a focused approach to your strength program.

The shift from the Transition Period to the Base Period brings with it a shift of focus from general strength training to Max Strength.

MAX STRENGTH PERIOD

Minute for minute, these are among the most important workouts of the year because they give you a boost in strength that pays off in many ways. Endeavor to arrive rested and excited for Max Strength sessions. Warm up well and give a good effort, especially with one-legged exercises like box step-ups, which will pay huge dividends in how your legs will feel churning uphill for hour after hour.

As a quick reminder: This is the stage where we increase the available pool of muscle fibers for the brain to choose from. Increasing Max Strength lays the groundwork for the conversion to Muscular Endurance. Following these prescriptions will produce large gains in strength, with no gains in body weight (often you will lose weight due to the resulting boost to your metabolism).

Pick two to four exercises from the General Strength Routine you were doing during the Transition Period to use for your Max Strength workouts. These should be ones that you feel need the most improvement or will be most useful in your climbing. As an example, for a climber aspiring to climb a long technical alpine route it could be wise to choose box step-ups, a pull-up variation (like Frenchies or typewriters), overhead squat, and one-arm isometric ice ax hangs.

Many variations of Max Strength training have been developed. Most rely on the basic principles outlined here. If you have a long history of strength training, and have stagnated in your strength gains, you may find it useful to explore some of the more esoteric methods. The best book we know of for additional very specific methods that have been well tested by athletes is *Special Strength Training: A Manual for Coaches*, by Yuri and Natalia Verkhoshansky. With careful reading and some imagination you can apply techniques that have produced multiple Olympic and World Champions. Otherwise you'll not go wrong following our simple prescriptions here.

The Max Strength workouts follow these principles:

- Use a load that would allow you to do no more than five reps. (Or use 85–90 percent of your one repetition max.)

- Use sets of one up to a maximum of four repetitions.

- Use four to six sets of each exercise per session.

- Allow three to five minutes of rest between sets.

- Do not go to muscular failure on any set. That will cause you to gain muscle mass.

- Do this twice a week.

- For isometrics like single arm hangs use the following method: Attain maximum muscle tension and hold that for six to eight seconds. Repeat this three to five times (reps) with one to two minutes between each rep. This constitutes one set. Repeat for four to six sets with five minutes rest between sets. By alternating arms you can be resting one while completing a set with the other.

Sample Max Strength Circuit Workout

	Reps	Rest between sets	Sets
Frenchies	4	3–5 min	4–6
Box step-ups	4	3–5 min	4–6
One-armed isometric ice-ax hangs	4 hangs, to near failure	3–5 min	4–6
Overhead squat	4	3–5 min	4–6

Special Strength Program Used for Pull-Ups

Who doesn't want to be able to do more pull-ups? Even if just as a party trick? As previously mentioned, pull-ups are the king of the upper-body exercises. While climbers can debate the applicability of pull-ups to hard climbing, there is no doubt that they're great for general strength training. They involve almost all of the body's muscle groups from the waist up.

The program to follow for making gains in pull-ups is simple and well tested. It has been used by many people who were either weak in pull-up strength or had reached a plateau in strength or endurance. All of them made dramatic improvements after following this plan for eight weeks. And they all did this without increasing their body weight. It can be adapted to movements other than pull-ups with a bit of creativity. If, for instance, you are trying to break through a strength plateau with a particular specific climbing move, model that move as well as possible, use supplemental resistance, and follow the same schedule.

It works and it is always fun to see fast progress. This routine has turned fourteen-year-old girls with noodles for arms into pull-up machines.

The principles of this special pull-up routine should be familiar to you since they follow the standard Max Strength prescriptions:

- Do this workout twice a week.

- Take at least three minutes' rest between sets.

- Lower slowly for five seconds on the last rep of each set.

- Before starting, do a ten-minute warm-up for your pulling muscles; use something like an assisted pull-up machine or a rowing machine.

- Do this religiously for eight weeks!

Special Max Strength Plan

Week	Workout	Sets	Reps	Rest
1	1	4	1	3 min
	2	4	1	3 min
2	1	1	2	3 min
	2	3	1	3 min
3	1	2	2	3 min
	2	2	1	3 min
4	1	3	2	3 min
	2	1	1	3 min
5	1	4	2	3 min
	2	4	2	3 min
6	1	1	3	3 min
	2	3	2	3 min
7	1	3	2	3 min
	2	2	2	3 min
8	1	3	3	3 min
	2	1	2	3 min

This seems so simple—how can it work? The catch is that you need to constantly adjust the load by adding weight (usually wearing a weight belt) to the point that you can only do the required number of reps. If the workout calls for three sets of two reps, you need to hang enough weight off yourself so that you can only do two reps.

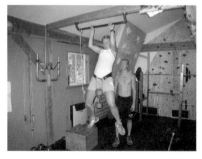

Before the start of a concentrated Max Strength pull-up program, Sadie Bjornsen could not do any pull-ups. Here she is using thirty-five pounds of added weight.
Photo: Scott Johnston collection

By doing this workout in a semi-circuit fashion you can move from one exercise to the next after a short break of thirty seconds to a minute. Alternating muscle groups like this should allow you three to five minutes before repeating the same exercise while also compressing the time needed to complete the workout. The correct amount of recovery time between exercises is important for getting the full benefits of Max Strength. Take as much rest as you feel you need to give your best effort on each set. With too little rest between sets of the same exercise you risk insufficient recovery and hence the loss of the maximal muscle fiber recruitment aspect that is necessary to this type of training. While our example exercises are simple, they work the major climbing muscles and will effectively prepare you for the conversion to Muscular Endurance phase, which comes next.

The One Rep Maximum—1RM

Knowing and constantly adjusting your load so that it reflects your newly gained strength is an important part of making strength gains. Some exercises lend themselves easily to finding your absolute maximum lift for one repetition. Others require some guesswork. There is also some risk of injury with young or poorly strength-trained individuals in lifting heavy weights to determine maximal strength. A simple way to determine your load for Max Strength training is to use a load that allows you to complete between three and five reps. This corresponds well to about 85 percent (five reps) and 90 percent (three reps) of your One Rep Max or 1RM.

Max Strength Outside

If you don't fancy the whole gym thing, that's OK. There are good ways for you to do most of the same training of the legs and lower body without lifting a barbell. This method will increase the muscle-fiber pool we talked about and improve the neural connections for the very specific movement of climbing a steep slope.

Improve Your Strength, Improve Your Endurance

Years ago a friend approached Scott with a dilemma: He'd been religiously training pull-ups for a year but had stagnated at a max of eighteen reps. He had tried many combinations of sets and reps in a futile attempt to break through this limit. When Scott suggested the routine outlined to the left, the friend was skeptical. How could doing fewer pull-ups help him do more? He seemed to be lacking endurance so in his mind he needed to increase the volume of pull-ups, not decrease it.

But he was willing to put his doubts aside and give this approach a concerted try. At no time during the eight-week program did the friend do any other pull-up training of any sort: no more days of cranking off as many sets of as many reps as he could manage. No more days of 400 to 500 pull-ups and the potential attendant elbow issues. By the end of eight weeks the friend had improved his max pull-up strength to his body weight plus seventy-five pounds. The very first workout in which he attempted to better his previous record of eighteen pull-ups he shot past his old record and sailed right up to thirty pull-ups. He was a convert, and you will be too. This is a great example of how improving strength improved endurance.

Hill Sprint Training

To execute this workout outdoors, first you need to find a steep hill with decent footing so you are not dodging roots and rocks and can sprint flat-out. The steeper, the better for our purposes. It should be at least 10 percent or a one-in-ten slope with 20–50 percent (two- to five-in-ten slope) being even better. A steep stadium can provide the needed steepness. If your movements are slow and cautious due to poor footing, you will not get the desired effect. The steep hill allows those who can't run fast to impose very high loads on their legs and hips without the higher impact of fast, flat running. This workout is incredibly simple and effective. It can also be combined with one gym Max Strength box step-up workout each week.

The principles of Hill Sprint Training for strength are as follows:

- Do this twice each week if this is your only strength training; once a week if combining with a gym strength workout.

- This is not meant to train endurance directly.

- Sprint at your maximum speed up this hill for eight to ten seconds at the most.

- Take a five-minute rest between sets.

- Speed of movement and explosiveness in the one-legged push are what give this the workout its desired effect.

- Walk back down and repeat six to eight times (six to eight reps up the hill) starting a new sprint every two minutes.

- As you build strength you'll be able to add sets.

- Stop the set when you feel your power drop.

- If you extend the length of the sprint beyond ten seconds, you will be training anaerobic endurance rather than maximum strength. You will also not be able to complete as many repetitions and hence the training effect will be less.

- The training effect occurs due to the number of reps, not the length of the individual reps, so keep them short (under ten seconds) and do more repetitions and sets.

To be clear: This workout would normally fall under the category of power training as opposed to Max Strength. Recall that power is a function of strength per time. It turns out that if you train for maximum power, you'll do a decent job of increasing maximum strength at the same time. Strength coaches will quibble over the efficacy of using this hill sprint workout in lieu of a more traditional Max program in a gym with 90 percent of 1RM. They'd

A Typical Progression for Hill Sprints

Week #	Sets	Reps	Duration	Rest per rep	Rest per set	Times per week
1–2	3	4	8 sec	2 min	5 min	2x
3–4	2	6	8 sec	2 min	5 min	2x
5–6	2	7	8 sec	2 min	5 min	2x
7–8	3	5	8 sec	2 min	5 min	2x
9–10	3	6	8 sec	2 min	5 min	1x
11–12	3	7	8 sec	2 min	5 min	1x

be correct of course, but this simple workout can have dramatic benefits in leg strength and its more sport-specific adjunct of leg power for those without gym facilities.

We have noticed that athletes who are unaccustomed to such high power training have difficulty even getting tired in the early weeks of doing this workout. That is because they move slowly due to their inability to engage enough of the fast twitch fibers needed to produce truly powerful movements. For most people it will take a few weeks before your nervous system begins to adapt to the point where you will get the full training effect of this regimen. Before that you'll likely be restricted to mainly using ST fibers, which don't get tired in eight to ten seconds. If you feel this workout in your breathing but not in your legs, don't be dismayed. In this case, this work will have the biggest benefits for you. Stick with it for a few weeks and see your leg power improve dramatically.

Even for top-level climbers, hill sprints are a simple, effective, specific, and best of all, highly portable. After the initial Max Strength Period we often advise people to do this workout one time each fourteen days for maintenance.

Don't have a steep, or even any, hill, or want some variations? Try dragging a tire. Steve used this very effectively during several of his recent training cycles. Another way to accomplish a similar increase in leg power that can be fun is to engage a few friends to push a car back and forth in a parking lot. You push one way and your friend pushes it back. Push on the front and rear bumpers so that you can really lean into it and get your big leg muscles involved. Take a few minutes of rest between short pushes of six to ten seconds and you'll see amazing results in leg strength. Some gyms may have steel sleds into which you can stack weight and you can then push the sled up and down a paved alley or across a grass sports field.

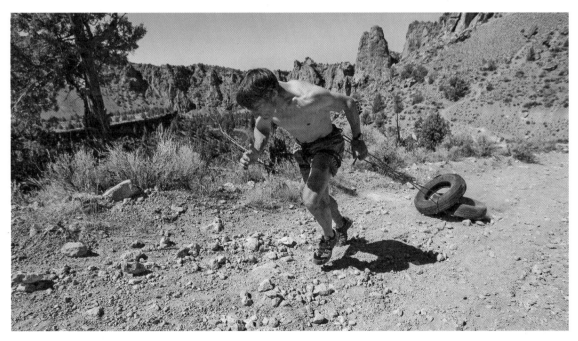

Steve dragging tires on the Burma Road at Smith Rocks in Oregon. This type of exercise can be used for both the short intense Max Strength and power training as laid out in the Hill Sprint description. But it also works as a Muscular Endurance workout for those who are limited in the amount of vertical terrain they have available to train on. Several, minute repeats of dragging tires on a less steep hill can be a very effective way to build muscular endurance. It is similar to the lower intensity but longer water jug carry repeats that we advocate in the Muscular Endurance section. *Photo: Ben Moon*

Upper-Body Power

You can execute a similar workout for your upper body by utilizing a simple overhanging ladder or the underside of a stairwell with open treads and doing a two-handed lunge from rung to rung going up and then back down again. This is very similar to a very high intensity campus board power workout using a two-handed dyno move from rung to rung. This campus workout is very demanding on finger strength. The ladder we built uses round rungs made from three-quarter-inch gas pipe so the stress is taken off the finger joints and allows you to overload the big muscles in the back and shoulders. As you get more powerful you can start skipping rungs on the way up and down. You can even use a weight vest.

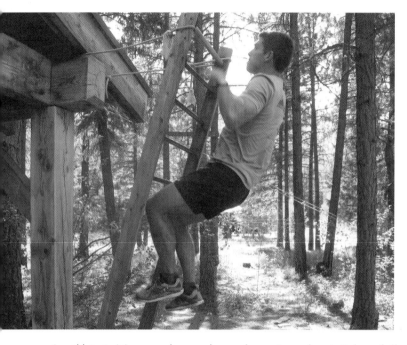

An athlete training on a cheap and simple homemade ladder. Let the ladder overhang by 10 degrees so that its weight will hold it in place. This one is portable and can be moved to various workout locations. Notice that his hands are off the pipe rung as he dynos up and then back down the ladder. This explosive upper body training is a very effective method of building powerful shoulders and arms that will provide a tremendous base for more climbing-specific muscular endurance work. After a couple of years this athlete has progressed to being able to skip rungs while wearing a 60-pound weight vest. Unweighted, he can jump from the bottom to the top rung and back again for eight repetitions.
Photo: Austin Siadak

Try to do at least five to six consecutive, well-executed, and controlled dynos in each set. Take a full recovery rest of three minutes between sets and repeat three to five times.

Maintaining Your Max Strength Gains

Experience in many sports shows eight weeks to be an effective length for the Max Strength Period. Longer and you tend to plateau. Shorter and you probably won't see the biggest gains unless you are very experienced at Max Strength training, in which case you'll see smaller gains and see them quicker. After this period you can maintain most if not all the gains you made for many more weeks with a simple and infrequent nudge to the neuromuscular system. You do not need to do a full workout to get the effect, so it won't leave you tired for climbing.

This can be as simple as doing a couple of sets of max ice tool hangs in a lock-off position or a car push once every ten days or so. This means that during a road trip you should take advantage of rainy days to spend fifteen minutes to crank off some weighted pull-ups or push your car around the laundromat parking lot. You can also use a shortened Max Strength workout as a warm-up for the Muscular Endurance workout, which we will describe in the next section.

CONVERSION TO MUSCULAR ENDURANCE PERIOD

After a good Max Strength phase you are ready to convert all the raw strength you have built over the past months into a more climbing-specific quality. In alpine climbing, endurance is one of the two main performance limiters, the other being technical skill. You know that burn you get in your legs when post-holing up the summit snowfield? We have a remedy for that.

Remember from the discussion about the physiology of endurance training that all training is muscle-fiber specific. Only those fibers that your brain recruits get trained. You select which fibers get trained by virtue of the intensity you train at. In the interest of full disclosure this is not 100 percent technically accurate since there is a bit of training effect occurring in the nonworking fibers if they become glycogen depleted during a workout.

The operative word in Muscular Endurance training is *endurance*. You want to improve the endurance of the main muscle groups used in climbing.

The Goal of Muscular Endurance Training

The goal of this phase is to improve the percentage of your maximum muscle power you can sustain for a longer and longer time. As you may recall from chapter 3 this is best done on top of a high strength base because the pool of recruitable muscle motor units will be larger than in a poorly strength-trained muscle. The theory goes that this bigger pool of fibers allows the brain to cycle fresh fibers into action as replacements for tired fibers, and therefore maintain that higher power output for longer. Hence, the bigger that neuromuscular fiber pool is, the more muscular endurance you have. A big aerobic base provides the metabolic support for operating at high percentages of your maximum muscle power for long durations. Here you can see the inextricably interlinked neuro-muscular and metabolic systems as they work together to contribute to maximal sport performance. We've been training these systems somewhat separately for efficacy, but in the real world of climbing they are partners in determining the physical limitations to your performance.

Muscular Endurance for the Legs

We'll start by explaining a plan for the legs since your legs are the main propulsion you have in the mountains—they include a large muscle mass and therefore need special attention. Then we'll address some strategies to help increase muscular endurance in your upper body.

There are many possible ways to accomplish improvements in Muscular Endurance. You can do it training in a gym with a demanding circuit-style workout much like the popular CrossFit style of training. Or you can lug a pack full of water jugs up a steep hill—which is our preferred method because of its direct transfer to alpine climbing. You can accomplish some of what we are trying to do by just carrying a heavy pack on the approaches to alpine climbs. All you have to do is graciously offer to your partner that you carry the lion's share of the gear. This is a bit of a random method and will not allow you to control the progressive loading and recovery that will maximize the benefits of this type of training, but it's better than nothing.

The Water Jug Carries

As simple as this workout is, it is amazingly effective if you have the right terrain for it. Water jug carries are designed to improve your muscle fiber recruitment scheme and keep those motor units cycling in and out of the pool of useable fibers during a state of high fatigue. By picking a steep and lengthy hill and ascending it with a weighted pack you can simulate, in a muscularly specific way, ascending moderate to steep alpine terrain. Your muscles won't know whether you are climbing a set of fire stairs in a high-rise or busting up that last snowfield to the top of the Cassin Ridge.

The advantage of carrying water as opposed to some other weight is that you can pour it out at the top of the hill climb and make a fast descent without trashing your knees. If you are doing multiple laps, try to find a water source at the base of your hill that allows you to refill. If you're lacking a handy stream, you can carry rocks and dump them out at the top, just bring extra padding for your back.

For the best training effect this workout should be done wearing boots similar to what you'll wear on your climb, not running shoes. Once you feel the difference between doing the uphill water carry in boots versus running shoes you will understand why we recommend boots.

Don't have any hills? Be creative—find a big stadium and use the stairs. Make friends with the building superintendent in a skyscraper. Andy Hampsten, two-time winner of cycling's Tour of Switzerland, and multiple-time winner of King of the Mountain in both the Giro d'Italia and Tour de France, both of which demand incredible muscular endurance on the mountain passes, grew up and trained for years in

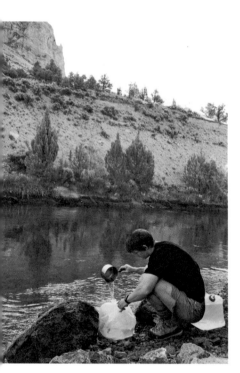

Steve House fills water jugs at the Crooked River, Smith Rock State Park, Oregon. Control the progression by gradually increasing the amount of water you carry. One gallon of water weighs eight pounds. *Photo: Ben Moon*

pancake-flat North Dakota. He once told Scott that he trained for hills while in North Dakota by doing laps on the interstate overpass ramps.

Here are a few things to understand before heading out to crank off some hot laps.

Intensity

How do you regulate the intensity? That's where our trusty nose breathing comes in again. You need to go at the top of your conversational pace.

While nose breathing is not a perfect physiological marker, it will help you keep the intensity in check. Your goal with this technique is a feeling of distinct fatigue in your legs even at relatively low heart rates. If you are able to hike fast enough to get short of breath, you need to add more weight or pick a steeper hill.

As your muscular endurance improves, say after six weeks, you can push the pace up to the point of breakaway breathing during occasional workouts. This is very demanding work and you'll need to have built a good base or these workouts will make you weaker, not stronger. By then you will be able to maintain that slow burn in your legs for many minutes at a time.

Steepness

To make this training most effective, the hill needs to be steep. The steeper, the better. You can get a training effect on a steeply graded trail, but you'll need a much heavier pack and you'll get much more specific training by seeking out steeps like a scree field or the fall line on a black diamond ski slope.

Length of the Climb

Ideally you will have access to a big/steep hill of at least 1,000 vertical feet (305 meters). If you don't have such a big hill to train on, you'll have to do more laps. As with steepness, longer is better, but you have to use what's available.

How Much Vertical?

How much total vertical will you climb on the route you're training for? As with all training, it depends on your fitness and your goals. You'd like to end this training cycle being able to cover at least the amount of vertical of your biggest potential day on your goal climb carrying a pack that is at least as heavy as you need on the real deal. As a guideline you should try to start this progression by climbing about

50 percent of your goal day's vertical with 0 to 50 percent of the weight you'll carry on that climb.

How Much Weight Should You Carry?

This depends on steepness as well as your fitness. You need to load up that backpack with water and go find out. If you've got well-conditioned legs, you'll need 20–25 percent of body weight to get that heavy-legs-while-going-easy feeling. If the most uphill hiking you do is to climb upstairs to your bedroom, then you may feel your legs as the limiter when using 10 percent of your body weight. **The point is to have your rate of climb be limited by your legs, not by your breathing.**

Hint: A gallon of water weighs eight pounds; one quart weighs two pounds.

An Option for the Vertically Impaired

So, you're in North Dakota and the highest thing within 150 miles is a hay barn. It can be very effective to do this type of weighted workout using only a twelve-inch box to step up and down off of. The boredom factor will become extreme, so you may want to arrange a source of entertainment, but it's easy to control the intensity and overall quantity of the training.

Muscular Endurance for the Upper Body

As with your legs, there are myriad ways to develop muscular endurance in the upper body. Imagination and access to some equipment will be the only limitations to what you devise. We are going to lay out several options that we have found useful, and then you can pick what seems to fit your situation best. Don't be afraid to try variations and mix these modalities for a little change of pace.

Note: Adding in a quick Max Strength session every ten to fourteen days will help you maintain strength, but more importantly we find that the sessions act as a very good recovery workout from these strenuous Muscular Endurance workouts.

Here's our list of options for the upper body:

Long Alpine/Ice Climbs

If you have easy access to climbing terrain that models your goal climb, you can get great benefits from an unstructured approach. Most of us do not have the luxury of large chunks of time for climbing trips so we are forced to design simulations that model the real thing in order to get a good training effect.

Climbing Gyms

Many people have access to this training tool but in order to use it to best effect for building muscular endurance you'll need to put aside some accepted practices. First, leave your rock shoes at home and wear your mountain boots. Next, take a pack and load it, starting with 10 percent of your body weight. Finally, leave your ego at the door and prepare to be heckled. You might consider going to the gym during their slowest hours so your friends don't see you.

What you are going to do is put in as much vertical as you can manage on routes you can do in boots with a pack. A self-belay rig like many gyms have will maximize your time spent climbing and not put your belayer to sleep. Climbing up and then down climbing the route is an especially good way to develop both the ME and the ability to reverse moves, which could save your life. Go for volume not maximum difficulty. Progress by adding time.

You may also find your footwork improving to the point where increasing the difficulty becomes possible. You will certainly gain new respect for the pre-sticky rubber accomplishments of the previous generations as well as respect for the edging ability of a good, stiff mountain boot. Be cautious about adding weight and never exceed 20 percent of body weight unless you have a good background of finger strength training. With high volume of specific training like this there is a high risk of tendon injury, and the skin on your hands will probably get very sore.

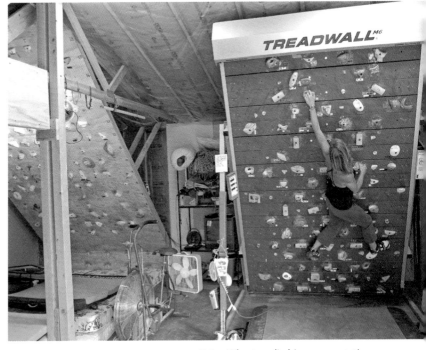

Rotating Climbing Walls

Rotating climbing walls have been around since the '80s, and some gyms have them. Treadwall is a brand of rotating wall that is currently in production; we even know of a few privately owned Treadwalls. This is a great training tool and it takes up relatively little space. You can basically perform the same sort of workouts as described above on a Treadwall.

Erinn Wharton climbing on a rotating climbing wall in her home gym.
Photo: Josh Wharton

Weighted Hill Climbs

To achieve the best results, take the time to lay out a gradual progression over at least eight, or better yet ten to twelve, weeks after you've completed a Max Strength Period and two weeks before you are planning your major alpine objective. Keep this in mind: This stuff is going to make your legs very tired and you will not be at your best till you have a good recovery period.

This workout should fit into the plan once or maybe twice in a week after a good general aerobic and strength base is laid. It will require a good recovery of seventy-two hours before the next demanding session. If your performance improves for the first couple of weeks, but then plateaus and drops off, you are doing too much and should drop down to one session per week.

Here are some examples of progressions we have used.

A 58-Year-Old Novice Climbing Mount Rainer's Disappointment Cleaver Route

Weeks	Elevation gain in feet/meters	% of body weight carried	# of times per week	Intensity
1–2	1,500/457	10	2	Zone 1
3–4	2,000/610	15	2	Zone 1
5–6	2,500/762	20	1	Zone 1
7–8	3,000/914	20	2	Zone 1
9–10	3,500/1,067	25	1	Zone 1
11–12	4,000/1,219	25	1	Zone 1

Notes:

- All of these workouts were done in Zone 1 which corresponded to her nose-breathing pace we described earlier due to the relatively low aerobic capacity of this climber.

- These workouts made up almost all of this person's vertical ascending for the weeks shown so she could do two sessions most weeks. If you are getting out climbing on the weekends and carrying a pack, then you may find that one session a week is plenty.

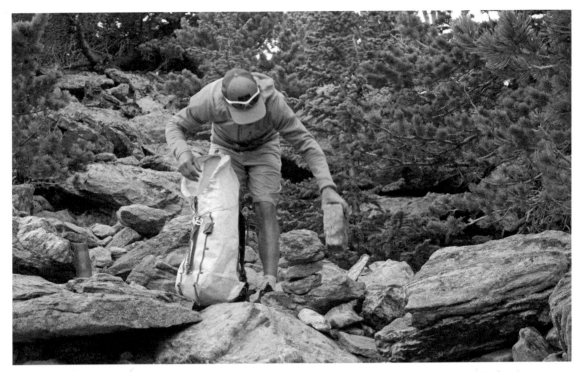

When a ready source of water is not available use what comes easily to hand. Most mountains are full of rocks. Steve House loading rocks in his pack near Rocky Mountain National Park, Colorado. *Photo: Eva House*

Steve's Preparation for the West Face of Makalu in 2008

Weeks	Elevation gain in feet/meters	Weight carried	# of times per week	Intensity
1–2	3,000/914	25 lbs	2	Zone 1
3–4	4,000/1,219	28 lbs	2	Zone 1
5–6	4,500/1,372	32 lbs	2	Zone 1
7–8	5,000/1,524	36 lbs	2	Zone 1
9–10	7,000/2,134	30 lbs	2	1x Zone 1, 1x at Zone 3
11–12	9,000/2,743	30 lbs	2	1x Zone 1, 1x at Zone 3

Notes:

- Steve gave this training a very high priority, so other climbing and workouts necessarily had to take a backseat to this demanding work.

- Due to his experience with these over several years he was able to get an added aerobic and muscular endurance benefit from including the higher-intensity work during the last month.

- Steve based his choice of weight to carry on his previous experiences with this training and started a little higher than the percentages recommended for climbers new to this method.

Conventional Treadmill Hand Walking

The only thing conventional about this workout is that it uses a popular piece of equipment found in many gyms, the treadmill. But it uses it in an entirely different way than originally intended. Turn on the belt to a slow speed like one mile per hour at first. Assume a push-up position with your feet on the floor and your hands on the side rails of the treadmill. Begin hand walking by stepping your hands out on to the moving belt. Hold a straight line from your head to your heels in a plank position and walk on your hands.

You will probably begin to almost immediately feel the effects of this strenuous movement. You must counter the tendency of your body to rotate while you move each hand forward. This requires significant core tension from your single hand all the way to your feet.

You may progress the challenge by:

- Elevating your feet

- By placing your feet on an exercise ball

- By lifting the opposite foot as you march your hands forward on the belt

- Adding a weight vest

- Speeding up the belt

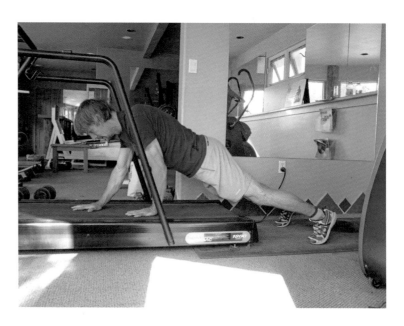

This is a very demanding core and upper body workout that can provide a very strong base of muscular endurance. Due to the intense nature of this workout you will need to use an interval protocol. See text for details.
Photo: Eva House

You'll get the best results by using an interval-type workout where you work for a period and stand to recover due to its demanding nature. Start with two sets of five reps of one minute with one minute recovery between reps, and five minutes recovery between sets. You will see rapid progress; we know of few better upper-body muscular endurance workouts. Despite its lack of climbing specificity, it has very good carryover.

BUILDING YOUR OWN BASE PERIOD ENDURANCE PLAN

Now that you have a working knowledge of the strength training component of the Base Period you will be better able to see how all this fits into an overall training plan.

Count only the aerobic volume when planning the progression of training. This is because you are going to progressively increase the volume of aerobic training. In strength training, time is not a good measure of the work done. So, strength training sessions will not become longer over the months.

If you have been using the full weekly training volume to build your progression don't worry that this is going to ruin your training plan. The basic principles of the book still apply especially the progressive nature of the training load. Keep in mind that the suggested weekly training progressions are not a magic formula or derived from extensive testing. They are general guidelines. There can, and will, be both intentional and accidental variations from these percentages. Real world training is not clean and formulaic. But despite these (sometimes large) variations and their impacts, as long as the general principles are adhered to—and you listen to how your body is responding to the training—things tend to work out well.

Training Plan for a Mountaineering Objective

The Base Period is where the training program for a mountaineer will diverge from that of a climber headed for a technical alpine route who needs to train his upper body's musculature just as much as his lower body's. Both climbers will place a heavy emphasis on developing aerobic endurance capacity but the climber headed for a technically demanding objective needs to balance time and energy spent

Marathon Pace

By Kelly Cordes

Three thousand feet (914 meters) up and we were flailing—failing and falling apart. The Kahiltna Glacier bent, flowed, and turned below us—its crevasses the size of city streets. We were done. Halfway up and nothing left.

I could faintly see the tent city at the landing strip down glacier. Scores of people were deepening the trench, single file, up Denali's standard route that very minute. A guy dragging a sled told us we were headed the wrong way when we started toward the north buttress of Mount Hunter a few days ago. Maybe he was right.

It was May 2002 and Scott DeCapio and I had plans to step it up. You always want to go bigger, to challenge yourself. We went to Alaska more fit and ready than we'd ever been.

But between the weather, the voodoo, and the internal and external conditions inherent to alpine climbing, you rarely get to pull the rope and try for a redpoint. So you'd better do it right the first time. Consciously I knew this—hell, I'd even remembered what Mark Twight wrote to me the summer before, in the front of my newly purchased and cherished copy of *Kiss or Kill*: "*Kelly, It's easy to be hard, but it's hard to be smart. Burn the torch!*"

Funny thing is, I thought I knew what he meant. Scotty and I had been working our way up the previous few seasons, building our skills and experiences, learning, moving into progressively bigger routes in lightweight, single-push style. In 2001 we'd raced up two 3,500-foot (1,067-meter) new routes with daypacks, heart rates redlining, go-go-go simul-climbing and falling in love, perhaps too in love, with the greatest joy I've ever known: moving freely in the mountains.

But not all routes are equal; some have short cruxes and long moderate sections, while others are more sustained, more physical. More exhausting.

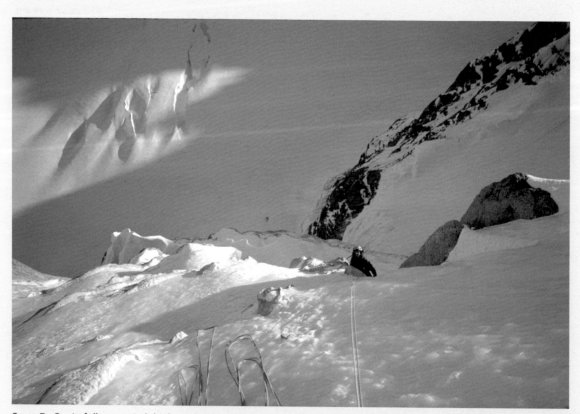

Scott DeCapio follows a pitch high on the French Route, Mount Hunter (14,573', 4,442m), Alaska. *Photo: Kelly Cordes*

So we were halfway up Mount Hunter's then-unrepeated 1984 French Route and we were spent. We'd sprinted through sustained ice and mixed terrain, simulclimbing between hanging belays, and then we sat on our empty packs on butt-seat ledges we'd chopped into the hard blue ice of the third ice band. Exhausted, delirious, feet dangling below. Our down parkas and the Alaskan sunlight kept us from shivering, and we gazed across the range in awe, as if we were on another planet. Scotty pulled on his insulated pants; I wrapped an ultralight tarp around me. I closed my eyes and leaned my head back, the sun bathing me with simple luxury. "*It wasn't that long,*" I remember thinking. "*I don't understand why we're so spent.*" We'd gained that height in twelve hours, before wasting another three looking for a rest spot. Scotty fell asleep belaying me as I led us astray, convinced from below that every rock had to be flat on top. No luck, rookies.

Twight's inscription was proving true.

Months later, in the reflection afforded by time, I thought about endurance athletes and how the best finely adjust their pace for the distance of the race.

In climbing I've heard something like you have to slow down to go fast, though I'm not sure I'd put it like that. Rather, you have to be fit and efficient and smart to go fast. You can't sprint a marathon.

Even the best marathoners aren't sprinting. You and I might not be able to run a single mile at a top marathoner's pace, but sprints and slogs can be relative things. Elite runners carefully redline their perfect pace for the distance, going as fast as they can without blowing up. I should have known better.

We slumped tight on our anchor, trying to recover, but deep-cell exhaustion crept beyond our muscles and bones, and stole our will. Alpine climbing departs from my race-pace analogy when we consider the consequences of mistakes; Scotty and I had crossed into sloppiness and left nothing in reserve. Shadows crept toward us. Bubbles from the stove instilled hope, but when the sun left we knew we'd have to move, up or down—or we'd freeze.

Down it would be. I drifted in and out of a dreamless world, oblivious to the lessons I was learning.

There's a time to run and a time to walk. But don't get me wrong: I'm not telling anyone to slow down. I've long viewed with suspicion the armchair directives barked at the young and driven, usually with the faux self-assuredness of someone who's never been there, about how they shouldn't push so hard, how they should go easy. I find beauty in charging into the unknown, armed with little more than a sharpened stick and unwavering self-belief. Beauty in dropping the excuses and *trying*, in making things happen rather than waiting for some imaginary time when you're good enough, wise enough, have a job that pays enough—a time that will never come if you're too busy waiting for it.

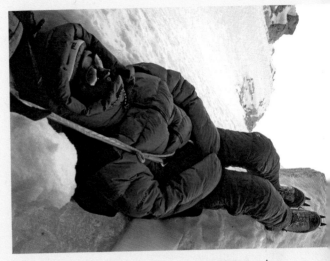

Scott DeCapio trying hard to recover some energy and willpower after going too hard for too long.
Photo: Kelly Cordes

There is also beauty in the wisdom of discipline, a wisdom that offers the sweet taste of knowing you did everything right. Then, instead of lying broken at the base, you might get lucky enough to stand on an obscure summit with just enough left to safely descend, breathing rarified air and feeling like some mystical powers of the universe conspired with everything you have, everything you trained for, and everything you sacrificed to get there.

And that, I am certain, feels far better than trying to sprint a marathon. But I guess that's the thing with alpine climbing—there is no recipe, rewards come hard, and sometimes it's hard to be smart.

Kelly Cordes is an accomplished alpinist, writer, and margarita artist who in 2004 with Josh Wharton established what is probably the biggest rock climb in the world, the Azeem Ridge on Great Trango Tower.

Modulating the Training Load

When I first began structured training for alpine climbing in 2003 I was taught to use a schedule of a three-week cycle: easy, medium, and hard weeks to create gradualness and modulation.

After using this model for one year, Scott taught me a more intuitive method, a method closer to what a true coach does with top athletes: going by how the athlete feels each day. This requires more monitoring and more flexibility. It is therefore best employed by athletes with more experience at what works well for them. The beauty of this system is that it allows for those periods when the stars are perfectly aligned and training is going like clockwork; then you can keep the pressure on, building a bit of fatigue on purpose for several days or a week when you know you can handle it. This is called over-reaching. When you recognize that the training effect has occurred, back off and recover for as long as it takes. For top athletes, this might only be a day or two of easy recovery work before they are ready to start another mini-buildup.

This approach allows you to take advantage of natural rhythms, which you may not understand. It is more attuned to the body but takes more body awareness and a flexible schedule to use successfully. The training plan becomes more of a suggestion or proposal rather than an ultimate dictate.

– Steve House

doing endurance training on foot with time spent honing his technical climbing skill and upper-body strength and endurance.

You should use a long-term general template such as the quarterly training log in chapter 7 that indicates the sort of average volume you are shooting for from month to month. From there it seems to work best to lay out more detailed training guidelines two, sometimes three, weeks in advance. This way you can target both the volume and the specific workouts you want to hit, without planning so far out into the future that your plan becomes an unrealistic shot in the dark that doesn't allow flexibility. This gives you enough lead time to schedule training and climbing partners around daily life.

Often when the training load is high you may not want to commit to the day's exact workout until the day itself and you've completed a warm-up and have an idea of how tired you are. If you've got a hard session planned, but are not feeling recovered for whatever reason, you should consider modifying that planned hard workout. As you will recall from chapter 2, if you are not recovered it can be counterproductive to yourself and the purpose of the harder workouts. It is also wise to allow yourself the freedom to change the workout while you're doing it; going a little longer if you're feeling good at the turn-around point or going back early if you're feeling tired and flat.

Remember that the purpose of the Base Period is to condition yourself to handle more work. This toughening up is what coaches sometimes call capacity training, increasing your capacity for lots of aerobic work and, in our case, climbing-related strength and endurance. As we've said before, expect to experience some persistent, low-level fatigue through your Base Period. Recovery will generally not be complete between workouts so do not to expect personal bests. If you have a particularly challenging climb you want to do, take a couple of days off beforehand. However if you schedule too many of these special climbs during the Base Period you'll spend too much time resting up for them and won't get the full benefits of this capacity-building period.

During a Base Period you have to do a lot of volume. The term a lot is relative, and while we have provided general guidelines based on how you handle the volume of the Transition Period, it can be tricky to find the right load that presses you but does not crush you. Steve and other climbers of his experience often do well over twenty hours training per week. In our training log we've left blanks for you to write down these and other ideas for workouts, trails you could run, loops you could ride, and of course routes to climb.

Base Period Plan for a Mountaineering Objective

As explained in some detail in chapter 3 this period is used to increase your ability to handle more and more work. In effect you are training so that you can train more and train harder later. The volume of work you do here is what will prepare you for the upcoming Specific Period. We cannot overemphasize the principles that you need to follow: **Continuity** in your training, **gradual** increase of the training load, and **modulation** of the training from hard to easy over days and weeks.

Bearing in mind that most mountaineering objectives have relatively low technical requirements it is wise to spend the majority of your Base Period training time in developing your ability to go uphill fast for a long time. This of course assumes that you do have the technical skills required. If you are new to walking and climbing moderate slopes in crampons, or if you lack familiarity with glacier travel or crevasse rescue, then you will need to spend time acquiring these skills to improve your efficiency. If on the other hand you are competent in mountaineering skills, this simplifies the training greatly.

The following plan will provide you with a general template to follow. You need to fit this into your life with the volume of training you can handle given everything you know about training.

Base Period Plan for a Technical Alpine Objective

A technical alpine objective presents a bigger challenge training-wise because it requires the same development of aerobic endurance and general strength as does the mountaineering plan but with the addition of at least maintaining (if not increasing) your technical climbing strength and skills. But it is a solid foundation of strength and aerobic endurance that, once on the climb, will allow you to fully exploit whatever your technical skill level may be. As Kelly Cordes told us, he and his climbing partner had to back off Mount Hunter not because they were technically deficient, but because they lacked the basic conditioning to attain their objective.

In practice most big alpine routes are executed at a technical level well below a climber's "home-crag" level. If you are training for the Cassin Ridge, a technical route, but you can climb several grades harder ice and rock at home, then the best strategy is to forget about training your technical skills in the buildup to the attempt and focus on your aerobic base.

As with the mountaineering example, if you are technically deficient you need to develop those skills first, or revaluate your goals until your goals match your skills. Most alpine climbs entail significant approaches and much of the basic aerobic capacity training can be combined with climbing days where you are maintaining your skills, but not pushing to new limits.

We are going to assume that you work a regular job or attend school but have most weekends free to get into the mountains. Full-time climbers such as guides can still use this same plan but will be able to substitute actual climbing for the less-specific workouts that we are recommending for the job-restricted climber.

Base Period Training Tasks for Weeks 1–8

Mountaineering objective	Technical alpine objective
2x/week Max Strength workout with Scott's Killer Core Routine as a warm-up.	2x/week Max Strength workout with Scott's Killer Core Routine as a warm-up.
One long Zone 1 workout comprising 25–30% of the total weekly volume on rolling, hilly terrain.	One long Zone 1 workout comprising 25–30% of the total weekly volume on rolling, hilly terrain. This can be an alpine route approach and descent.
One Zone 1–2 workout comprising 20% of total weekly volume on sustained steep terrain. Make this workout Zone 3 in weeks 5 through 7.	One Zone 1–2 workout comprising 20% of total weekly volume on sustained steep terrain. Make this workout Zone 3 in weeks 5 through 7.
Make up the rest of the volume with Zone 1 or recovery aerobic.	Make up the rest of the volume with Zone 1 or recovery aerobic.
	One day of technical alpine climbing or the best approximation.
	One day cragging two grades below your current onsight ability.

Example Training Schedule for Week 1

	Monday	Tuesday	Wednesday	Thursday	Friday	Saturday	Sunday
AM	Off	Zone 1	Zone 2	Off	Off	Climbing	Long Z1
PM	Strength	Climbing	Recovery	Strength	Off	Off	Off

Notes for Weeks 1–8:

- The goal here is to begin to challenge several of your body's systems at once. To put them into a crisis state as referred to in chapter 3.

- Initial volume will be 10 percent more volume than the last high-volume week in the Transition Period.

- Weeks 1–3: Increase training volume 10–20 percent each week.

- Week 4: Reduce training volume 25–35 percent from week 3. This is a recovery week to allow you to absorb the previous training.

- Weeks 5–6: Hold volume constant at week 3 level. This allows your body to adapt to the new higher workload.

- Week 7: Increase training 25 percent from week 6. Reduce Zone 3 workout time by half. Limit strength training time to a maximum of three hours a week. As overall volume rises the percentage of strength volume drops.

- Week 8: Reduce training volume 50 percent from week 7. This is an important rest week before launching into the next cycle.

- For the technical objective you should continue to climb, but below your maximum level in these early weeks.

- When adding in climbing time something has to give in the volume of training. Long approaches to alpine climbs will be part of your Zone 1 or even Zone 2 work.

Recommendations:

- Get in the mountains for the long Zone 1 sessions if you can. Include climbing, scrambling, hiking, ski touring, or trail running.

- Find a sustained hill for your harder Zone 2 aerobic workouts, even if it's the fire stairs in a high-rise building (for the mountaineering program, the technical program will incorporate technical climbing).

- Find a very steep hill if you are doing hill sprints.

Relative Volumes by Training Modes – Weeks 1–8 Base Period: *Mountaineering*

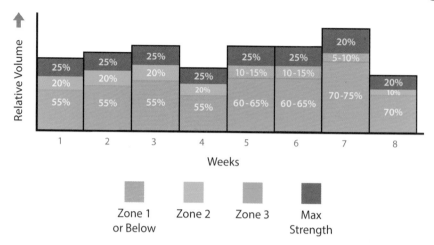

Each bar represents the volume of weekly training. In that week you will do the recommended amounts of training in the specified zones. As an example if Week 1 had 10 hours of training, 5.5 of those hours would be done in Zone 1 or below. In this plan we assume that the climber's technical skills are already fully sufficient to meet the needs of the planned climb(s). That frees up the bulk of this block of training to be used for increasing your work capacity. This plan can also fit the needs of the technical alpine climber whose skills already surpass those needed on the goal climb. Note: The chart shows the low end of the weekly increases in volume we recommend in the notes for weeks 1–8 above.

Relative Volumes by Training Modes – Weeks 1–8 Base Period: *Technical Alpine*

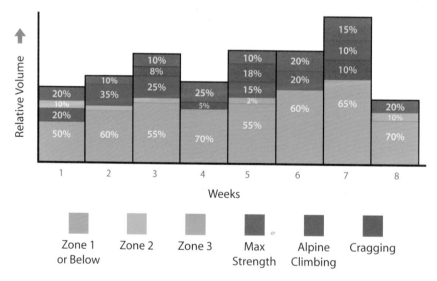

This plan follows the same basic approach as the mountaineering objective, but includes some time spent developing or maintaining technical skills. This will benefit a beginning mountaineer that needs to learn to walk on moderately steep terrain without hooking crampons on pant legs, and it can also help a strong alpine climber maintain his climbing skills and strength. Nonetheless, the main objective of this period remains to build work capacity primarily in a general and non-climbing-specific way. As such, actual climbing must take a back seat to the other training. Note: This chart shows the high end of the weekly increase in volume we recommend in the notes for weeks 1–8 above.

Base Period Training Tasks for Weeks 9–16

Mountaineering objective	Technical alpine objective
Begin Muscular Endurance 1–2 times per week.	Begin Muscular Endurance 1–2 times per week.
One day per week continue with abbreviated Max Strength routine. Later it will become 1x/2 weeks as a warm-up for ME.	One day per week continue with abbreviated Max Strength routine. Later it will become 1x/2 weeks as a warm-up for ME.
Use Scott's Killer Core Routine 1x/2wks for maintenance.	Use Scott's Killer Core Routine 1x/2wks for maintenance.
Two long Zone 1 sessions each week. One 30% and one 20% of weekly volume.	Two long Zone 1 sessions each week. One 30% and one 20% of weekly volume.
One Zone 3 hill climb/uphill hike workout. 10% of weekly volume.	One Zone 3 hill climb/uphill hike workout. 10% of weekly volume.
Make up the remainder of the volume with recovery or Zone 1 aerobic training.	Make up the remainder of the volume with recovery or Zone 1 aerobic training.
	Two days moderate alpine climbing including long Zone 1 approaches.
	One midweek climbing session: Ice, indoor, or cragging two grades below your max.

Notes for Weeks 9–16:

- The goal of this period is to build upon weeks 1–8 by taking advantage of the base fitness you have developed, which will allow you to absorb a higher training load.

- Get into the mountains for long hikes, runs, and approaches, preferably off trail and moving smoothly over rough terrain. Even better yet, get on snow. It's OK to combine the two Zone 1 workouts into one long day out.

- If you have not been, now is the time to begin to carry weight on the two long Zone 1 workouts. Start at 10 percent of your body weight. Increase weight 5 percent every other week. Don't exceed 30 percent of your body weight.

- Initial volume is determined by the highest volume during weeks 1–8. Adjust accordingly depending on how you handled that level. Shoot for week 9 volume to be around week 7 volume. This could be as high as 50–80 percent greater than where you started 8 weeks before.

- Weeks 9–11: Increase volume 5–10 percent per week.

- Week 12: Recovery week. Reduce volume by 50 percent from week 11.

- Weeks 13–14: Volume remains steady at week 11.

- Week 15: Volume overload week. Increase 20 percent from week 14.

- Week 16: Volume drops 50–70 percent from week 15.

- This is a big period of overload, and you will get tired. Do not expect to perform at your best during this block of training. Take advantage of the rest weeks 12 and 16. Take days off from training if you need them. Pay close attention to your recovery to ensure you don't get sick or injured. No partying. Eat well. Get lots of sleep. We cannot overstate the need to monitor your recovery. Do not blindly follow any program into your grave.

Relative Volumes by Training Modes – Weeks 9–16 Base Period: *Mountaineering*

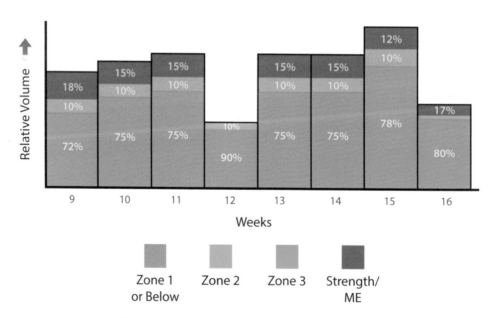

The chart shows relative percentage of the various modes of training that are used during this block of training. Aerobic endurance dominates again because we assume the climber is already in possession of the required technical skills needed for the climb. Note that as the volume of endurance activities becomes large, the percentage of the total volume devoted to strength training shrinks. The actual hours of strength training will remain fairly constant, however. The big drops in load during weeks 12 and 16 are an important part of the plan. Do not think that by fudging hours there you can make up for lost time in previous weeks. Training does not work like that.

Relative Volumes by Training Modes – Weeks 9–16 Base Period: *Technical Alpine*

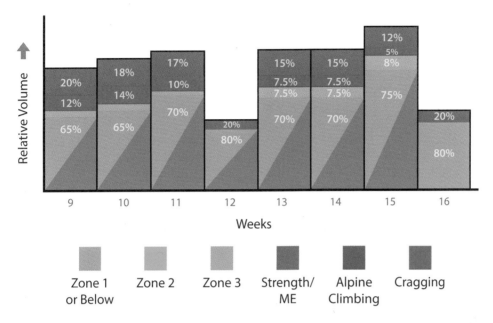

This chart shows the relative percentage of the various modes of training that are used during this block. Include the approaches to, and the moderate alpine routes you do into the Zone 1 percentage. Be sure to keep up on the strength training and once again do not expect to put in record-breaking results during this heavy overload block. You'll be carrying some fatigue through much of these 8 weeks. Take the recovery weeks for what they are intended to be. They are not about increasing your capacities but about restoring all your body's systems.

Base Period Training Tasks for Weeks 17–20

Mountaineering objective	Technical alpine objective
On even weeks continue with one Max Strength and one Muscular Endurance workout.	On even weeks continue with one Max Strength and one Muscular Endurance workout. Include exercises specific to upper body as well as lower body.
On odd weeks do only the one Muscular Endurance workout.	On odd weeks do only the one Muscular Endurance workout. Include same split of upper-body and lower-body exercises.
Two long Zone 1 aerobic workouts. One 30% and one 20% of weekly volume each week.	Two long Zone 1 approaches with long, technical climbs. Climb also done at Zone 1 exertion. One at approximately 30% and one at approximately 20% of weekly volume each week.
Remaining volume will be done as recovery or Zone 1 distance.	Remaining volume will be done as recovery or Zone 1 distance.

The goal for this period is to consolidate the fitness gains made so far and allow for the full adaptation to the stress you've been imposing.

Notes for Weeks 17–20:

- Week 17: The same volume as week 15.

- Week 18: The volume is 25 percent less than week 17.

- Weeks 19–20: The volume is same as week 17.

- All Muscular Endurance workouts will be done in Zone 3 and will be very tiring so allow plenty of recovery between.

- Both the mountaineer and the alpinist should get into the mountains for only the long Zone 1 days, preferably on terrain that is similar to your goal climb.

- Most of the Zone 1 work should be done as easy aerobic training or recovery workouts to account for the very high workload of the muscular endurance.

- Alpine climbers should drop cragging workouts during this period so that more time can be spent on muscular endurance and alpine climbs.

Relative Volumes by Training Modes – Weeks 17–20 Base Period: *Mountaineering*

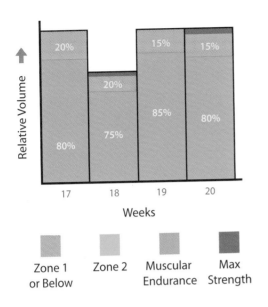

In this block of the Base Period priority is given to the Muscular Endurance workouts. The bulk of the other training will be easy aerobic, either in the mountains or in recovery workouts in flat terrain. Done correctly this preparation will set you up for some of the strongest days you have ever had in the mountains during your specific preparation.

Relative Volumes by Training Modes – Weeks 17–20 Base Period: *Technical Alpine*

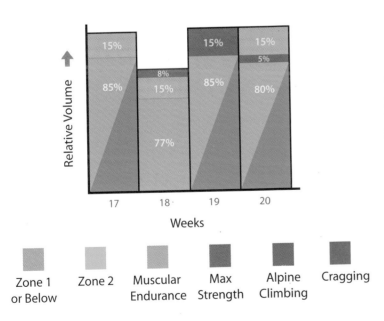

The Muscular Endurance training you do during this block of training is critical and will be very fatiguing. Allow plenty of recovery workouts. Notice that most weeks the Zone 1 percentages are heavily weighted away from alpine climbing and towards actual easy training. This is to allow you to get maximum benefit from the muscular endurance work, which will pay off big when you begin your more specific training in the next period.

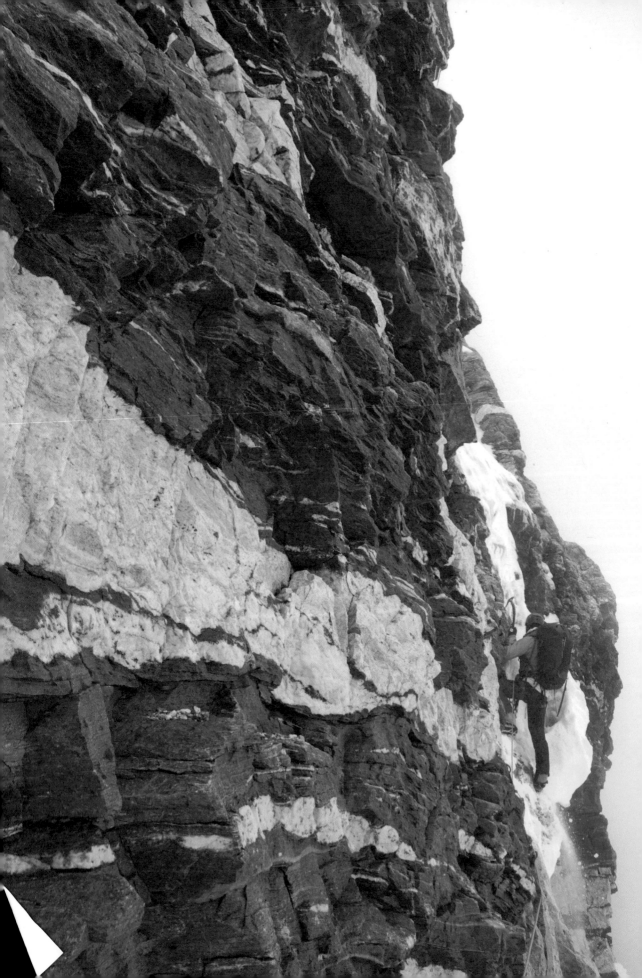

Chapter 9

Climb, Climb, Climb

"A few hours mountain climbing turns a rogue and a saint into two roughly equal creatures. Weariness is the shortest path to equality and fraternity—and liberty is finally added by sleep."

— FRIEDRICH NIETZSCHE

PLANNING THE CLIMBING-SPECIFIC PERIOD

After establishing a good level of general endurance and strength over the course of the Base Period, you will be ready to focus on climbing-specific training activities. And, as we've stated before, for less well-conditioned climbers a Base Period of sixteen to twenty weeks, or more, will be helpful. Remember the bank account analogy described in an earlier part of the book? You need to have as big of a bank balance as possible before you enter this period. The more hard work you are capable of doing, the better the results from this climbing-focused training will be.

Unless you have put in an absolute minimum of twelve weeks of good base training, skip this Specific Period and keep building your base right up until your trip. Many climbers on compressed timelines,

Opposite: Marko Prezelj climbs on day one of an attempt on the west face of Makalu (27,825′, 8,481m).
Photo: Steve House

four months or less, or with less training background, will not do this period. Despite its direct application to climbing, this is actually the least-critical stage of the training and the one most dependent on the work before it being done correctly. Don't worry—it won't matter much whether or not you can onsight 5.12 M10 at the crag if you're exhausted by the time you reach the crux of a long route.

For elite-level climbers, the training load in any single one of these training sessions can be very high. All the training that has taken place up to this point was done to give you the ability to tax several systems simultaneously to near-maximum and as specifically as possible. In a very real sense all prior training has been done in order to support this training: **You have been training to train.**

During this period, almost all nonspecific workouts will be done for recovery with only a few workouts that act to maintain basic qualities like strength and endurance. This will allow you to get maximum benefit from the specific workouts. Cycling and other fun non-weight-bearing aerobic activities that may have made up part of your Base Period conditioning will now be used only for recovery. From this point on, most hard training needs to be as similar as possible to the climbing you are targeting.

The length of this Specific Period is not cast in stone. It can range from a couple of weeks for less-experienced climbers to two months for those with years of training behind them. Steve built his 2005 pre–Nanga Parbat conversion period around a five-week expedition to Peru.

Specific Training by Climbing Trip

For Steve preparing for Nanga Parbat, specificity meant technical alpine climbing at altitude for many consecutive days. The Nanga Parbat ascent took eight days round-trip carrying packs that started out at thirty-two pounds per climber. Because of his previous attempt on the Rupal Face he knew how much load he would need to be able to handle so he could target his conversion phase to achieve exactly that state of readiness.

Steve decided on a pre-expedition trip to Peru with longtime partner Marko Prezelj. Upon landing in Peru Marko and Steve quickly moved up to a camp below La Esfinge, a beautiful granite wall with a base camp at 15,100 feet (4,602 meters). They free climbed several routes on this granite wall, its summit lies at 17,470 feet (5,325 meters). They spent eight days there, allowing ample time to acclimate.

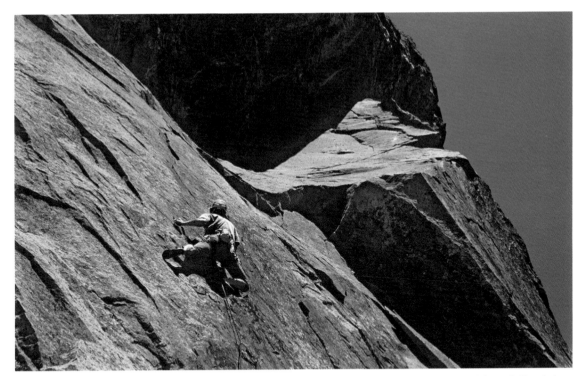

Steve House onsights a 5.12a pitch on Cruz del Sur at 15,500 feet (4,724m) on La Esfinge (17,470', 5,325m) in Peru. *Photo: Marko Prezelj*

The pair then returned to town for a day's rest and repacking before approaching the 14,435-foot (4,400-meter) high base camp for Cayesh. There they spent a day in bad weather before moving camp up to an advanced base camp at the edge of the glacier at 16,235 feet (4,948 meters). The following day started in the dark and they climbed a difficult seventeen-pitch new route to the 18,758-foot (5,717-meter) summit.

After a rest day they spent one full day hiking out with heavy packs, returning to town to rest for a couple of days before approaching the north face of Huascarán, the area's highest summit. After counting seventeen rock fall incidents in forty-five minutes, they decided to return to town. With only a week left, they made what is usually a three-day approach to Taulliraju in one big day and spent the next three days climbing the French pillar, with a bivy on the summit at 19,122 feet (5,828 meters), and descended having completed the first free ascent.

Examining this trip and these climbs, you can see that they each increased in intensity, length, and load—each climb was harder, longer, and higher than the one before it. Steve and Marko recovered for one to four days between each ascent. While none of the climbs they did was an exact model of the Rupal Face, they combined enough of the elements of what Steve knew he would have to deal with to give him the confidence that he was well prepared. If the partners had struggled with these preparatory climbs Steve would have needed to reassess his goal.

In 2011, Steve went to Makalu to attempt a new route on the west face with Marko. On their final acclimatization round they left a bivy at 21,325 feet (6,500 meters) on the route they were attempting and hoped to climb and descend a minimum of 2,300 to 2,600 feet (701 to 792 meters) that day with light packs. They turned back after climbing only 1,650 feet (503 meters) in eight hours. Their pace was too slow, and they knew it. They came back again for one final attempt in the hope that their acclimatization had made them faster. It hadn't, and they did not start the route. This is an example of testing oneself against a facsimile of what you expect a route to require, not measuring up, and deciding against further attempts until you can come back more prepared.

Let's summarize the priorities during a climbing-trip–specific period:

- Choose test or training objectives as similar to your goal climb as possible.

- Each climb should be more difficult than the last. Training outings should build in difficulty and duration.

- Ideally, each peak should be a bit higher in elevation than the previous summit.

- Get adequate recovery between climbs.

Scott Johnston approaching Mount Robson (12,972', 3,954m) en route to making an early ascent of the difficult Emperor Ridge.
Photo: Scott Johnston collection

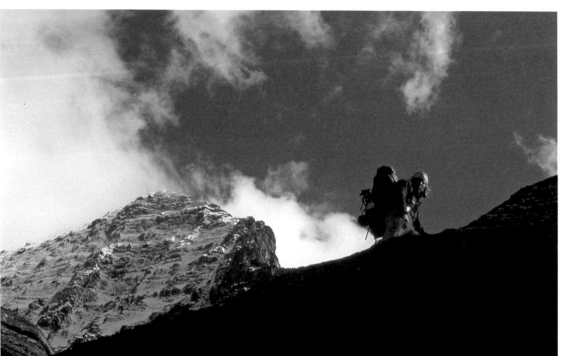

Specific Training Period without Leaving Home

Most people don't have the luxury of going on an expedition as preparation for an expedition. As an example of how to execute a good conversion close to home, we'll examine Scott's preparations for his expedition to K2 in 1995. With a very full work schedule, Scott used three key workouts per week for maximum recovery between hard efforts.

According to the principles of the specificity period, Scott designed workouts that would induce training adaptations that would mimic as closely as possible the stress of the actual expedition. All his training during the rest of the week was devoted to recovery and included two strength maintenance sessions. Since steep hiking and climbing at an easy technical level would be the main focus on K2, where he was to attempt the Abruzzi Spur, this type of training needed to be the main focus of his Specific Period.

Scott had three main workouts that he did on Saturday, Sunday, and Wednesday. Let's look at what he did:

Saturday: Heading to Smith Rock State Park, Scott utilized a very steep game trail directly up the fall line of a steep hill. The trail started at the shore of the Crooked River and ascended 1,500 vertical feet (457 meters). Scott would hike up this steep slope wearing mountain boots and carrying water jugs. On top he'd empty the jugs and descend quickly to refill them at the river for the next lap. He used a progression in both the number of laps and in the weight he carried so that the load became greater each workout. The final workout on this hill entailed 7,500 vertical feet (2,286 meters) carrying thirty pounds, and was done at his breakaway breathing point, meaning at the top of his aerobic zone. This was the first time Scott used the water carry method we describe in this book.

Sunday: Every Sunday Scott would do an all-day, low-intensity ski tour often with an alpine climb or with an easy mountaineering objective included. This workout was designed to maintain his basic aerobic foundation. Stacking this workout on the back of the more intense one on Saturday is thought to have the desirable effect of enhancing fat metabolism.

Wednesday: After work Scott would drive to the local ski area, don alpine touring skis, and ski 2,800 feet (853 meters) up the alpine runs to the summit. Initially he did this with a light pack, but soon began to add weight in the form of gallon jugs of water, which he dumped on the summit. These workouts were done in the dark and even in the nastiest weather conditions—for training mental toughness. The intensity progressed by increasing the weight carried on the ski up and typically took about forty-five minutes. The purpose of this workout was to improve his speed at his lactate threshold and was again done at breakaway breathing point.

Let's summarize the priorities during an at-home/full-time-job conversion-to-specificity training block:

- Two Zone 3 workouts per week on moderate to steep uphill terrain carrying an alpine-weight pack. These are Scott's Wednesday and Saturday workouts.

- One big day per week that involves a lot of vertical gain and loss, and a long time spent moving continuously at a low intensity. Ideally this includes moderate technical climbing if that is part of your goal.

- Easy days leading up to and following these special workout days allows recovery before and after so that the training effects can be maximized.

- Maintenance of Max Strength is done in a gym two evenings per week.

- Include technical climbing if your objective requires it.

- Further maintenance of the aerobic base is to be done via easy recovery workouts like jogging, fast hiking, or easy swimming.

- Include an overall high percentage of recovery workouts.

Here is Scott's program outlined for two weeks.

Specific Period Example: Two Weeks of Training

Saturday	AM: Uphill water carry at Smith Rock. 4,500' of gain/loss with 24 lbs
	PM: Recovery run ¾ hour

Sunday	AM: Ski tour with ice climbing, 8 hours

Monday	AM: Off
	PM: Muscular Endurance strength workout in gym if recovered

Tuesday	AM: Long-distance run or XC ski 2 hours at Zone 1–2
	PM: Indoor climbing for 2 hours or Muscular Endurance in the gym, if not done on Monday
Wednesday	AM: Easy recovery run, 1 hour
	PM: Ski up Mount Bachelor w/24 lbs water
Thursday	AM: Recovery XC ski 1.5 hours
	PM: Muscular Endurance
Friday	AM: Easy run
	PM: Off
Saturday	AM: Hill repeats at Smith Rock 4,500' w/30 lbs of water
Sunday	AM: Long ski tour, 7,000 vertical feet (2,134 meters) of gain/loss
Monday	AM: Off
	PM: Muscular Endurance gym workout
Tuesday	AM: Easy XC ski or run
	PM: Off
Wednesday	AM: Easy run, 1 hour
	PM: Ski up Mount Bachelor with 30 lbs of water
Thursday	AM: Easy run or XC ski, 1.5 hours
	PM: Muscular Endurance gym workout
Friday	AM: Easy run, 1 hour
	PM: Off

Keep in mind that these weeks of training would be impossible to replicate by someone with less base training than Scott. Note that

Training to Perform

By Will Gadd

In 2010 I decided to climb ice for twenty-four hours straight in Ouray, Colorado. In every event, climb, or competition I enter I'm there to have the best possible performance, and that needs to be defined or it won't happen. I set my goals: to survive, still be climbing ice when the twenty-four hours has ended, and climb at least 12,000 vertical feet (3,658 meters). Without defined goals, appropriate training cannot even be envisioned, and what cannot be visualized is impossible.

So, how to keep climbing on near-vertical ice for twenty-four hours? Put another way: What will stop me from reaching my goals? I made a long list of possible problems ranging from sheer muscular failure to electrolyte imbalances down to elbow tendonitis, and ranked them according to what I felt the probability of each occurring was. I then developed a plan and response for each potential problem. I was prepared to duct-tape my tools to my hands if they cramped up too badly, or tie my elbows in place if my tendon problems became too severe. I had a nurse on call to give me an IV if my electrolytes got too screwed up. I had dozens of batteries and lighting systems. I organized very solid belayers who switched out every hour so they would be fresh and could guard my life as my mind decomposed—survival first. I solved every single problem I could think of.

I did all this before I even swung an ice tool or lifted a weight for the season. Training is preparation, and good preparation is to consider a goal in its entirety, not just the physical requirements.

I needed to begin to establish a base of volume, but in August there's not a lot of ice to climb so I built a sixteen-foot (five-meter) high pegboard with footholds in my backyard that I could train on with my ice tools. It was deadly boring climbing hundreds of laps, but even that was good mental training for the actual event. I also climbed long, moderate rock routes at speed.

When the ice came in, I was climbing well and feeling strong, but belaying became a challenge. Nobody wants to stand there for two hours straight pulling on a rope at minus twenty; it's just hard work. My partners and I developed a twenty-on-twenty-off routine, so we each climbed as many laps in twenty minutes as we could, then switched. This allowed us to stay warm and also taught us a lot about belay systems, rope wear, lowering, and other specific skills required for twenty-four hours of ice climbing. The biggest training day I had was about 5,500 feet (1,676 meters), and I was wrecked after it.

When the clock finally ticked twenty-four hours in Ouray I had survived, done over 1,000 feet (305 meters) of climbing in the last hour alone, and climbed over 25,000 feet (7,620 meters) in total. I had to switch boots four times, I puked once, and my fingers were bleeding, but overall I was in pretty good shape—and safe. I had actually climbed far more than I thought was possible. As I look back at the climb, I could have done better. Each training season brings more knowledge, but only if examined carefully. I'm now sure that 40,000 feet (12,192 meters) of ice climbing in twenty-four hours is possible.

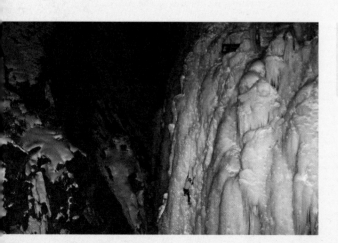

Will Gadd is a pioneer of hard, bolt-protected mixed routes as well as an accomplished paraglider pilot, kayaker, and father.

Right: Will Gadd climbing big ice in Eidfjord, Norway.
Photo: Christian Pondella

Left: Will Gadd during the Endless Ascent project to raise money for the dZi Foundation. www.dzifoundation.org
Photo: James Beissel

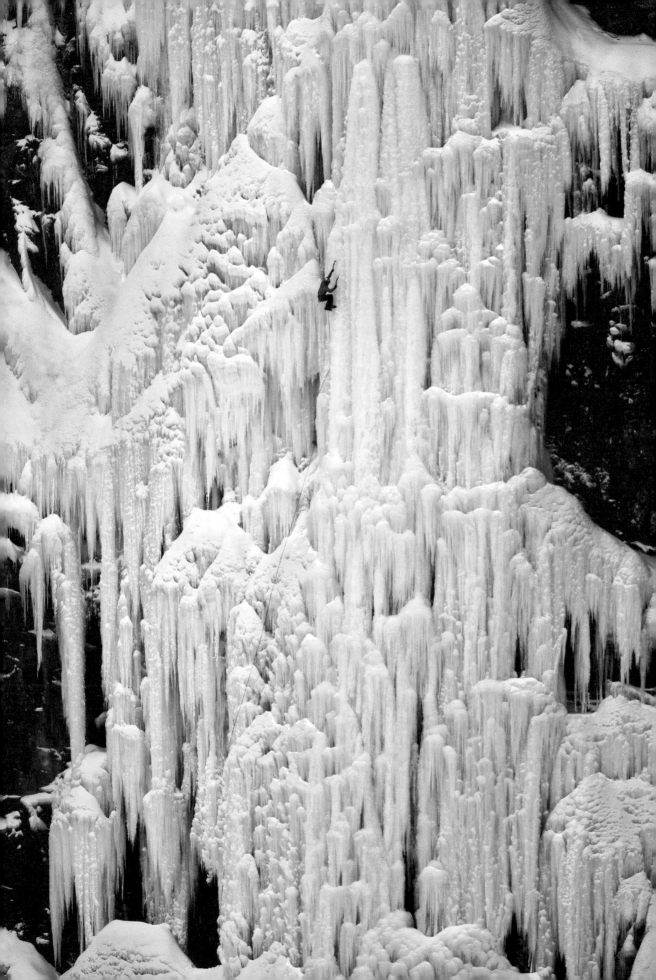

ascending over 7,000 feet (2,134 meters) with thirty pounds of weight is close to double the distance of the biggest day he'd encounter on K2. However, K2 is at very high altitude.

Scott included no technical rock climbing in this conversion period because there is minimal rock climbing (to 5.7) on his goal climb, and his climbing skills didn't need to be trained to manage that.

As a general rule for this period, these hard days should be at least as hard, and ideally significantly harder than, the big days of your big climb. The difference is that in training you allow for recovery. On a big climb, you don't have the luxury of good food and a comfortable bed.

Scott's final hard training session for K2 was to climb and ski a steep route on the west face of Mount Jefferson near his home in Oregon. This route involves 7,000 feet (2,134 meters) of thirty- to forty-five-degree cramponing on neve, a couple hundred feet of low fifth-class rock climbing to the summit, and then a ski descent of the same route. The climb/ski was completed with a training partner who was a two-time Olympian in cross-country skiing, and the round-trip took the pair a mere three and a half hours. While neither the altitude nor the duration of the route were identical to what he'd encounter on K2, the fact that they could knock off this climb in time to be home for lunch and not get too tired gave Scott confidence that the training had been effective and that his preparation was complete.

BUILDING YOUR SPECIFIC PERIOD PLAN

After years of structured training, Steve still consistently finds the Specific Period to be the most exciting, and the most frightening. This is when it would be so nice to have a coach to dictate your workouts, record them, monitor your recovery, and prime your motivation. In fact it is in these workouts that a coach in a conventional sport imposes the most control, often to the extent of altering the workout while it is in progress based on the response he observes in the athlete. The workouts are hard from the start, and the hardest of the period can destroy you to the point that all you can do is go home, eat, and fall asleep on the couch.

Do these well and you'll have a new appreciation of what it means to be an athlete, trained and in your prime. The period after these weeks is when you'll be in the best shape of your life. It's an amazing feeling. This gives you the confidence boost you need to climb a route that would have been unattainable before.

The increase in training intensity is what distinguishes this period from the Base Period. This increase comes from either climbing harder and faster, or imposing climbing-specific training loads at the top of your aerobic zone. General conditioning and building your resistance to fatigue are no longer your focus. Now you must create specially designed workouts that put several components of climbing-related fitness together into one workout.

Note that the overall volume of training will plateau in the early stages during this period as the intensity increases due to either more challenging workouts or harder and longer climbs. Volume will actually begin to drop as intensity and duration of your climbs, or individual simulated-climb workouts, increase even more. These are hard workouts; if it doesn't take a mighty act of will to complete these, they may be too easy.

What follows is a template for a four-week Climbing-Specific Period. We assume that you have access to good-sized mountains within a day's travel, but will be living and training from home.

Specific Period Training Plan for a Mountaineering Objective

Goal: To convert general fitness and resistance to fatigue into nearly endless endurance and greater speed and comfort on a big mountain.

Week 1: Training volume equals 80 percent of your last Base Period week (week 20 volume).

- One big day (40–50 percent of weekly volume) in the mountains with 100 percent as much vertical as the biggest day you expect on your climb. Carrying 50 percent of the most weight you will carry on your goal climb.

- One sustained (may be done as repeats on a smaller hill) Zone 3 hill climb, wearing mountain boots, covering 50 percent of the vertical of the goal climb's biggest day. Carry 75 percent of the most weight you'll carry. Go hard.

- One Zone 1–2 day midweek at 15 percent of weekly volume.

- One Max Strength maintenance workout as warm-up for core routine.

- All other training hours are performed at recovery level.

Week 2: Volume equal to 75 percent of your last Base Period week (week 20 volume).

- One big day in the mountains (50 percent of your weekly volume). Climb 100 percent of the vertical you expect on your biggest day of your goal climb with 60 percent of your expected biggest weight.

- One sustained Zone 3 interval hill climb, wearing mountain boots, covering 50 percent of the vertical of your biggest goal climb day carrying 75 percent of the max weight you expect on the goal climb.

- One Zone 1–2 midweek aerobic workout, 15 percent of weekly volume.

- All other training hours are performed at recovery level.

Week 3: Volume equal to 70 percent of your last Base Period week (week 20 volume).

- Two big days in the mountains, back-to-back, that total 75 percent of the weekly volume and 150 percent of your biggest goal climb day's vertical, using 100 percent of the weight you expect to carry.

- One sustained Zone 3 hill climb, wearing mountain boots, covering 75–80 percent of your biggest day on the goal climb with 100 percent of the weight you expect to carry.

- One midweek Zone 1–2 aerobic maintenance workout, 10 percent of weekly volume.

- One Max Strength maintenance workout as warm-up for core routine.

- All other training hours are performed at recovery level.

Week 4: Volume equal to 70 percent of your last Base Period week (week 20 volume). Graduation week!

- This is a consolidation week to allow this very high training load to be absorbed fully.

- Two big days in the mountains or one super-big day amounting to 75 percent of this week's volume and 150 percent of the goal climb's biggest vertical single day carrying 100 percent of the weight you expect to carry.

- One sustained Zone 3 uphill interval workout, wearing mountain boots, covering 80–90 percent of your goal climb's biggest vertical day and carrying 100 percent of the weight you expect to carry. This should now feel relatively easy.

- One Max Strength maintenance workout as warm-up for core routine.

- All other training hours are performed at recovery level.

Notes for the Specific Period weeks:

- Training becomes concentrated on the most specific methods that model as closely as possible the actual stress of your goal climb.

- This period requires careful recovery because the imposed stress of the main workouts is very high.

- Done properly, this block of training will set you up, both mentally and physically, for success. Done improperly, this will bury you.

- After this you are ready for a Taper Period.

- If you do not have big mountains nearby, your job will be harder from the specificity standpoint. At the minimum you'll need to find some hilly terrain, which you are going to become intimately familiar with. Then you'll have to adjust these workouts to fit your options.

Specific Period Plan for a Technical Alpine Objective

As for the mountaineering objective, the goal for this period is to create mini-simulations of the challenges you will face on your goal climb. By doing so, you will convert the basic fitness and climbing skills you've been developing over the past months and years. You will become an alpine climbing machine. It is during this period that you will develop the confidence and mental power to tackle new objectives. With your new, enhanced physical powers you will be in a position to shatter your old limits. This is not hyperbole; if you've done everything well to this point, you will be stronger than you've ever been in your life.

There are two ways to execute a Specific Period. The first is where a climbing trip is possible, such as what Steve did in Peru before his expedition to Nanga Parbat. A second, more common, method in which our hypothetical climber is tied to his home territory, is like what Scott did before heading to K2. We have already outlined the climbing trip plan by describing Steve's preparations for Nanga Parbat earlier in this chapter so we will instead focus here on the person who is tied to a home base.

Home-Based Conversion Period

Most climbers will be restricted to staying close to home for this period. Many will be simulating the vertical gain of their climb by hiking uphill, and often the technical climbing must be done at a crag, usually combining these on the same day. We've had the best results by climbing first and then hiking in the afternoon.

For example, let's say your goal is to ascend Denali's Cassin Ridge and you expect to be on the route three days. The biggest day aerobically will be 4,000 vertical feet (1,219 meters) of steep snow climbing to the 20,320-foot (6,194-meter) summit, but no technical climbing. The most technical climbing would likely be seven to twelve pitches wearing a heavy pack at the start of the route. None of the climbing is harder than a short section of 5.8 rock or seventy-degree ice.

Example of a Specific Period Training Plan for the Cassin Ridge

Week 1

- Two days, each involving 100 percent of the vertical gain by steep hiking or scrambling, *and* 100 percent of technical climbing of the biggest single day on your goal climb. These workouts take however much time you need to complete that task. These two days must be separated by at least seventy-two hours of recovery.

- Your pack should weigh 50 percent of the weight you expect to carry.

- One Muscular Endurance maintenance workout or cragging day where you climb five to ten pitches as close to your limit as you can do safely.

- All other training hours are performed at recovery level.

Week 2

- Two days, each involving 110 percent of the vertical gain by steep hiking or scrambling, *and* 110 percent of technical climbing of the biggest single day on your goal climb. These workouts take however much time you need to complete that task. These two days must be separated by at least seventy-two hours of recovery.

- Your pack should weigh 50 percent of the weight you expect to carry.

- Each climb should be separated by two or three rest days.

- One Muscular Endurance maintenance workout or cragging day where you climb five to ten pitches as close to your limit as you can do safely.

- All other training hours are performed at recovery level.

Week 3

- Two days, each involving 120 percent of the vertical gain by steep hiking or scrambling, *and* 120 percent of technical climbing of the biggest single day on your goal climb. These workouts take however much time you need to complete that task. These two days must be separated by at least seventy-two hours of recovery.

Ueli Steck climbing on the north face of the Mönch (13,474', 4,107m), Switzerland. *Photo: Jonathan Griffith*

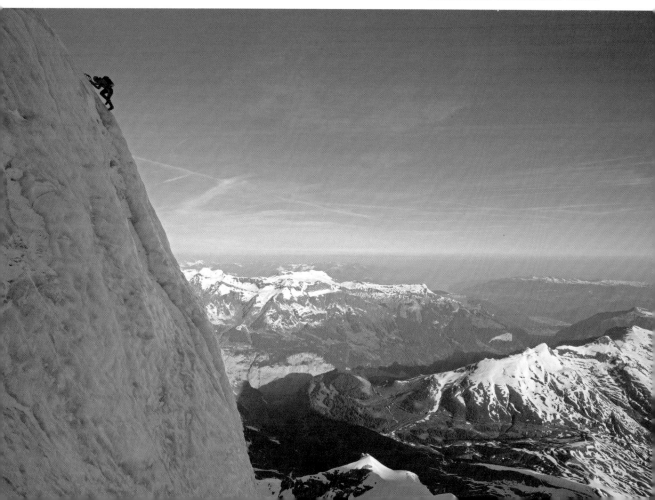

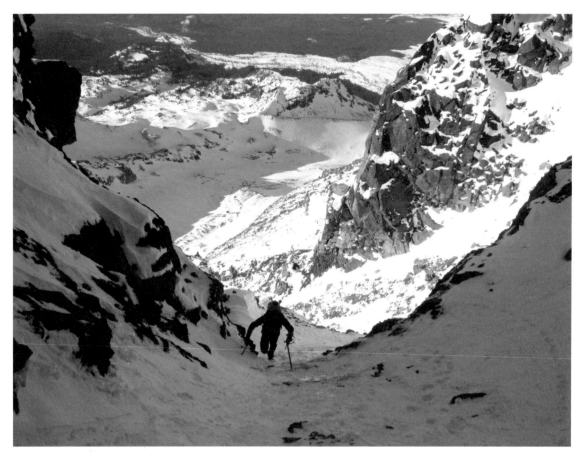

Many people have all-day mountaineering objectives within a day's travel from their homes such as this peak, North Sister in the Central Oregon Cascades.
Photo: Steve House

- Your pack should weigh 50 percent of the weight you expect to carry.

- One Muscular Endurance maintenance workout or cragging day where you climb five to ten pitches as close to your limit as you can do safely.

- All other training hours are performed at recovery level.

Week 4

- This is a consolidation week with the same loading as the previous week, allowing your body a chance to absorb this very high training load.

- Two days, each involving 120 percent of vertical gain steep hiking or scrambling, *and* 120 percent of technical climbing of the biggest single day on your goal climb. These workouts take however much time you need to complete that task. These two days must be separated by at least seventy-two hours of recovery.

- Your pack should weigh 50 percent of the weight you expect to carry.

- One Muscular Endurance maintenance workout or cragging day where you climb five to ten pitches as close to your limit as you can do safely.

- All other training hours are performed at recovery level.

Alternate Week 4

Take a weekend road trip and do a graduation climb. Ascend a peak that is as similar to your goal climb as possible. Also consider doing something that will be technically harder, but at a lower elevation. For the Cassin Ridge you could plan a one-day ascent of Liberty Ridge. In the San Juan Mountains of Colorado, a good objective would be to link two ascents of two different routes on the north face of Mount Sneffels in one day or do one of the routes starting from the trailhead and back in a day. The aim of these is to challenge yourself physically, mentally, and technically so that you are at your peak for your goal.

Notes:

- The ideal Specific Period would involve a lot of time spent climbing that is as similar to your goal climb as possible.

- The idea is to acclimate your mind to the technical difficulties, risk management, and complexity of alpine climbing.

- You are trying to imitate your goal climb as closely as possible, but on a smaller scale.

- Ideally these climbs should be of the same nature as your goal climb. Climbing in Yosemite is appropriate if you're heading to Patagonia for alpine rock climbs. If you are heading to Alaska, the Canadian Rockies are an excellent warm-up.

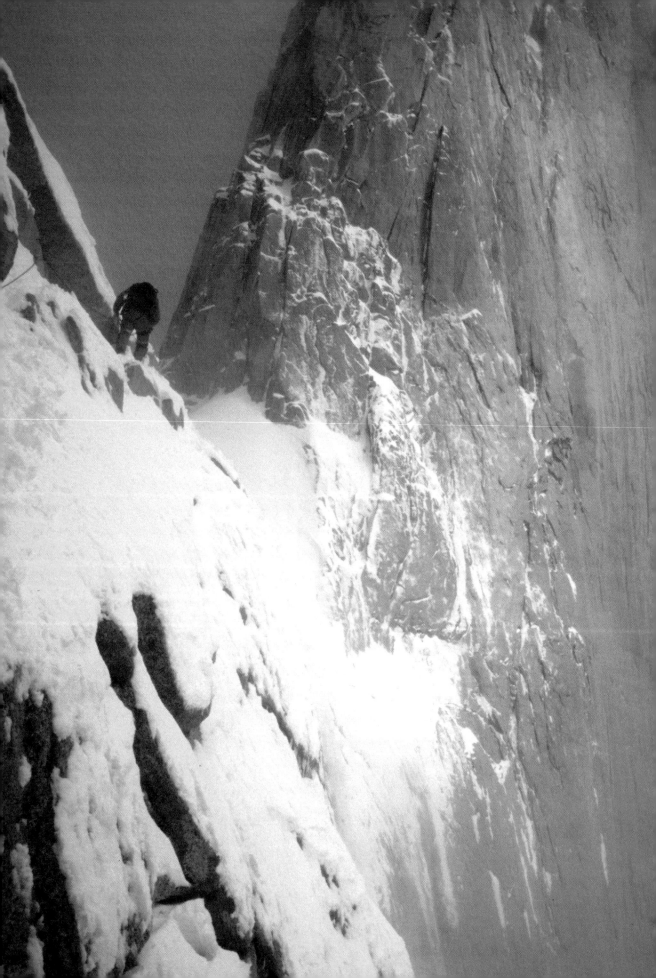

Chapter 10

Tapering

"Firm rock, rich in good holds. Up I go, no need
for pitons here. There is nothing finer than this
kind of unprotected climbing, with the abyss ever-
deepening below."

—HERMANN BUHL, climbing pioneer

TAPER TIMING

The purpose of the Taper Period is to allow your body to fully recover
and realize a maximum state of supercompensation from the long-
term stress of training. As you are coming off the intense Specific
Period and into the Taper Period you will dramatically drop both your
volume and intensity of training. This will result in the peaking effect
and you will reach your best fitness for the year.

The amount of time it will take for that supercompensation to
produce your peak will vary depending on the length and intensity of
your past training and the quality of your recovery. If you have done a
good job with your training up to this point, this will take about two
weeks of tapering to achieve peak fitness. If you engaged in continuous,
progressive training for a short time, less than four months, your Taper
Period may be much shorter, on the order of four to seven days.

Opposite: Alessandro Beltrami
reaching the Col of Patience and the
base of Cerro Torre's southeast ridge.
To the right is the east face of Cerro
Torre. *Photo: Rolando Garibotti*

Once at your peak, a maintenance program can keep you there for up to six weeks.

Taper Period Activities

This is a critical period and you've invested a lot to get here. Now that the training is over and the money is in the bank (so to speak), your job is to stay healthy and be rested. Illness and overexertion can derail months of preparation and destroy any chance of success.

It takes much less effort to maintain a level of fitness than it does to achieve that state in the first place. As you may recall from chapter 3, aerobic capacity is the first aspect of fitness to be lost. Studies have shown that after five days of bed rest, mitochondrial mass decreases as much as 50 percent. This doesn't mean that your aerobic capacity is lost this quickly; it is made up of more than just the density of mitochondria. The good news is that those precious mitochondria respond quickly to continued training bouts, and a light load of aerobic activity during the Taper Period will keep them on duty.

You will need to do one or two long, easy aerobic Zone 1–2 outings per week to keep your aerobic capacity tuned. As a climber your taper will likely include travel or approaching your climb, in which case you may have enough activity. If you are travelling at the beginning of a longer expedition you will likely be more sedentary, but as you will almost always be starting a long, slow trek to higher altitude, don't worry about it. It's certainly not worth the various health risks of running in Kathmandu to try to save a few mitochondria. Regular aerobic-level activity allows you to extend the taper and peak climbing fitness for several weeks.

Earlier we looked at the example of Scott's specific preparation for K2. His taper lasted only as long as the travel to base camp, about two weeks' worth of flights, repacking, jeep rides, and trekking. During this period his training volume dropped by close to 50 percent and the week-long trek to base camp served the purpose of maintaining the aerobic base while allowing time for acclimatization and recovery from the very high training load he had been carrying before leaving for Pakistan. It was crucial that while dealing with the stress of traveling half-way around the world and adjusting to a new time zone, different food, and high altitude, he didn't impose any additional training load. He arrived in base camp rested, healthy, and at peak fitness.

When Steve returned from his Peru expedition with Marko, which served as his specific preparation period before Nanga Parbat he rested completely for four days at home before going on a week-long trip to the beach where he relaxed at sea level, except for one all-day run/hike. Returning home, he spent the remaining three weeks before climbing the Rupal Face on Nanga Parbat in a maintenance cycle, which meant one long, easy hike per week, one to two water-carry workouts per week, and twice-weekly strength training to preserve his Max Strength and Muscular Endurance gains. At the end of these three weeks, he had a further week of rest during the travel to Pakistan and base camp.

While this may seem like a long Taper Period, it served the purpose of making sure he was absolutely rested. The risk of getting sick, even a cold, en route to base camp is very high. The demands placed on your body by acclimating to climb an 8,000-meter peak are significant. This substantial Taper Period was, in our opinion, a significant factor in the success of that expedition.

Prolonging the Peak and Dealing with Stagnation in Performance

To prolong your peak season beyond six weeks, create a period of time where you can return to training both your aerobic and strength base for two to three weeks.

After you experience a peak or a highpoint of fitness you will start to regress. This is easily observed in sport climbing, the all-too-common scenario being that a climber working a project stops making progress, or is unable to reach a previous highpoint. Barring mental factors, this would be the indicator to take time off from specific fitness (meaning, that climb), go back to basic strength and fitness work for a couple of weeks, and then return to the project.

If you are on an extended climbing trip and want to extend your peak, simply return to two weeks of structured, high-volume endurance and strength training.

In alpine climbing this could happen when you're attempting several climbs near your limit. In 2004 Steve spent six weeks attempting, and eventually succeeding, in climbing K7. Bruce Miller, along with Doug Chabot, also climbed K7 during that same expedition. After a two-week rest at low altitude, which included some adventure travel, Steve and Bruce started up Nanga Parbat for an attempt on the Rupal Face. They should have realized that they had peaked on their

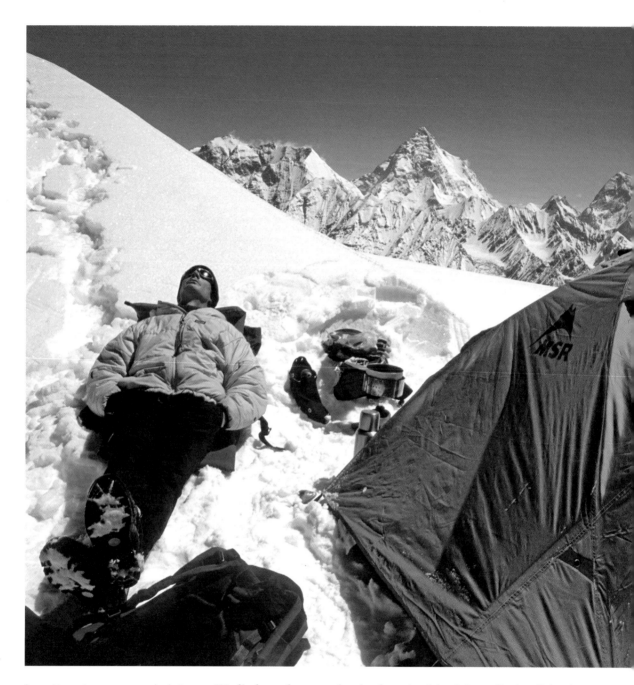

Steve House in recovery mode during the first days of an expedition to Masherbrum (25,659', 7,821m). K2 (28,251', 8,611m) and Broad Peak (26,414', 8,051m) can be seen across the valley. *Photo: Marko Prezelj*

K7 climbs and expected to be de-trained (and de-acclimiated) by the time they felt rested enough to attempt Nanga Parbat.

Ideally, they should have rested for one to two weeks, then executed two weeks of solid base training had they wanted to try to create a second peak for Nanga Parbat. This is a problem with the multi-peak expedition where you attempt to climb several mountains on one trip. If the climbs are too far apart, while you may consolidate gains in acclimatization, the de-training effect will be significant.

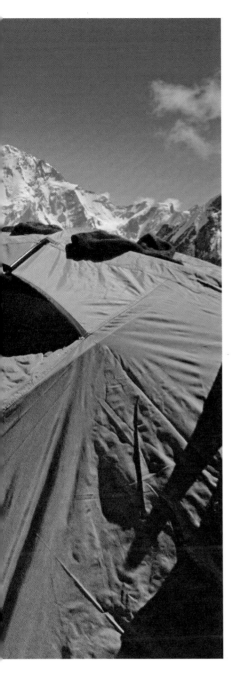

Taper and Altitude

Altitude and acclimating to high mountains presents many unique challenges, which we discuss in detail in chapter 13. Being aerobically fit will help you to keep your heart rate as low as possible during all outings. Use your breathing as a governor; stay at a conversational pace, something that will come naturally after completing hours of training at this exertion level.

A common problem for inexperienced alpinists is that the approach to, or the first days of, the objective climb is as hard or harder than much of the training they have done. The approach should be a fun and relatively mellow experience.

You cannot consider the trek to base camp as physical training. If you are expecting to get fit on the approach, then you have missed the point of this book. The scenario of climbers erring by going too hard on the approach and exposing themselves to illness and fatigue has played itself out many times in the great ranges.

Taper and International Travel

Shifting time zones creates its own stress. The first days you arrive in Kathmandu, for example, are some of the most important days for your expedition; many crucial decisions will be made during that time. These are also days where it is easy to get sick.

The rule of thumb is to allow one day of for each hour of time change before expecting to feel normal again. In distant time zones,

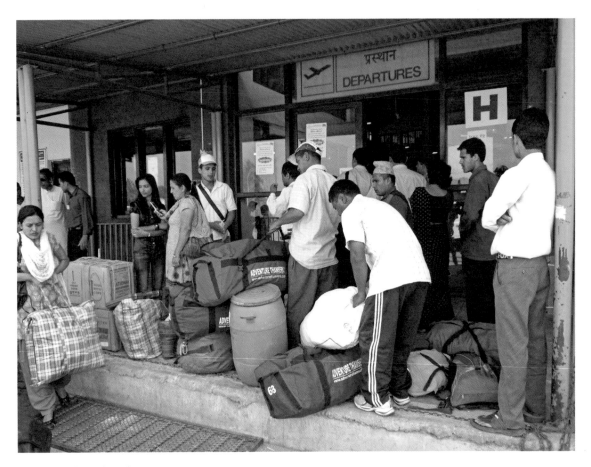

International travel can be more chaotic and stressful than restful.
Photo: Steve House

sleep aids can be useful to help adjust your sleep pattern to the new nighttime.

Experts recommend setting your watch to the destination time upon boarding the plane and only napping when it is night at your destination. If you bring your own food onboard you can time your in-flight meals to meal times at your destination. The timing of in-flight caffeine and alcohol should also be adjusted so they are consumed during the appropriate time at your destination.

In adjusting to your new time zone it helps to understand that large delays of the body clock are easier to achieve than large advances. To delay your body clock would be to fly from New York City to Los Angeles. For a New York denizen to stay up until midnight, in Los Angeles your body clock would be at 3 a.m. This is easier to accomplish than the reverse, in which case if your bedtime in New York is 10 p.m., your body clock will say it's only 7 p.m. and you can't fall asleep.

Sleep experts recommend that you should try to advance your body clock when flying eastward only when you cross eight or fewer time zones. After a flight to the east for more than eight time zones, avoid sleeping during the flight so that you can sleep on arrival. If this is not possible stay indoors upon arrival, avoiding sunlight. In this example, you're trying to delay your body clock.

After a flight to the west across more than eight time zones, get out and about upon arrival to get used to the new schedule of light exposure. Naps the first few days after arrival can be useful and do not have to be avoided as long as they are not long enough to hinder nighttime sleep in the new destination.

Jet Lag

Flying East (Less than 8-hour shift)	Flying East (more than an 8-hour shift)	Flying West (any amount of time shift)
Body clock must be advanced	Body clock must be delayed	Body clock must be delayed
Avoid morning light at new destination; seek afternoon light at new destination	Get outside as soon as possible in the new daytime	Get outside as soon as possible in the new daytime

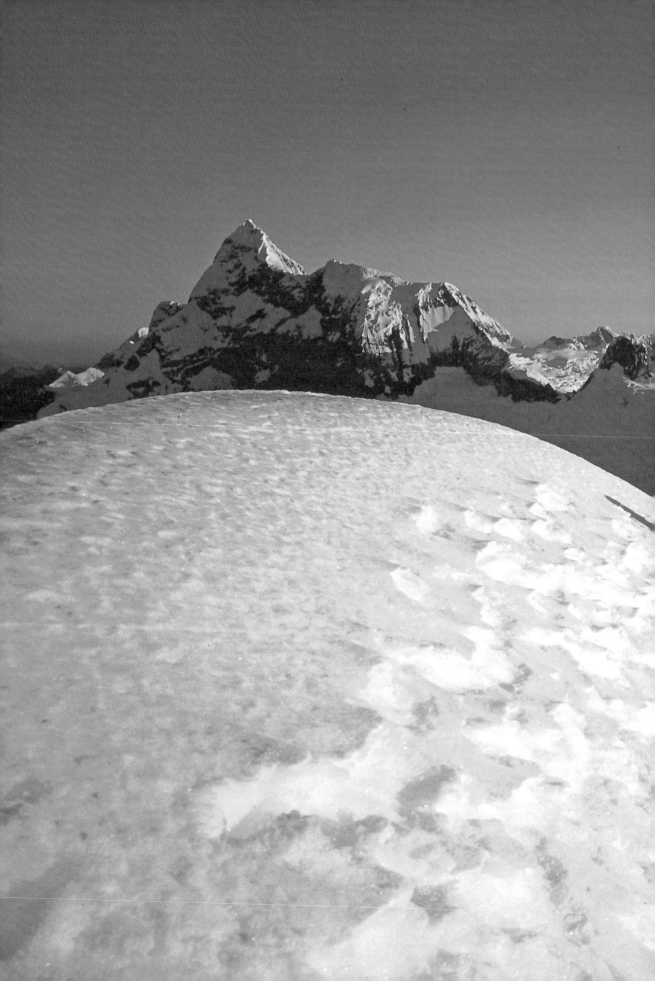

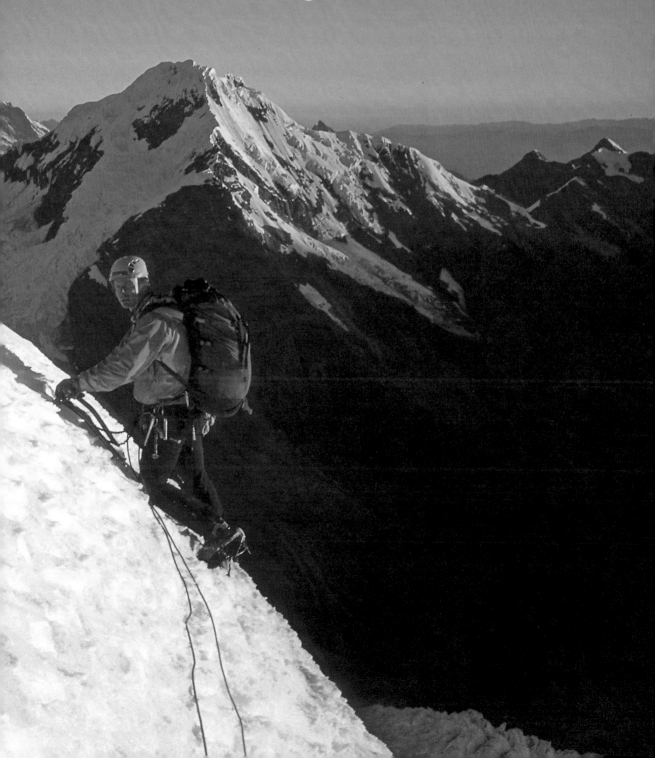

Section 3

Tools for Training

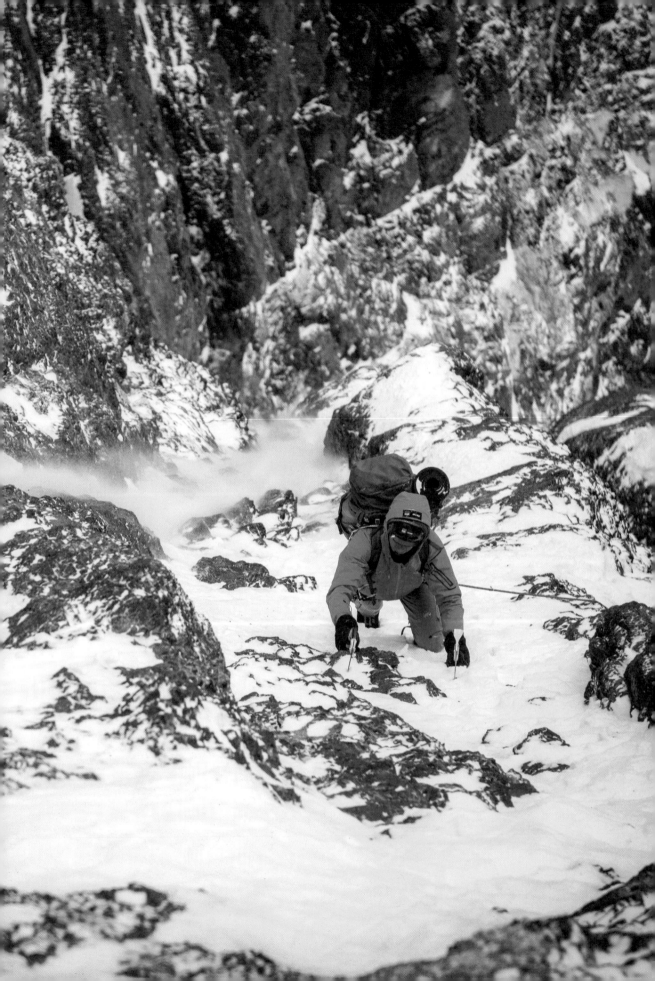

Chapter 11

Nutrition: Eating with Purpose

"Eat Food. Not too much. Mostly vegetables."

— MICHAEL POLLAN, author of
The Omnivore's Dilemma and food-guru

EATING FOR CLIMBING PERFORMANCE

Eating with a purpose is key to increasing your capacity for any sport. We believe it is one of the most important aspects of climbing performance. We've heard fitness experts claim, though it is difficult to put science behind this, that our bodies are 60 percent the food we eat and 40 percent the exercise we do. Regardless of the numbers, nutrition is hugely important to health and performance. When taken as a whole, shopping, cooking, eating, and washing-up is also one of the most time-consuming aspects of training.

THE COMPONENTS OF FOOD

Eating while training, eating while on an expedition, and eating while on a route are all different and are governed by the differing

Opposite: Stephan Siegrist climbs above the Exit Cracks of the 1938 Route on the north face of the Eiger (13,025', 3,970m). *Photo: Thomas Senf*

Previous spread: Steve House descends from the summit of Cayesh (18,760', 5,719m) during a preparatory expedition to Peru shortly before climbing Nanga Parbat in 2005. *Photo: Marko Prezelj*

circumstances and demands of each circumstance. Before diving into the minutiae, we need to understand food as its three macronutrient components: carbohydrates, protein, and fat.

Carbohydrates

Carbohydrates include familiar staples such as pasta, bread, potatoes, and rice. All carbohydrates contain four calories per gram. But the carbohydrate group also includes starchy vegetables and sugary foods such as fruit, soda pop, honey, and chocolate, as well as savory snack foods like corn and potato chips. Your digestive system breaks all carbohydrates down into glucose. Glucose is the simple sugar that fuels your brain, your entire nervous system, and much of your physical motion. Most climbers we know consume plenty of carbohydrate-rich foods because they are cheap and plentiful.

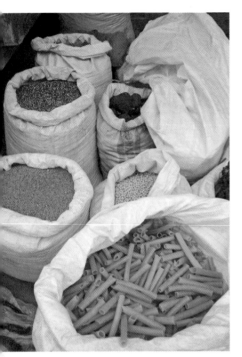

Pasta, lentils, and beans are common food staples available in just about any market in the world. *Photo: Steve House*

Recently, some people have become somewhat anti-carbohydrate and put themselves at risk of consuming too few carbs in their diet. As we will see, this is just as bad as eating too little protein or too little fat. In a recent study on Everest in 2012, measured carbohydrate intake was about 3 g/kg (grams of carbohydrate per kilogram of body weight). Minimum recommendations are 5 g/kg; at high energy, expenditures are likely to be 7–10 g/kg.

Carbohydrates vary widely in quality with regard to athletic performance. It is useful to understand that some carbohydrates are considered sugars, others as starches. Sugars (simple sugars) include most candy, soft drinks, condiments, processed and enriched breads (such as white bread), cakes, and jam, but also some healthy foods such as fruits. Sugary foods generally are ones that give you a quick rush of energy and then subsequent low as the carbohydrate gets used up. Starchy foods (complex carbohydrates) include vegetables and whole grain foods such as brown rice and pasta. Starchy sources of carbohydrates give you a longer-lasting source of energy.

Proteins

Aside from water, protein is the most abundant molecule in the body and is the major structural component of all cells, especially muscle. Proteins contain four calories per gram. Your digestive system breaks protein into amino acids. Amino acids are the building blocks of new cells and important for repairing damaged tissue and maintaining immune function.

Meat and poultry do not contain carbohydrates. Foods such as eggs, hard cheeses, avocado, nuts, or oils contain very small amounts of carbohydrates, but nutritionists consider them as protein or fat foods. Foods without any carbohydrate component have little effect on your blood sugar levels in the first hours following your meal. High fiber also slows the post-meal rise in blood glucose.

How Much Protein?

We have heard many climbers wonder how much protein they should consume when climbing hard. Indeed, a lot of research has gone into attempting to answer this question for athletes. The American and Canadian daily dietary reference intake guidelines recommend 0.8 grams of protein per kilogram of body weight for a person of average activity level.

If you're climbing and training for climbing, you exercise more than the average person.

The most recent research concludes that endurance training, defined as training that lasts two to five hours, causes the athlete's protein intake requirement to increase. Current guidelines suggest a range of 1.2 to 1.4 grams of protein intake per kilogram of body weight per day for endurance athletes, 50 to 85 percent more than the recommendations for non-athletes. For ultra-endurance distance athletes, those training for and competing in events lasting over five hours, the recommendation is 1.2 to 2.0 grams per kilogram, the higher value being for those starting out with endurance training and those engaging in high volumes of training.

In many mountainous areas the main protein sources often consist of live goats, sheep, and sometimes yaks. As there is no food for these animals on the glacier they have to be slaughtered and consumed quickly.
Photo: Marko Prezelj

The reasoning for this increased protein intake is based on two factors: First, 5 to 10 percent of an endurance athlete's total energy typically comes from digested protein, and that needs to be replaced. Second, protein is required for repairing the muscle and tissue damage inherent to endurance sports. Endurance athletes do not build much new muscle except in the early adaptive years when beginning real training. However, your body is always replacing mitochondria, capillaries, nerves, and other cellular structures.

High-Protein Diets

Some climbers follow a high-protein, low-carb diet, which for many helps them feel lean. This works because protein is a thermogenic nutrient, which means that it is less likely than carbs or fats to be stored as body fat. In addition, the body has to work hard to break down protein; 20 to 30 percent of its already-low caloric value is lost in digestion.

As of the time of this writing there are no scientific studies that have been published in a peer-reviewed scientific journal that demonstrate any performance benefit of a high-protein diet. This type of diet can be of concern if an athlete is eating high protein and low carbohydrates because a low-carb intake could then lead to depleted glycogen stores, which will cause reduced performance in exercise lasting longer than half an hour. The second downside of the high-protein diet is the high environmental cost of producing meat. We, along with the current sports-nutrition science consensus, recommend replacing high protein diets with ones containing balanced levels of carbohydrate, protein, and fats.

Fats

As Steve's experience in his "Learning to Fuel" story illustrates, athletes frequently undervalue dietary fat as a contributor to performance and health. There are four types of dietary fat, more precisely fatty acids: saturated, monounsaturated, polyunsaturated, and trans. All fats contain nine calories per gram. While the types of fat are more related to long-term health, as an athlete you need to be aware that just because you're highly active does not give you carte blanche to eat anything you want. Heart disease occurs in athletes too.

KEY NUTRITIONAL KNOWLEDGE

Mixing Foods

Most of the time we eat meals composed of all three macronutrient components. By mixing fats and proteins with carbohydrates, say chicken with rice topped with some fresh avocado, you effectively balance the macronutrients, which explains why eating just rice can leave you feeling hungry, but chicken and rice is a satisfying meal. Snacking on high-fat foods, such as nuts, that also contain significant amounts of carbohydrate also leaves you satisfied for longer. Adding fiber to a meal is another way to experience the *full* effect.

Learning to Fuel

By Steve House

I began a slow jog around the dirt track on the edge of the Central Oregon Community College campus. Nearby, in a pre-fab building partially hidden by the morning fog, two exercise physiologists prepared their lab. A treadmill, engineered for training horses and modified for humans to cross-country ski on with roller skis, stood underneath breathing masks and wires. I was due to hike, and eventually run with ski poles, in a simulated cross-country skiing motion, while hooked up to machines measuring the gases in my exhalations and my heart rate, and be needle-pricked every three minutes to measure blood lactate.

The results of that day put me at a VO_2 max of 61.5ml/kg, not horrible but not world class, either. In most endurance sports you'd need a score of 75 to be considered decent. I did come away with an accurate measurement of my ideal heart-rate training zones, which would be helpful in my quest to climb the Rupal Face of Nanga Parbat. But what was most interesting from this experiment was that, by measuring my steady-state exercise respiratory exchange ratio (the volume of CO_2 divided by the volume of O_2 I exhaled), the physiologists could see that I was relying almost entirely on carbohydrate for fuel.

Dr. Julie Downing, the head physiologist, asked me to keep a food journal for two weeks and return. Two weeks later, as she leafed through the pages of salad, eggs, skinless chicken breast, kale, and cabbage, I heard her say to herself, *"Where's the fat?"* Indeed, I had been avoiding almost all foods containing fat in an effort to stay light for climbing. Dr. Downing estimated I'd been getting 5 percent of my calories from fat with my diet and suggested that I needed to get approximately 30 percent of my calories from fat. After that, my new breakfast included an entire avocado, and I began using olive oil generously. I took fish-oil supplements and upped my intake of red meat from one to two or three servings per week. Armed with this new regimen I continued training.

Two months later I returned. After warming up, I weighed in. I was a whopping 170 pounds, the heaviest I'd been in my life and six pounds heavier than before. I was immediately disheartened. VO_2 max is a measure of how much oxygen you process per kilogram of body weight, and with my extra weight, I was sure to score worse now. But as the treadmill spun faster, I felt strong, steady, and energetic. The track got slowly steeper, but I kept up the pace, feeling powerful, until suddenly I struggled and in a flash, I was off the back. The stop button was pushed, I donated one last blood sample and then went out to do a few slow laps around the track while the data dumped out of the computer.

"Great news," piped Dr. Downing as I reentered the lab. *"You increased your VO_2 max by 10 percent!"* As we went through the numbers, everything was up, and my new VO_2 max was a more respectable 68.5ml/kg. This was extra encouraging given my weight gain. My body fat had remained exactly the same, 5.6 percent, the six pounds I had gained in muscle allowed a very significant increase in my aerobic work capacity. In the earlier test I had run out of fuel at sixteen minutes; this time around I held onto my energy stores for a full twenty-three and a half minutes, 50 percent longer, a result she attributed to my increased, now more balanced, fat intake and the related increased calorie intake that supported a healthier muscle mass. She considered this proof that I had been consuming too few calories for my activity level, and especially insufficient fat, creating a low-level starvation that negatively affected my athletic capacity.

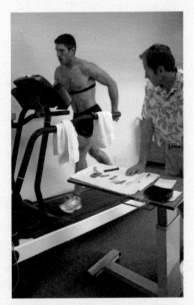

Scott Johnston looks on as Sam Naney completes a lactate threshold test on a treadmill. *Photo: Scott Johnston collection*

Types of Fatty Acids

Fat	Found in	Example foods	Comments
Saturated fat	Meat and dairy	Beef, milk, coconut oil, butter, cream, half and half, hard margarine, bacon	Required to build certain hormones, but should be limited due to its effects on cholesterol and arterial plaque build-up.
Monounsaturated fatty acid	Vegetables and nuts	Olives, olive oil, peanut oil, canola oil, avocado, peanuts, almonds, hazelnuts, pecans, pistachios	Most fat calories in your diet should come from this group.
Polyunsaturated fatty acid, including omega-3	Fish, some nuts, and certain vegetable oils	Fish, corn oil, flaxseed oil, sunflower oil, soybean oil, squeezable margarine, mayonnaise, walnuts, flax seeds	May help fight inflammatory diseases such as arthritis and heart disease. Omega-3s may decrease inflammation.
Trans fatty acid	In nearly all fatty foods in small amounts	Mostly in processed and fast foods	Mostly a long-term health concern. Often labeled as "hydrogenated oil." Trans fat lowers good cholesterol and raises bad cholesterol levels.

The Role of Insulin

Eating food, and in particular food that contains carbohydrate or protein, triggers your body to secrete insulin, a hormone that regulates carbohydrate, protein, and fat metabolism. This affects the body in three important ways.

First, insulin can be thought of as the key to the door through which glucose passes into your cells for metabolism.

Second, insulin has an anabolic effect. This means that it triggers (turns on) your body's signal to build new protein structures, in particular repairing and building new muscle.

Third, the level of insulin in your body controls how glycogen (future fuel) and fats are stored in your muscles and liver after you've digested your food.

Key points to remember:

- Sugars burn quickly, starches more slowly.

- The presence of sugar and amino acids trigger your body to produce insulin.

Fat Is Our Fuel

The body has very large fat stores, in terms of energy. An average fit athlete has 2,000 kcals of energy stored as carbohydrate intramuscularly and in the liver. In comparison, the same fit athlete has over

Exercise Intensity and Fuel Source

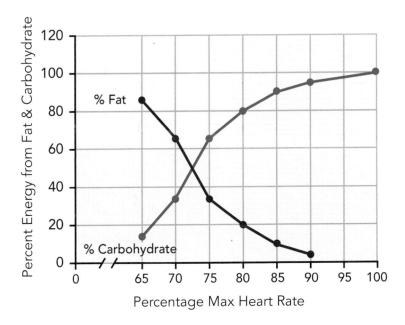

This graph shows how the intensity of exercise affects the muscles' choice of fuel in a well-trained endurance athlete. Low to moderate intensities (as measured by heart rate) rely predominately on fat as the fuel source. As the intensity rises the need for rapid ATP synthesis demands more and more contribution from glycolysis which requires the breakdown of carbohydrates to supply the needed sugars for fuel. The downside to the high-intensity work is that the body's glycogen stores are very limited, so these rates of work cannot be sustained for the times that are meaningful for alpine climbers. Since alpine climbs are typically done at intensities that average in the 60–70 percent range of max heart rate, alpine climbers are best advised to train so as to enhance their reliance on fat. Source: Wikipedia commons.

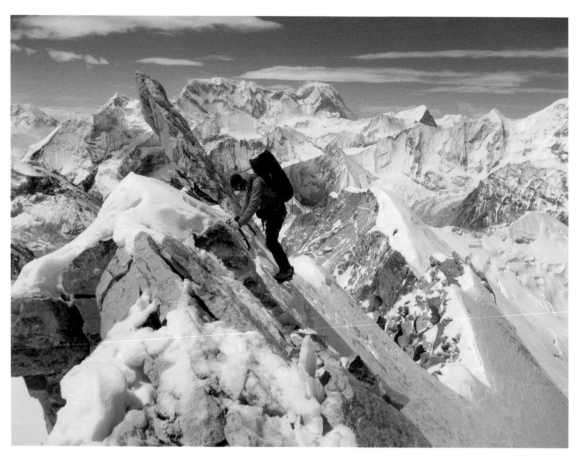

Marko Prezelj fat-burning during the first traverse of the Chago Ridge (up to 22,440', 6,640m), Makalu Himal. *Photo: Steve House*

100,000 kcals in fat stores, mostly in adipose tissue (the fat under your skin). Theoretically, that's enough energy for a runner to run for 100 hours (assuming the runner could rely solely on fat metabolism). As alpinists, it serves us well to tap into those energy reserves as much as possible. The food bag in your pack is heavy, yet we already carry lots of energy with us all the time. The trick is to train your body and eat strategically so that you burn this energy source and need less food.

Proportionally, we burn a greater percentage of our total calories as fat at rest, during low-intensity exercise, and during long-duration exercise (greater than one hour). As exercise intensity increases, our fuel source tilts towards carbohydrates.

Carbohydrate Ingestion, Insulin, and Your Ability to Burn Fat

Carbohydrate ingestion during the hours before exercise, even in relatively small amounts, reduces fat oxidation during exercise largely through the action of insulin. Eating simple-carbohydrate-rich foods such as energy gels, energy bars, or candy bars before or during training or alpine climbing impacts your ability to burn stored fat as a fuel and negatively affects long-duration, low-intensity performance.

The reason for this is that carbohydrate ingestion causes the release of insulin, and when you have insulin in your bloodstream this effectively blocks a minimum of 30 percent of the use of free fatty acids as an active fuel source. However, both exercise and epinephrine (adrenaline) suppress insulin output. Once you start exercising, insulin gets mostly shut off and you can begin to use fat as a fuel. The thing to note here is not to eat a gel or bar right before training or climbing at low intensity. A small snack with a balance of carbs and fats is best immediately before starting to climb (to the degree to which your stomach can tolerate it).

The exact degree to which mid-exercise carbohydrate ingestion affects moderate- to high-intensity performance is an area of ongoing debate among sports nutrition scientists. Probably the adaption is highly individual and dependent on fitness. What is very well understood is that at a certain level of high-intensity exercise, fat oxidation is decreased, carbohydrate becomes the main fuel source for exercise, and at the same time digestion nearly ceases.

Exercise Duration and Fuel Utilization

An important reality of nutrition and exercise is that the longer your exercise period lasts, the more you must rely on fat as a fuel. You simply burn through those 2,000 calories or so of stored carbohydrate and you become dependent on fat as a fuel. Depending on the individual's fitness, their diet, and their exercise intensity, after about sixty to ninety minutes of exercise you need to start replacing carbohydrates that are needed in the fat metabolism process in order to continue to provide fuel for aerobic metabolism. Without feeding you will eventually bonk.

Fuel Utilization Trainability

It is important to reiterate that this "sweet spot" of fat-burning intensity is highly trainable. Recall from our earlier discussions of physiology that you can significantly raise both your aerobic and anaerobic thresholds through training and, by extension, significantly raise the exertion level at which you can rely primarily on fat as your fuel source. Much of this adaptation is thought to be due to the increased number and size of the trained muscles' mitochondria. As you become more fit, you develop the ability to use more fat at a given exercise intensity which in turn allows you to stretch out those precious glycogen stores. This incredible adaptability explains why well-trained athletes are capable of such mind-blowing feats of endurance.

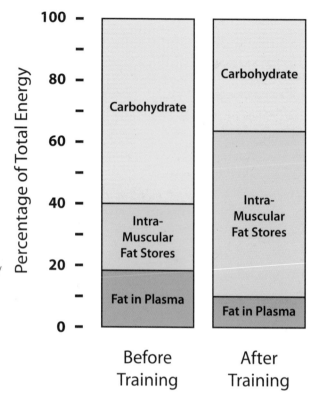

The Trainability of Fuel Usage

This chart shows the effects of twelve weeks of endurance training on the body's selection of preferential fuel use measured during thirty minutes of endurance exercise at an intensity of 64 percent of the athlete's VO_2 max. This is an intensity that corresponds to that which an alpine climber will mainly use. Through proper training you can train your muscles to utilize more fat for the same rate of work. Source: Martin et al, 1993.

It is important to remember that all long-duration aerobic exercise requires some carbohydrate for lipolysis, the biochemical process of converting stored bodily fat into fuel. This means we always need to be providing our bodies with some carbohydrates while climbing; it becomes a question of when and how much.

EATING WHILE TRAINING FOR ALPINE CLIMBING

Before we examine the best foods to eat while climbing, let's look at what we should eat throughout training. Combining good dietary choices with exercise will give you the best results in your training. We also want to keep in mind that as climbers, our strength-to-weight ratio is crucial. Our philosophy about eating for training can be summarized in the following points:

■ Eat early: A big breakfast with a lot of calories from all three sources (carb/protein/fat) is the best way to fuel a big day. If it's been more than two hours since breakfast, eat a simple-carbohydrate pre-work-out snack twenty minutes before you begin in order to top up your glycogen stores.

- Experiment: Training is the time to find what foods work best for you in different circumstances.

- Eat often: Feed on small snacks throughout the day. During low-intensity training sessions, mix snacks containing a balance of macronutrients in with predominantly carbohydrate snacks. During higher-intensity training sessions, eat predominantly carbo-hydrate snacks only. Or sip on a carbo-hydrate-rich drink mix.

- Balance: Include carbohydrate, protein, and small amounts of healthy fats in all meals.

- Immediately after exercise, consume carbohydrates and fluids.

Before Training

Start every day with a full breakfast consumed two to four hours before train-ing. This is important. Not only do you have to replace the liver glycogen depleted while you were sleeping, you have to lay in extra glycogen for the coming training. It is not an exaggeration that breakfast is the most important meal of the day; this is especially true for athletes.

The Slovenian alpinist Marko Prezelj, a true endurance machine, invariably takes a lot of time to eat a huge breakfast. When he goes climbing he goes all day with little to eat or drink, but without suffering from flagging energy midday. He rarely takes a lunch at all, and drinks only plain water, usually a half liter or less during the day. This regime works for him; experiment and find out what works for you.

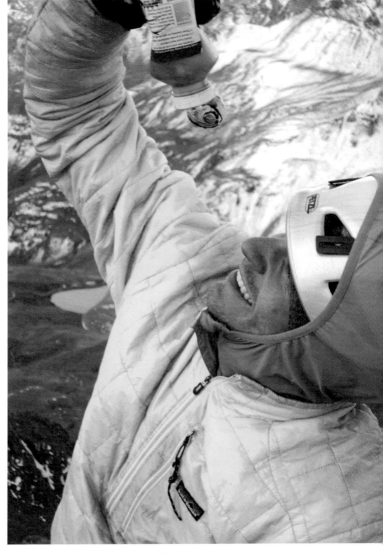

If you choose to use energy gels on a cold day, be sure to keep them someplace warm. *Photo: Steve House*

Skillet or Blender?

If Steve has a big training day planned he gets up early enough to eat a big breakfast, typically three eggs scrambled in a large pan full of spinach or kale cooked in olive oil, plus a whole avocado and three or four pieces of homemade amaranth-flour bread with butter.

His second favorite breakfast is the same bread toasted with butter and avocado topped with mild-tasting cold cuts.

If he doesn't have time for these, he'll put apple cider, fresh kale, spinach, ginger, bananas, and whatever other vegetables he can find combined with an oil supplement and twenty to twenty-five grams of whey protein in the blender. Whey is the most bio-available form of protein; it contains leucine (an important amino acid) and it's cheap. It is derived from milk so some people may not tolerate it as well as a vegetarian source such as soy. If you do go with the blender method you'd be wise to include an oil supplement (Udo's Oil is a good and popular supplement) or take a fish-oil supplement to balance fat with the protein and carbohydrates in your daily diet. It is also good to add oil if you need to add total calories to your diet; omega-3s are thought to help control inflammation.

Eat Often

When training for more than 120 minutes, it is important to eat during your workout. Not only so you have a good workout, but also for good recovery.

Ideal Levels of Carbohydrate Intake for High-Intensity Activity

For athletes engaged in high-intensity exercise for thirty to sixty minutes or longer, sport science recommends consuming thirty to seventy grams (120–280 calories) of carbohydrate per hour. This is based on numerous studies that suggest endurance athletes perform best ingesting 1.0–1.2 grams of carbohydrate per minute, which is the maximal oxidation rate of carbohydrate. To get that much carbohydrate, you'd have to consume one of the following *each hour* evenly over the hour:

- 1 liter of sugary sports drink (6–8% carbohydrate)

- 1.5 Power Bars

- 1.5 Clif Bars

- 3 medium bananas

- 3–4 energy gels, depending on the brand

We can't, and don't, typically eat that much while training. The one and a half Clif Bars or three energy gels per hour may be a viable goal on a road bike or in an organized foot race with support stations. In climbing you can't just let go and grab a snack, and it's rare to have time to eat so much.

One important aim of eating while training is to prevent the depletion of glycogen stores in the muscles and liver so you recover as quickly as possible. You don't want to bonk while training; that's counterproductive. Also, you need to provide sufficient calories plus raw materials for repairing tissue damaged by the act of training.

We know we have to eat frequently and consume more than what is reasonably possible. Where is the balance? From our own experience and the recommendations of the American College of Sports Medicine, we've learned that for training lasting for more than one hour we should:

- Consume a minimum of 100 calories per hour. When we have the chance, we'll eat more.

- The higher the intensity, the more carbohydrate.

- The longer the duration, the more balanced carbohydrate/protein/fat intake. Eat when you get to a belay or at the start of periods where you'll be less active and have time to digest before starting up again.

- The higher the intensity, the more difficult it will be to eat. In this case you might try fluids instead of solid food. Remember: Digestion is hindered during exercise.

- Eat what you plan to eat while climbing. If you don't know what you will eat while climbing, use this time to find out.

Opportunivores

For all-day exercise at 50 percent of VO_2 max or less, it is believed that given sufficient time, humans can adapt to many different diets. We are opportunivores. Consider that climbers culturally predisposed to a high-fat/high-protein diet, think Russian, Polish, Kazakh, and Slovene, excel at technical, high-altitude climbing. However, Sherpas

Experimentation

One thing that we've experimented with, that worked for us, is training while fasting. If your training day is going to be less than two hours, wake up, drink black coffee (or tea) and water, and go train. The idea is to adapt your body to preferentially burn fat. This is often used in cycling—road cyclists may have invented the idea. There is evidence that it works to adapt our bodies to oxidizing fat for energy, a process aided by the caffeine, as long as the duration of the exercise is less than 120 minutes and the intensity is low.

The first dozen times you try this, you may feel yourself bonking after thirty to sixty minutes. This is especially likely if you are adapted to a high-carbohydrate diet and frequently include sugary drink mixes in your hydration. Remember what we said about at-rest carbohydrate intake altering fat metabolism; more than likely you're experiencing that phenomenon at work when you bonk after such a short time.

You do have to be careful that this method, or other experiments you may conduct on yourself, doesn't negatively impact your workout. If you can't complete your workout with the intensity and duration desired because you don't have enough energy, then you need to address this and eat more.

Research has found that while this type of training does work, it doesn't translate into increased performance. These studies have been conducted on conventional athletes who are operating at higher intensities and hence higher metabolic rates than alpinists. In climbing, one might argue that an increase in performance could result from having to carry less food or being able to sustain the low-intensity work for longer.

This is not a recommendation, rather something we've tried in our efforts to go longer on less food. It is outside of what current nutrition science recommends. However, training is the place to do these self-experiments.

and Tibetans, who typically eat a vegetable-based, low-protein/low-fat diet, are also high-performing high-altitude climbers, but are the dietary opposite.

Keep in mind when you read studies—sometimes propaganda—telling you what to eat while training and climbing, that most other athletes are working at much higher exercise intensities than most climbers, and so the results can be difficult to extrapolate to alpine climbing. A ski-mountaineering racer may operate at 85 percent of his max heart rate for most of the day. That athlete will need carbs to fuel. An alpine guide who ascends and descends Mount Rainier twenty times each summer can climb Rainier eating just about any food because the effort of climbing Mount Rainier is so easy for her. Take that same guide, and ask her to significantly increase her speed (intensity) on a climb, and she will no longer tolerate a sausage-and-cheese bagel for breakfast.

SUMMARY OF EATING DURING TRAINING

Evidence clearly suggests that for moderate-intensity exercise, such as most alpine climbing, the best daily diet is one with balanced fat, carbohydrate, and protein content. While exercising, you need consistent feeding of carbohydrates, but the longer the duration, the more you rely on fats as a fuel. Trained athletes have been shown to metabolize intra-muscular fats much better than untrained individuals and this aspect of your physiology is highly trainable. This reinforces the high value of establishing a large volume of low-intensity training in the Transition and Base Periods. Experiment with food while training and whenever possible try to train on the actual foods you will eat on an alpine climb.

Three Sisters in a Day on Only M&Ms

By Scott Johnston

While it may be open to debate whether Peanut M&M's are in fact nature's most perfect food, it is certainly beyond question that they are one of the tastiest and easiest snacks to carry. But could they provide enough of the nutritional needs for a fast, all-day outing in the mountains?

My pal and regular training partner Ben Husaby, a two-time Olympian in cross-country skiing, and I hatched a spur-of-the-moment plan to traverse all three of central Oregon's Three Sisters volcanoes in a day. Only North Sister contained any sort of technical difficulties with a bit of third- and fourth-class terrain. By going from North to South Sister we'd put that behind us early in the day while we were still fresh. This would leave the long expanses of snowfields and scree on the Middle and South Sisters for the afternoon.

We had no idea how long the day would be, and I didn't expect it to be quite as big a day as it turned out to be. Not a stickler for careful planning in general and especially on spontaneous occasions like this, I grabbed a one-pound bag of the Mars candy company's finest at a convenience store on the early-morning drive to the start of our adventure. I figured I'd just tough it out if I ran out of food.

The early hours of that July morning went smoothly as we quickly ran from the Three Creeks trailhead and gained the south ridge of North Sister. The scramble to the summit flew by and we were soon bombing head-long down the huge scree slopes toward the Collier Glacier. We raced over the top of Middle and glissaded down into the Chambers Lake Basin. Ben was snacking on a six-pack of bagel sandwiches with peanut butter. My bag of M&M's seemed to be doing the trick . . . until about halfway up the west side of South Sister when my gas tank went dry. I didn't even have fumes to run on. I went from chatting happily about the beer and burgers awaiting us back in Bend to a weaving, stumbling bumbly in two to three minutes. I was reduced to a

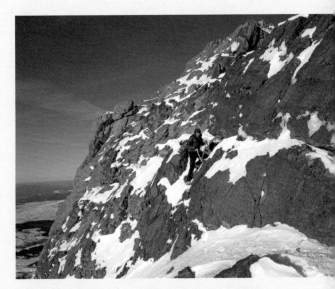

Mark Postle descends from the summit of North Sister (10,085', 3,074m) in early winter conditions, Cascades, Oregon. *Photo: Steve House*

literal crawl, needing my hands to steady myself on the touchy scree boulders.

Ben, who gains strength the longer the outing, quickly began to feed me the remains of his bagel stash. With one hand on my fanny pack to keep me steady, he pushed me up the slope. With the other hand he broke off pieces of bagel as quickly as I could stuff them into my mouth.

Within a few minutes I was back in the game and we pushed over the summit and raced down to the Devil's Lake parking lot and to our awaiting burgers, having learned a valuable nutritional lesson the hard way.

For such a long, demanding day in the mountains I would have been much better off eating a more balanced mix of simple and complex carbs, fat, and protein, as Ben chose.

POST-TRAINING NUTRITION

The most important time to fuel your post-exercise recovery is the thirty to sixty minutes right after you stop training. During this period you need to eat both carbohydrate and protein, and drink water, and include electrolytes in either your food or fluid.

- Carbohydrate: A 150-pound climber needs 270–400 calories of carbohydrate during this post-exercise window. For best recovery repeat this every two hours to re-stimulate glycogen resynthesis for up to six hours.

- Protein: Consuming protein after a workout is useful to help the body repair damaged muscle, but studies are inconclusive about whether or not the timing is as important as it is for carbohydrate consumption.

- Fluid. Drink water and replace electrolytes. Adjust your intake to match the temperature and the amount you've sweated.

The table on the right summarizes recommended eating practices before, during, and after training and climbing.

The Rest of the Day

Because your strength-to-weight ratio is so important for your climbing you must consistently make good food choices. Each day you are training you're investing between one and twelve hours in working out. That leaves up to twenty-three hours of the day where you can torpedo your training by making bad food choices or simply overeating. It may be tempting to overeat, grab a Twinkie, or drink too much alcohol. When we are tempted to make bad food choices we consider the hard work we've been doing, and ask ourselves if we want to disrespect that work. Occasionally, it pays to give yourself a rest from the discipline. Some people take food holidays and give themselves one day a week when they eat whatever they want. This likely pays off in longevity; you don't need to be 100 percent hardcore 100 percent of the time.

If you want to lose weight and convert excess fat stores to muscle, your body has to enter a negative energy balance for a sustained period until you reach your ideal weight. Your energy expenditure (exercise) has to exceed your energy intake (food you put in). We don't think it is necessary to recommend a specific weight-loss program because almost everyone following the precepts outlined in this book will lose

Eating Before, During, and After Training or Climbing

Period	Carbohydrate intake	Protein intake	Food examples
3–5 hours before training/climbing	1–4 g/kg, or 0.5–1.8 g/lb, or 50–300 g	15–20 g	• 1 c milk, 2 c cereal, 1 banana, water • 1 bagel, 2 Tbsp peanut butter, 1 apple, 10 oz milk • 1–2 poached eggs, 2 pieces toast, 1 orange, 10 oz milk • 2 c of pasta with tomato sauce, 1/2 c cottage cheese, water
30–60 min before training/climbing	30–50 g	10 g before strength training session	• 1 energy bar, 1 c water • 1 fruit yogurt, 1/2 c cereal, 1 c water • 1 bagel, 2 slices turkey with mustard, 1 c water • 2 c sport drink • 1 c milk, 1 c of cereal, 1 c water
Fueling during training/climbing	1 g/min or 30–60 g per hour	No intake	• 2 1/2–4 c sport drink • 2–2 1/2 c sport drink, sports gel or bar, water • energy bars
Within 30–60 min of training session or post-climb, especially important for two-a-day sessions or successive climbing days	1 g/kg, or 0.4 g/lb, or 50–70 g	10–15 g	• 2 c sport drink, 1–2 c water, sport bar • 2 c sport drink, 1–2 c water, peanut butter sandwich • 2 c sport drink, 1–2 c water, turkey sandwich • 2–3 c water, 1 c low-fat chocolate milk, 3 graham crackers • 2 c sport drink, 1–2 c water, 1 fruit yogurt

Carbohydrate Content in Foods

Foods containing 25 g of carbohydrate	Foods containing 50 g of carbohydrate	Sports foods
1 piece of fruit	1 c rice	**Bars (g)**
1 thick slice of bread	1 medium potato	PowerBar (45)
3/4 of 10" flour tortilla	1 1/2 medium sweet potato	PowerBar Harvest Energy (45)
1 c plain yogurt with fruit	1/3–1/2 c dry couscous	Balance Bar (22)
2 c of skim milk	1 1/2 c of cooked pasta	Luna bar (27)
2 c of berries or watermelon	1 c dry oats	Clif Bar (51)
1 c of lima beans (frozen)	2 c Honey Nut Cheerios	Clif Mojo (25)
2/3 c of cooked black beans	2/3 c granola	PowerBar Pria (16)
2/3 c of hummus	4 thin slices of bread	PowerBar Bites (32)
1 1/2 Tbsp of honey	1 1/2 flour tortilla (10")	
1 granola bar	1 large bagel or 1 1/2 medium bagels	**Drinks (g)**
3 Chips Ahoy! chocolate chip cookies	1/2 c of raisins	Gatorade (14g/8 oz)
2 1/2 Fig Newtons	1 c unsweetened apple sauce	All Sport (19g/8 oz)
1/2 c of frozen yogurt or ice cream	2 pieces of fruit	Powerade (19g/8 oz)
3/4 c of unsweetened pineapple	10 pieces of small pretzels	Accelerade (26g/12 oz)
12 pieces of baked Lays potato chips	2 c of apple juice	Endurox (53g/12 oz)
10 Doritos tortilla chips	2 c of orange juice	
1/2 bagel with 1 Tbsp jam	2 slices of pizza	**Gels (g)**
1 c of Cheerios + 1 c skim milk	3 large carrots	Gu (20)
3/4 c of fruit yogurt	2 c of stir-fry vegetables	Clif Shot (24)
1/2 c of Ben and Jerry's Ice Cream	2 1/4 c of butternut squash cooked	
	1 c cooked garbanzo beans	

some weight, many will maintain their already healthy weight, and no one will gain weight.

If you would like to lose some of the weight you currently have, consider your choice of exercise. Running burns more calories per time spent than cycling. Mixing in more high-intensity exercises such as strength training with your endurance will ramp up your metabolism, resulting in more calories burned.

If, in training or climbing, you get into a negative energy balance, your body will catabolize muscle to make up the deficit. When this happens, it will impact your training. Eating too little compromises your potential fitness gains just as much as eating too much. This is why climbers are usually so weak after high-altitude expeditions; eating is a challenge at altitude. We'll discuss this in detail in the next chapter.

Calculate Your Carbohydrate Needs

Training	g carb/lb
60–90 min/d	2.3–3.2
90–120 min/d	3.0–4.5
CHO loading	3.0–4.5
Ultraendurance	4.5–5.5

Body wt = _____ lbs
Training = _____ g/lb
_____ lbs x _____ g/lb
= _____ g/day

Meeting your needs?
How does your intake
compare to your needs?
_____ g/d

How Much Food Is Enough?

Let's return to the question of recovery and eating to fuel your training: How much you should eat after training? The answer will surprise many climbers, especially those subscribing to high-protein or calorie-restricted diets. Tables in the appendix summarize various food sources of carbohydrate and protein and will help you calculate the correct amounts of these nutrients that an athlete in training needs to consume daily. The tables on the left and on the next page will allow you to calculate your carbohydrate and protein needs based on your training load and weight.

EATING WHILE ALPINE CLIMBING

By the time you get on your climb, your food plan should be familiar. The main difference, especially on expeditions, might be the availability of foods you took for granted at home. Fresh fruits and dairy products in particular are nonexistent on extended trips.

The Day Before Climbing

Many of you have heard of carbo-loading for marathons. This can also be done for climbing. We find that a higher-than-average carbohydrate diet in the days leading up to the start of a climb produces the best energy on the morning we start out. In a study done on trained cyclists, those on a moderate carbohydrate diet (40–50 percent of total calories from carbohydrate) had about 1,000 calories available for lower-body exercise. Those on a high-carbohydrate diet (60–70 percent of calories

Protein Content in Foods

Plant-based foods	grams	Animal-based foods	grams	Combination foods	grams
2 Tbsp peanut butter	9	1 c skim or 1% milk	8	1/2 c rice & 1/2 c beans	7.5
1/4 c soy nuts	12	1 c 2% chocolate milk	8	1/2 c vanilla yogurt & 1/4 c Grape-Nuts	9
1/4 c of almonds	9	6 oz Yoplait yogurt	10	1/2 c vanilla yogurt & 1/2 c Wheaties	7.5
1/4 c peanuts	8	1 Dannon fruit yogurt	9	2 slices of bread & 2 oz turkey sandwich	11
1/2 c garbanzo beans	6	1 Dannon nonfat fruit yogurt	8	2 slices of bread & 2 Tbsp peanut butter/jam	11
1/2 c of black beans	5	1/2 c low-fat cottage cheese	12	2 slices of bread & 1/4 c hummus	8
1/2 c of kidney beans	6	1 string cheese	8	1 c couscous w/pine nuts	7
1/2 c hummus	6	1 oz swiss or cheddar cheese	7	1 tortilla & 1 oz mozzarella cheese	11
3.5 oz extra firm tofu	11	1 egg	3.5	1/2 c cottage cheese & 1 small baked potato	15.5
1 veggie burger	8	1 egg white	6		
1 Boca burger	14	3 oz tuna, canned	19	**Sport Foods**	**grams**
1 c pasta	6	3 oz salmon	20	Luna bar	10
1 c couscous	6	3 oz halibut	22	Clif Bar	12
1 c soy milk	7	3 oz chicken breast	26	Clif Mojo bar	8
1 soy yogurt	4	3 oz steak	22	PowerBar	10
		3 oz pork loin	22	PowerBar Pria	5
		3 oz hamburger	22	PowerBar Bites	8
		3 oz turkey burger	23	PowerBar Protein Plus	15
		2 oz deli turkey	9	PR*Bar	14
		2 oz deli ham	9	PowerBar Harvest Energy	7
		2 oz roast beef	10	Balance Bar	14
				Exceed ProteinBar	12
				Accelerade (12 oz)	6.5
				Endurox (12 oz)	13

from carbohydrate) had double the stored caloric energy, 2,000 calories, and the high-carb-diet group cycled further and produced more power than the moderate-carbohydrate-diet group.

When you are on an expedition it's impossible to eat enough at three sit-down meals a day, so make frequent snacking a priority. Walking into the mess tent of a Slovenian expedition two hours after breakfast you're likely to find the table spread with sliced dry sausage, hard cheeses, red onion, and garlic. Steve brings instant meal-replacement shakes that he can mix with water for days he is feeling too lazy to snack but wants to get some calories down regardless. Be sure to pack lots of easy-to-access foods such as canned fish, canned fruit, nuts, dried fruit, and nut butters.

Steve's favorite pre-climb meal in Asia is good old lentils and rice washed down with a sugary drink. In Alaska, where it's much colder, he finds that a simple, protein-centered meal, like tuna-mac-and-cheese followed by a chocolate bar, is better.

The Alpine Start

To consume a big breakfast really early in the morning, with nerves aflutter and the alpine clock ticking down the minutes until nightfall comes, is a serious challenge. If you've had a very short night, say you're waking at midnight, we suggest an energy gel or two and some coffee or tea.

If it's a little later, say after 2 a.m., it's important to get real food in your belly. In this case we recommend eating instant oatmeal or porridge mixed with raisins, butter, protein powder, or maybe an egg if you have it. If you want to be quick out the door, mix a meal-replacement shake that contains roughly equal portions of carbohydrate, protein, and fat.

Alpinists often find themselves in the situation of eating solid meals shortly before starting a climb. Because it's hard to eat and then exercise, always treat the first sixty to ninety minutes of any approach or climb as a warm-up; stick to conversational pace. If you go out too hard this scenario can cause a dip in your blood sugar at sixty to ninety minutes that can leave you feeling undermotivated. If you can't seem to escape the ninety-minute dip, then try not eating until after you start climbing and then eat only small, frequent amounts of gels or other easy-to-access foods. If you haven't had time to figure out what works best for you, we recommend eating according to our suggestions, and adapting your diet as dictated by your own observations and experiences.

Calculate Your Protein Needs

Athlete	g pro/lb
Growing	0.7–0.9
Endurance	0.6–0.7
Strength	0.6–0.8
Adult Upper Limit	0.9

Body wt = _____ lbs

Athlete = _____ g/lb
_____ lbs x _____ g/lb
= _____ g/day

Meeting your needs?
How does your intake
compare to your needs?

_____ g/day

The Slovak Direct: What Not to Do

The day before Mark Twight, Scott Backes, and I set off to climb the Slovak Direct on Denali it fell to me to prepare the evening meal. I decided to cook spaghetti with tomato sauce heavily laden with big chunks of salami and an extra helping of Parmesan cheese. I was cooking for calories, and I succeeded. That night, none of us slept too well, due to the heavy meal and dry mouth caused by the salt we'd ingested. We laid awake half the night sweating, sleeping bags open, waiting for the alarm to go off.

Since that experience, I try to eat a lighter meal before bedtime. If I have the luxury, I make my pre-climbing-day noontime meal my biggest and then have a lighter meal for dinner. This seems to set me up for the best rest the night before a big climb.

– Steve House

The Duration of Exercise versus Muscle Glycogen Stores

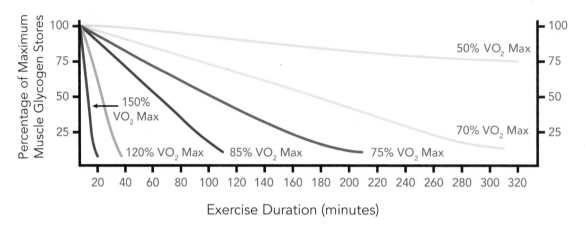

The above figure shows the rate of muscle glycogen depletion at various exercise intensities. The top green line shows that at a low intensity the exercise duration can last for over five hours with only a 25 percent drop in glycogen stores. Pick up the pace and you'll be consuming glycogen at a much faster rate and may almost completely deplete your glycogen stores in a couple of hours as indicated by area around the dark blue and purple lines. Most alpinists will spend the bulk of their approach and climbing time in the range near 60–75 percent of VO₂ max. At these intensities it will still be necessary to refuel in order to avoid a dramatic slowdown that results when the percentage of glycogen stores dip too low. Reprinted with permission from *Lore of Running* by Timothy Noakes, MD, PhD.

In the world of competitive endurance sports, athletes aim to eat a large meal three hours before their start time, then thirty minutes before start time they have a light carbohydrate snack such as a rice cake or energy drink. It doesn't pay to eat while running a marathon or doing anything at very high intensities—in some cases speed climbing—as your gastrointestinal system will be shut down.

The figure above shows that when you start with maximum levels of intramuscular glycogen, after five hours of exercise at an average of 70 percent of VO₂ max that intramuscular glycogen has dropped to almost 10 percent of its starting level. We have to replace that carbohydrate to be able to continue to think and move. As you know, many climbing days extend much beyond five hours of constant climbing time.

On the Route

In an ideal world we'd eat seventy grams of carbohydrate per hour to replace the roughly 400–800 calories per hour we're burning while climbing. This equates to eating a minimum of four gel packets every hour. Alpine climbing is far from an ideal world. For athletes with aid stations along their route, seventy grams per hour is possible. For climbers, it's not, and the lesson is that even one hundred calories (one typical gel package) per hour is really insufficient. In fact, for events lasting longer than five or six hours physiologists suggest that you should aim to replace at least 50 percent of the calories you are burning each hour.

Low Intensity, Long Duration

On a long all-day or multi-day effort you have to stick to conversational pace most of the time. In this case, plan to eat frequent small amounts of food balanced with carbohydrate/protein/fat such as a sandwich or wrap. Trail mix is also a nice balanced source of macronutrients. Gels and bars can work as well. Drink a bit every time you feed.

High Intensity, Extreme Altitude

For high intensities and above 18,000 feet (5,486 meters), and for all intensity levels above 23,000 feet (7,010 meters), stick to carbohydrates. If you choose this path, you must remember to maintain strict discipline to the one-gel-per-hour-minimum rule. We reinforce this rule by using a watch alarm and an accessible supply of gels and water in jacket pockets. When possible, eat as many as three gels per hour. More than three will likely cause you to vomit, especially at high exertion levels. Gels cannot be replaced with the popular chews. The chews taste like candy because they are candy. Their predominance of simple carbohydrates will invite blood sugar spikes followed by the inevitable lows.

Because carbohydrates are all you can effectively metabolize in high altitude situations, if you stop or get lazy and don't eat enough carbs, you will bonk. You will lose your motivation, your coordination, and your endurance simultaneously—an extremely dangerous situation for an alpinist.

Gels and meal-replacement shakes seem to work best for us while moving, and simple foods are preferred for bivouacs. Everyone seems to have a different tolerance for high-calorie shakes and gels. For those that can't tolerate this type of food well, try alternating simple real foods (rice balls, wraps) with what we call "science foods" while climbing. When resting go with natural real foods; eat unsalted roasted nuts, dried fruit, low-sodium soups, plain ramen noodles, rehydrated stuffing, or sugary milk tea: all are simple, easy to digest, carbohydrate-rich foods.

Caloric Values of Common Climbing Foods

To help you to choose your training and climbing foods, we've compiled tables in the appendix of various foods that climbers typically eat,

Hitting the Wall

By Vince Anderson

It's our third day climbing on the Rupal Face, and I am ready to throw in the towel. I can hardly move. The altitude is crushing me. Steve says I should eat—I haven't in a long time—but I decline. My low energy must be a result of the altitude. We've been climbing for eighteen hours today and I've just followed Steve up another three pitches of simulclimbing at 20,000 feet (6,096 meters).

Steve and I have shared the same food and water bottles. He knows I have not come close to finishing today's rations. He has been done with his for quite some time.

"Eat a bar!" he demands, reading the thoughts of doubt written on my face. I agree and chow on one of our raw food bars and wash it down with some high-calorie meal-replacement drink.

As Steve leads out again, I feel my energy return. After twenty minutes or so, a new man emerges. I have my second wind and we continue climbing another six hours into the night to our bivy. Three days later I reach the top of Nanga Parbat at 26,660 feet (8,126 meters).

I bonked hard and failed to recognize the signs. I guess it was not the altitude after all. I failed to follow the rules of proper climbing nutrition by eating and drinking on a schedule. I didn't follow the plan. Fortunately, I had a good partner who saw this and helped me avoid derailing a great alpine climb.

I have done plenty of long days on minimal food where recovery is simple: Eat a big meal afterward and then go back out a few days later. That doesn't work on a multi-day effort where the food you eat now is for your climbing now, as well as for the climbing to come tomorrow. The calorie deficit I ran up that morning made me pay dearly that afternoon. So much so, that I really thought I needed to quit the climb and descend. Sometimes it's hard to recognize your own foolishness and mistakes.

Vince Anderson is an AMGA–IFMGA certified mountain guide and founder/owner of Skyward Mountaineering, www.skywardmountaineering.com. Vince loves his juicer and is highly competitive in single-speed mountain bike stage races, in addition to being a husband and the father of three well-fed boys.

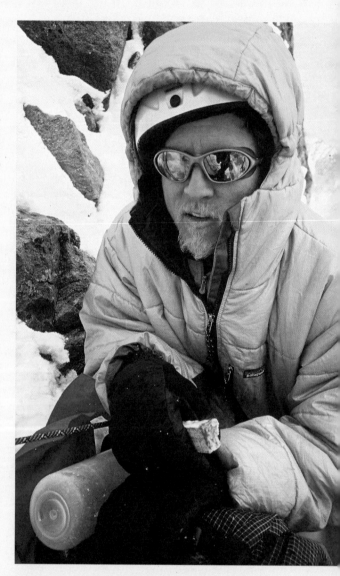

Vince Anderson eating a bar early on day three of the ascent of the Rupal Face of Nanga Parbat (26,660', 8,126m) in Pakistan. He hit the wall about six hours after this photo was taken. *Photo: Steve House*

organized by meal and by caloric value per one hundred grams of weight. As we've pointed out, a frequent dilemma in alpine climbing is that food, no matter the form, is heavy. Exactly how much food do you need to provide enough energy to get you up the route? How much can you eat on the go? A healthy dose of experience, and the physiological adaptation to rely on one's already-stored body fat, can save you lots of food weight in the rucksack. The tables in the appendix are provided to help you choose weight-efficient, palatable foods so you can build appropriate menus now that have the macronutrients you need to eat before, during, and after training and climbing. Training is the time to experiment, the time to find a nutrition strategy that works best for you.

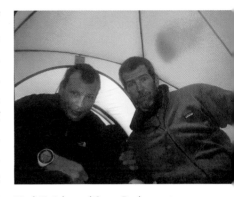

Mark Twight and Scott Backes not looking relaxed at 8 p.m. the night before starting our sixty-hour ascent of the Slovak Direct route on Denali (20,322', 6,194m), Alaska.
Photo: Steve House

HYDRATION

We dehydrate normally, through breathing, peeing, defecating, and sweating. At altitude you dehydrate more than normal through respiration; it's also common to lose significant amounts of fluid through vomiting and diarrhea. Sweating while alpine climbing indicates that you've made a mistake in your clothing system—you should consider sweating a waste of fluids.

It is our experience that many people overhydrate both when training and climbing. If you are eating frequently while training or alpine climbing, you probably don't have to think about extra hydration as long as you drink a little bit every time you eat. Despite the common dictum of *clear and copious*, the ideal color of your urine is straw-yellow, assuming you're not ingesting vitamins or foods that may change its color. The rule of thumb we like was put forth by the ultra-endurance athlete, doctor, and author of *Lore of Running*, Tim Noakes, MD, PhD. He states that while training and racing ultra-length endurance sports it is best to consume only plain water, and to drink only to thirst.

The American Dietetic Association and American College of Sports Medicine is more traditional in their recommendations. Their hydration guidelines are as follows:

- Four hours before exercise drink 5–7 milliliters of fluid per kilogram of body weight. That means 350–500 milliliters (1.5–2 cups) of fluid for a 150-pound climber.

- During exercise your goal is to avoid any fluid loss greater than 2 percent of your body weight. For a 150-pound climber, that means losing no more than three pounds of weight during exercise, or one and a half quarts of water.

A Few Case Studies in Eating While Alpine Climbing

By Steve House

These ascents were three of my best climbs, in no small part because my partners and I got our nutrition mostly right. And what we got wrong, we survived. I share these examples because, though no two routes are exactly the same, the thought process and problem-solving that went into these different examples will be nearly universal.

Nutrition for Sixty Hours
Nonstop on the Slovak Direct

The Slovak Direct route is the most sustained, difficult route on Denali ascending 8,000 vertical feet (2,438 meters) with the first 5,000 feet (1,524 meters) being technical snow, ice, and mixed climbing. In 2000, Mark Twight, Scott Backes, and I succeeded in our goal of climbing the route with no bivy gear, taking a total of sixty hours to ascend from our glacier camp to the top of the south face.

We based our nutrition strategy on the advice of Dr. William Vaughan, who co-created PowerBar in 1986 and created GU energy gel in 1989. He advised Mark that we should each consume one GU gel every sixty minutes. We packed 146 GU packages, assuming one per person per hour for forty-eight hours. We finished the climb with a bunch of GU left over, having not met our goal. We all bonked hard late during the second night near the top of the technical climbing, in part because we'd stopped eating often enough. Our approach was not optimal, the result of the imperfect reality of a hard climb and less-than-perfect discipline.

During our ascent we stopped to brew, eat, and rest four times at somewhat irregular time intervals. Drinking cold water and experiencing nausea from the exertion and altitude, it became hard to get the cold, viscous gel down my throat. If I had it to do over I would change a few things:

- The bottom part of the route is easy, so you can start fast. This would have been the time to eat gels only.
- At the rest stops, besides tea and soups, I would have some meal-replacement shakes with balanced carb/protein/fat ratios. Or I would eat some real foods such as a quick-cooking pasta dish with protein and fat added.

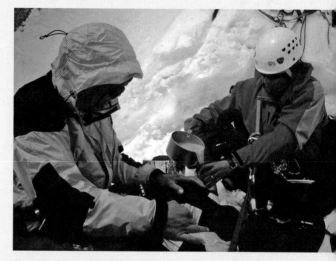

Scott Backes and Mark Twight hydrating with sweetened tea (with added dried milk) after the first eight hours of climbing. *Photo: Steve House*

- During the hardest climbing, which came during the first night, I would stick to balanced, whole foods because the pace was slow.
- During the difficult early-morning hours I'd have caffeine on hand; chocolate-covered espresso beans would have been welcome.
- I'd have a lot of caffeinated gels for the last 4,000 vertical feet (1,219 meters) of steep hiking that finish the route to the summit. I would force as much gel into myself as I thought I could without puking—probably around five or six over four hours.

If you were to attempt to ingest 300 calories per hour, following the seventy gram/hour rule, that would have meant a total of 540 gel packets for three guys for forty-eight hours, and would weigh over forty pounds: clearly an impossible load given the amount of technical climbing. Not to mention the insurmountable task of eating three gels per hour for forty-eight hours. Of course this begs the question, if you ate three gels per hour and went as fast as possible, could you climb the Slovak Direct in

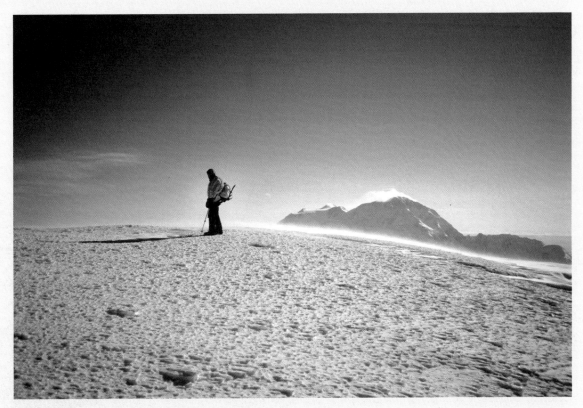

Rolando Garibotti near the summit of Mount Foraker (17,402', 5,304m) twenty-five hours after starting the climb. The previous fastest ascent had been seven days. *Photo: Steve House*

fifteen hours? I believe someone will do just that; but instead of more food, they will be fitter, move more efficiently, and simply need fewer calories.

Race Pace on Mount Foraker

When Rolando Garibotti and I climbed the Infinite Spur route in Alaska in 2001, I wore a recording heart-rate monitor. The monitor I had at the time could record maximum, minimum, and average heart rate for up to forty-eight hours. Our climb, from a camp near the base of the route, to the summit, down the Sultana Ridge, over Mount Crosson, and back to Kahiltna Base Camp took us forty-five hours. My average heart rate for this period was 146 beats per minute, close to my aerobic threshold. During the climb we fed entirely on gels except at a rest break where we consumed instant mashed potatoes flavored with olive oil and instant soup. It is clear that without constant carbohydrate refueling it would have been metabolically impossible for me to finish that climb much faster than we did.

Max Heart Rate on K7

On some of my attempts on K7 in Pakistan in 2003 and 2004 I wore a heart-rate monitor. Unfortunately that monitor was a cheaper model and did not record. Though perceived exertion was very high, I had real difficulty getting my heart rate above 135 beats per minute at over 20,000 feet (6,000 meters). At higher altitudes your body simply does not allow higher heart rates; we'll discuss why in the next chapter. On the successful ascent I was climbing above 50 percent of my max heart rate over the forty-one hour round-trip climbing time.

I consumed almost all carbohydrate gels on my K7 attempts and climb because the effort was so intense. I again ate instant mashed potatoes enhanced with olive oil (store it in doubled Ziplocs because it hardens in the cold) and instant soup at rest beaks on K7.

- It is normal, and OK, to return from a climb somewhat dehydrated. We usually count on that. We will explain how to exactly measure that in the next section.

- For events lasting longer than one hour, use a drink mix that provides 6 to 8 percent concentration of carbohydrate with electrolytes.

No matter whether you measure your water loss with a scale or let thirst guide you, taking consistent, small drinks is best. The most water you can absorb through your digestive system is 800 milliliters (3.4 cups) per hour in ideal circumstances. Cool water is absorbed by the digestive system more readily than warm or hot water; this is the likely reason why you crave a cold drink over a hot one when you're thirsty.

Measuring Fluid Loss

It's remarkably easy to measure how much water you lose on a given training day. Weigh yourself before and after you train. Assuming you did not consume a large amount of food while exercising, the difference in your weight before and after exercise will tell you the weight

House-Made Bars

Below are a few simple recipes for no-bake bars that Eva House has been making for the last few years. They are cheaper than store-bought energy bars, you can adjust them to your tastes, and they contain simple, nutritious ingredients. Use these recipes as starting points and modify them as you like. All you need is a food processor or blender, wax paper, and your ingredients. It takes about thirty minutes to make one batch. Enjoy!

Protein Heroes

½ cup (roasted) almonds
½ cup cashews
16 dates
8 figs
1 tsp bee pollen, optional, for vitamins and minerals. Omit if you have

allergies to bees or pollen.
Salt/pepper to taste
Directions: Put all ingredients in a food processor and grind well. Place on wax paper, cover with wax paper, and compress into one big slab. Cut into bars and wrap in paper or foil. Store in the refrigerator.

Protein Chocolate Heroes

½ cup cashews
24 dates
2 Tbs chocolate powder
2 Tbs dark chocolate chips
1 tsp bee pollen, optional, for vitamins and minerals. Omit if you have allergies to bees or pollen.
Salt/pepper to taste
Directions: As above, but add the chocolate chips last and mix them in by hand.

Carb Champions

2 cups oat flakes
¼ cup chopped cashews
8 dates
¼ cup raisins
¼ cup agave syrup
¼ cup peanut butter
2 tsp bee pollen, optional, for vitamins and minerals. Omit if you have allergies to bees or pollen.
Salt/pepper to taste
Directions: Slowly heat agave syrup and peanut butter in a small pan on the stovetop. Blend dates and raisins in the food processor. Then add all other ingredients and pulse the food processor a few times. The ingredients should be well mixed, but not ground. Place on wax paper, cover with wax paper, and compress into one big slab. Cut into bars and wrap in paper or foil. Store in the refrigerator.

of the water you lost. Since water weighs eight pounds per gallon, if you lost two pounds during exercise that means you lost a quarter of a gallon, or a quart of water during your workout.

It is good to measure this because people vary greatly in how much fluid they need. It's also a quick way to check how much water you need to replace after any workout.

Fluid Loss at Altitude

To our knowledge, fluid loss to respiration at altitudes above 20,000 feet (6,096 meters) has never been directly measured. But in our experience we find that climbers can function very well on about four liters of fluids per day and can get by on two liters per day even above 23,000 feet (7,010 meters). Some experts recommend six liters per day at extreme altitudes, but the practical considerations of getting so much snow melted and water swallowed while alpine climbing makes this an impossibility, as we will discuss in the next chapter

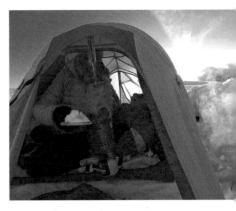

Vince Anderson melting snow and getting hydrated the evening before climbing a new route on the northwest face of Kanchungtse (aka Makalu II, 25,190', 7,678m).
Photo: Steve House

The Dangers of Overhydration

On the first expedition to Denali where Steve worked as a guide, one member of the team was complaining of weakness, loss of appetite, fatigue, and poor coordination. They thought he was showing early signs of altitude illness since they were at 14,200 feet (4,328 meters). After getting a thorough history, they decided that he had hyponatremia, a condition of dangerously low serum sodium levels. It was revealed that he had been religiously downing six liters of mostly plain water each day for a week. He had peed off enough that his body's electrolytes were out of balance. They began feeding him soup, salty foods, and putting sports drink mixes in his bottles. He was back to his strong self within a day and a half, and summited Denali five days later.

Due to the amount of water we drink on expeditions, consider it mandatory to regularly (but not necessarily always) add electrolyte drink powders to your hot and cold drinks while in base camp. Due to the short duration of most climbs, usually less than a couple of days, there is no need to carry electrolyte powders above base camp. Exceptions would be when you need to make bad-tasting water palatable and on climbs like Denali by the West Buttress where you are above base camp for two weeks or more.

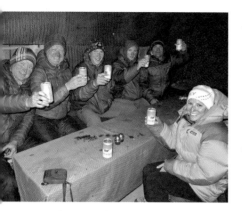

The 2011 Slovenian-American Makalu Expedition celebrates with a high-altitude beer after climbing Mera Peak (21,247', 6,476m) in Nepal. *Photo: Steve House*

Alcohol

Most climbers we know like to drink alcohol. Nutritionally speaking, alcohol is a non-nutrient, but it does contain seven calories per gram. Most of us enjoy the taste of beer or wine with a meal. While training try switching to light beer—it has less alcohol—and limit yourself to one per day. Eliminating all alcoholic beverages may be a good idea while training and climbing. Alcohol suppresses the immune system and may actually decrease muscle protein synthesis. For an athlete in training, one of the surest ways to get sick is to drink three or more alcoholic beverages.

In base camp it is traditional to keep liquor on hand, presumably for a summit celebration, though it never seems to last that long. Some drinking in base camp may be worthwhile: You have to take care of your mental state as well as your physical state. A nightcap with friends is a great way to relax before a good night's sleep. Or, as we've heard it said: You can't put a price on morale.

VITAMINS, MINERALS, AND SUPPLEMENTS

Many climbers consume vitamin and mineral supplements in the belief that they will help prevent injury, illness, speed recovery, or simply improve performance. Despite the financial backing of the $28 *billion* per year dietary supplement industry, no peer-reviewed scientific studies have shown that doses of vitamins or minerals in excess of the U.S. recommended daily allowances (USRDA) improve performance. To the contrary, there have been numerous studies that show vitamin turnover in our bodies to be unaffected by exercise.

Vitamins from Food

The best source of vitamins and minerals is always food. Generally speaking, those who eat a well-balanced diet do not need to supplement with vitamins and minerals, because those of us who exercise more generally eat more. It follows that when you eat more food you also get more vitamins and minerals. However, for anyone on a calorie-restricted diet, travelling, or on an expedition where nutrients are not as available, it may be prudent to supplement with vitamin pills. We do.

Vitamins for Climbers

Climbers may have some specific needs that make it wise for them to take a vitamin supplement.

- Eating the same, nutrient-poor foods on long trips.

- An attempt to counteract the damage of free radicals, especially at higher altitudes and under greater workloads.

- Expeditionary climbers are likely to be susceptible to potassium deficiency because potassium is found only in dairy or fresh fruit. Diarrhea and diuretic drugs such as acetazolamide, a drug commonly used to aid acclimatization, deplete potassium. Potassium deficiency is very common among athletes of all types.

- Iron deficiency is found in 21 percent of women, and training seems to increase the risk of deficiency. Iron and calcium should be closely monitored by female athletes and their doctors. Iron is essential for oxygen transport and utilization at the cellular level; it is important to all of us. On expeditions we are again deprived of the most common sources of dietary iron: leafy green vegetables and meats. The one advantage we do have is access to iron-rich foods like dried fruit and legumes.

- We recommend that people get their serum ferritin (blood iron levels) checked before leaving on a major expedition since there is significant evidence that low iron levels may slow acclimatization to high altitude and impair exercise performance. This occurs with iron depletion, the stage before iron-deficiency anemia. Most doctors will be looking for iron-deficiency anemia unless you specify that you are looking for iron depletion with the testing. Just checking hemoglobin or hematocrit will not give you the information you need to assess your iron status.

- There is some indication that B vitamin needs increase to support large amounts of exercise, but as long as you are eating enough carbohydrates, you should be fine. Also, all sports bars are fortified with B vitamins.

Choosing a Multivitamin Supplement

Check for the following when looking for that perfect supplement for your diet.

- A supplement containing 100 percent of all the USRDA recommendations of vitamins and minerals.

- Avoid supplements with an excess of any one ingredient, as that ingredient may compete with another ingredient for absorption. An example is calcium and iron; iron will inhibit calcium absorption. Ideally try to supplement your minerals in separate doses at different times of the day since most minerals compete with each other. It is generally accepted that a mineral or multi-vitamin supplement will not be 100 percent absorbed.

- Look for the United States Pharmacopeia (USP) stamp; this guarantees that the vitamins are of a type that dissolve properly in your body.

- Vitamin A: The main source should be beta-carotene, The main source should be beta-carotene (not actual vitamin A, aka Retinol).

- Vitamin C: There is no evidence that doses in excess of 250mg/day are beneficial.

- Vitamin E: An important antioxidant supplement that you can't get from your diet without eating a lot of fatty foods. Do not to exceed 100–200 IU per day.

- Take your vitamins with food.

- Over the age of 50: Look for iron-free formulas with Vitamin B6 and B12 during training. During a high-altitude expedition go ahead and take an iron-containing supplement to ensure your body has sufficient iron available for the new red blood cells that are produced as you move to altitude.

Recommended Supplements for Climbers

Caffeine!

Caffeine is surely the most common performance supplement used by climbers, and for good reason. A large number of studies have shown increased endurance capacity and increased time to exhaustion on the order of 10 to 20 percent. This was originally thought to be related to caffeine's ability to conserve glycogen by enhancing fat oxidation. However, recent research suggests caffeine may work via activation of the central nervous system. Cognitive function and reaction time is also increased during and after exercise.

Studies on dosages have shown that increased dosages do not have an increased positive affect. More is not better. Contrary to popular belief, no studies have shown that habitual users of caffeine have different performance changes from non-users. Studies have demonstrated that moderate intake of caffeine does not affect urine loss or hydration status, and there is no diuretic effect with *moderate* intake. This may seem to be contrary to most personal experience, but realize that moderate caffeine intake is defined as 140–210 mg for an average 155-pound (70 kilogram) athlete. Most people we know exceed that amount daily. For reference, one short drip coffee from Starbucks has 180 mg of caffeine.

Vitamin I

The second most common supplement for climbers is non-steroidal anti-inflammatory (NSAID) medications such as ibuprofen and naproxen. NSAIDs should be avoided except to deal with acute injury. There is evidence that they interfere with muscle regeneration and growth, not to mention kidney health concerns not directly related to training. In females, it may increase susceptibility to dangerously low serum levels of sodium known as hyponatriemia. To get these negative affects you would likely have to consume a lot of NSAID daily for weeks or months at a time. For most of us, NSAIDs are a staple of our diet at one time or another.

Supplementing with Protein

BCAAs, or branched-chain amino acids, are found in protein powders and many commercial post-exercise recovery drink products. There is evidence that consuming BCAAs, particularly leucine, during and after exercise promotes optimal muscle protein synthesis and muscular recovery. This is especially true in the cases of low-calorie, weight-loss diets and at high altitude where muscle wasting is a problem.

Whey protein blended into a carbohydrate-rich fluid, such as fruit juice or an energy drink, during the second half of long workouts, immediately after workouts, and once or twice a day while trekking and at base camp has shown good results. These drinks are tasty, easy to digest, and good supplemental mini-meals when you're working hard. Studies have shown that supplementing with BCAAs is associated with faster recovery and reduction in muscle damage and soreness, but the mechanism is unclear and scientists are currently doing more research in this area. It is thought that because BCAAs are a fuel source of skeletal muscle they are oxidized more readily with exercise. They are also utilized more when glycogen stores and carbohydrate sources of energy are low. Leucine, one type of BCAA, in particular seems to turn on the switch for muscle protein synthesis, though the doses required are thought to far exceed what most bars and gels contain. Supplementing with leucine is difficult in part due to its bitter taste. Whey protein is a good source of leucine. Vegetarian athletes especially should consider supplementing with BCAAs.

Antioxidants

Many climbers supplement with antioxidants, especially vitamins C and E. Vitamin E is probably the one necessary vitamin/antioxidant supplement because we don't get enough of it without eating a lot of animal fats. However, do not exceed 100–200 IU per day; there is evidence that muscle cells adapt to increased free-radical activity associated with training, and you don't want to inhibit these adaptations because they may protect muscles from future bouts of normally damaging free-radical activity. It is widely thought that these adaptations play a role in maintaining cell viability.

Recently science has backed away from the value of antioxidants to the point of saying that free-radical damage at the cellular level is a normal part of what triggers the body to repair damaged tissue. The study that started the anti-antioxidant trend fed one gram of vitamin C to experienced cyclists who then demonstrated reduced endurance capacity.

In short, there is no research to support any benefit in exercise performance except, possibly, at altitude. Some recent research shows that the scenario of low food intakes, increased oxidative stress, combined with the demands of exercise indicate an overall positive benefit by supplementing with antioxidants. Do we take antioxidants at altitude? Yes. Do we recommend them to others going to altitude? Yes. Do you need them if you are *not* at altitude? Probably not. Better to get them from fresh fruit and veggies plus some sunflower seeds for the vitamin E since most people are very low in vitamin E intake.

Probiotics

We always take probiotics with us when we travel, and not just on expeditions. Gut atrophy is a common problem when you're sedentary during travel as well as at high altitude. Anything to promote the good bugs in the gut will be helpful. It is also helpful with mitigating diarrhea and helping your gut recover from antibiotics if you have taken those to recover from an intestinal illness. We have not found any research on this topic related specifically to altitude (although there are plenty of research studies in other populations), but we have found using probiotics helpful many times.

Special Nutritional Considerations for High Altitudes

Generally speaking, the best foods for high altitudes are the ones you can eat. Eating is a huge challenge at elevation. All the science in the world fails us when we're struggling to eat something, anything, and keep it down. Travel packets of cream cheese, packets of frosting, tins of Spam, potato chips. We've seen lots of strange foods being consumed up high. Some will argue that they are better than nothing. Our opinion is that eating bad foods—foods that are high in fat, sodium, or are otherwise difficult to digest—add stress to your body, which is worse than eating nothing.

Nutrition scientists recommend that athletes on a calorie-restricted diet consume at least 1.5 grams of protein per kilogram of body weight to minimize muscle loss. A group of these scientists have an ongoing study to see if this amount of protein, enriched with leucine, would help prevent muscle wasting at altitude as well. The study is not complete, but we think leucine enrichment is likely to help.

We know that most altitude veterans, including the authors, recommend sticking to simple, natural foods when at really high altitudes.

EAT WITH PURPOSE

You can build the perfect machine, but if you can't fuel it, it will go nowhere. As important as training is to better climbing and increased safety in the mountains, nutrition plays a vital role. Today's alpine climber should understand nutrition in ways that climbers of the past did not. This is one key to unlocking the next levels of difficulty in your climbing.

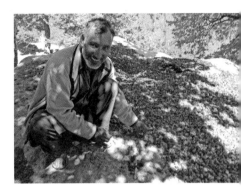

Baltistan, the region of Pakistan where its highest peaks reside, is famous for its apricot and apple orchards. Local dried fruits are a delicious carbohydrate-rich trekking and high altitude food.
Photo: Steve House

A Conversation
with Peter Habeler

By Steve House

In November 2012, in a guesthouse in Lienz, Austria, I spent two and a half hours talking with one of my personal climbing heroes, the Austrian mountaineer Peter Habeler. Habeler is best known as the climbing partner of Reinhold Messner when the two made several breakthroughs in alpinism: a ten-hour ascent of the Eiger North Face in 1969 (apparently still the record for a roped party), the first alpine-style ascent of an 8,000-meter peak (Gasherbrum I in 1975), and the first climb of Everest without supplemental oxygen in 1978. The Habeler I met is a fit 70-year-old with a thick shock of gray hair. He talked animatedly and arranged our meeting at this particular guesthouse because he claimed they had the best goulash in Tyrol. (It was delicious, spicy, and served with polenta.) What follows are excerpts from our conversation.

Peter: "I would train a lot in the Ziller Alps [Habeler was born and lives in the Ziller Valley in Tyrol] and I would do these very long mixed ridges. This is why I could move fast on mixed terrain. For me, there is nothing better than that for training. You have to be careful, you learn the best route-finding, you learn to deal with loose rock, and so on. I had also done all of my mountain guide exams, which resulted in safety, good rope technique, knowledge about glaciers and avalanches, and so on. On the other hand, I had hard climbing routes with other people, such as Messner.

"In my days the training was nothing other than running up a steep hill, fast. And coming down fast again. And ski touring. I did a lot of ski touring. We didn't have heart-rate monitors, no computers. Now the poor guys have a hard time, they have to look up the weather, they have to text their friends, download something to their computer afterwards. We could concentrate on the mountain, which was good.

"I didn't do anything else but climbing. Of course my private life was more or less in shambles; I had ladies, but when they were asking, 'Me or the mountains?' I would say, 'The mountains, I'm sorry.'

"I was always light. I am still the same weight as when I was at sixteen years old, 63 kilo. I think this helps at altitude, not to be too big. [Jerzy] Kukuczka and [Kurt] Diemberger, those guys both would put on some weight before expeditions. I never liked this, I never did this.

"I was against big expeditions, big teams, with the exception of Everest. On Everest, Messner and I were part of a bigger Austrian team, but we were the only expedition allowed on the mountain that season. During the expedition we only saw four trekkers in base camp. On all my expeditions, I always had only one partner, at the most three, which was on Kanchenjunga. I was very fond of small teams. I was very fond of doing things simple. Simple.

"I always used ski poles for mountaineering and trekking, it made my knees last. I was guiding all the time, always using ski poles. I was the first person I know that used ski poles for approaching and descending the mountains.

"On Hidden Peak, in 1975, we didn't care about the outcome. We had doctors around that were telling us we would get brain damage; that when we came home we wouldn't recognize our wives anymore, or our own homes, and so on. I was not interested in their opinions. Since the early years we always had one doctor, Dr. Raimund Margreiter. He said, 'Peter, come on, you can do this.' He came to Everest base camp with us in 1978. And of course we knew the Sherpas had been high on Everest not using oxygen, the Swiss had been high on Everest not using oxygen. Fritz Wiessner had been very high on K2 in 1938 not using oxygen. Hermann Buhl in '53 climbed Nanga Parbat without oxygen. Matthias Rebitsch, who was very high on Nanga Parbat in 1953, also told us we could do it.

"So with all these heroes telling us we could do it, it meant that we should try it! We were unsure if we could climb Gasherbrum I quickly enough, or Everest without oxygen, but we trained hard. Not in a scientific way, not compared to now. But I truly believe that my training was fantastic. It made it possible for me to do all of these things, and it made it possible for me to stay alive. Of course, luck was on our side. Luck, good friends, good partners; that's the biggest part of the game.

"Success builds you up. Success lifts you.

"Reinhold and I didn't talk at all about our training for Everest. He did whatever he thought was good. He was running. Reinhold is not so much the skier.

"Before Everest [1978] I was training very hard. I was working at the ski school, there were about 150 instructors, and I was the head instructor; I had to make the

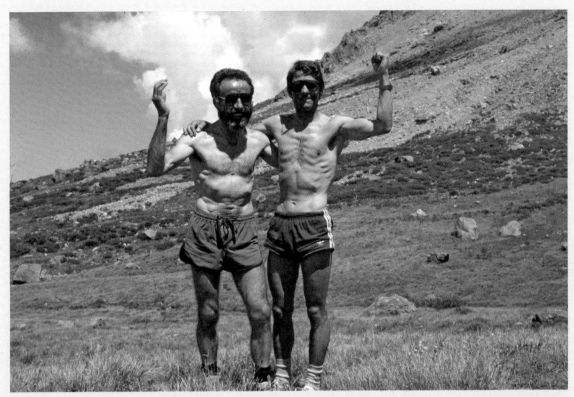

Michael Dacher and Peter Habeler after climbing Nanga Parbat (26,660', 8,126m) in 1985. *Photo: Peter Habeler collection*

assignments every day. My boss gave me the entire winter off from work so I could train. I didn't have to work, but he paid me in full and checked my training log. Almost every other day I did a ski tour that had a 2,000-meter [6,562-foot] gain, a special route I could do even when the weather was bad. Every three or four days, my boss would check my training, ask to see my log of what I did, but he gave me full pay. I owe my fitness on Everest to that man.

"We stayed in base camp at Everest; we were there three months in total. We were the only expedition on the mountain. We went to Camp 3 at 7,200 meters [23,622 feet] before our final summit attempt. We were very well acclimatized. It took us about six hours from the South Col to the summit. We only used a rope on the Hillary Step, we carried a twenty-meter [sixty-six foot] length of rope that we used to belay each other.

"On Everest I was afraid. I was scared. I had married the year before and we had a baby at home. I remember once we went through the Khumbu to a camp at 6,100 meters [20,013 feet]. The next day started off good and we went up to the Western Cwm, and we set up a tent and the weather got bad, it was a whiteout. We couldn't fix the tent properly, the wind was blowing so hard. All night we sat inside holding the tent around us. I was scared to shit. I thought, 'If it's like this higher up, I won't go.' The next day the weather cleared, but I promised myself that on this mountain, I will be careful.

"When we were on Everest in '78, which was a long time ago, we were the first to have plastic boots, and they were the lightest boots available. The inside of the boot was Aveolite foam, but it was very difficult to shape this foam; it was quite thick. These were Kastinger boots. The Koflach boots that came later had much thinner foam, but they were not as warm. The boots they use on Everest now are much heavier than what we had. We went very light to the South Col. When we went to the summit, I left my rucksack—I had no thermos, no water, only a camera. We wore down suits; light, warm like hell! Then we had sealskin overboots and boiled wool mittens from Dachstein, Austria; very warm.

"I was not very comfortable on the summit; I left after fifteen minutes. I came back down by glissading, but glissading takes you too much toward the Kangshung Face, so I would stop every once and a while and walk to the right and then glissade again. It took me one hour from the summit to come back to the South Col. That night was not very comfortable, Reinhold had burned his eyes because he'd spent so much time filming without sunglasses. After a bad night, no sleep, we went down.

"On Everest, I didn't feel like this was a historic thing for climbing. Maybe Reinhold was aware, but I was not aware of this. We knew that the Swiss were high on this ridge before. Wiessner in the 1930s would have climbed K2 without oxygen, definitely. He was physically strong,

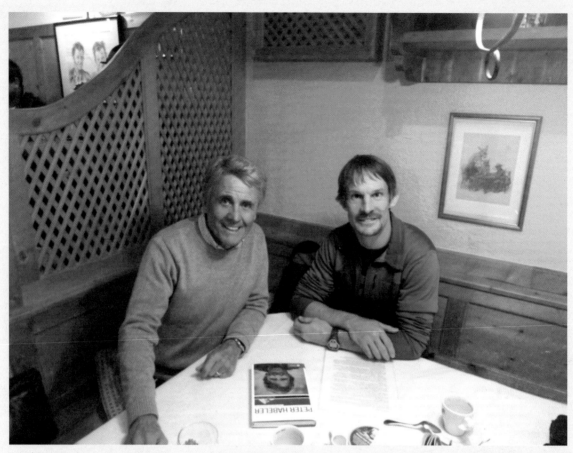

Peter Habeler and Steve House post-goulash in a Tyrolian *gasthaus* (restaurant) in Lienz, Austria. *Photo: Steve House*

he was fast, and his mind was strong. I was lucky to meet him many times. Wiessner was a fantastic guy. That was a remarkable thing he did on K2.

"When we came back from Everest, we had this big test in Zurich in the hospital at the University of Zurich. There were several of us who had been on the summit, some using oxygen. The night before we drank I don't know how many bottles of wine, and the next day we went to the test. Before we got on the treadmill, they did a muscle biopsy from our legs, it was painful and we couldn't run after that. It was hilarious, we were just making jokes, and finally we got on the treadmill and did the tests. When the results came back, Reinhold was the worst. They then put us into this chamber that they de-pressurized, we started at 6,000 meters [19,685 feet]. We were de-acclimated by then of course. We just had to keep signing our names as they took us up to 8,500 meters [27,887 feet], or something, and then they stopped. We came out of the chamber and they showed us the results. By the end we couldn't write our names. But when we were in the chamber, they asked us if we thought we had written our names correctly, and we said, yes of course. So you see

what could have happened to us.

"On hard routes I remember I usually took an apple and a carrot. My friends, they had ham-and-cheese sandwiches. When we climbed the Eiger we carried no rucksacks. We had one rope, four or five pitons, some ice screws, and some cashews and raisins in our pockets. No water, there was lots of water on the face. I am a bad eater—I don't eat much. [True to his word, Peter did not finish his goulash and polenta.]

"I would encourage people to use all the means you have now. I always listened to my body. Our training methods were certainly not always right because it was always full power, and when this became too much, we would slow down a bit and when it was better, full power again. Sometimes we would get deadly tired. Now all these tools make it possible to see your heart rate, your elevation gain, everything. Now I would use all these things.

"What I got out of climbing is a very strong belief in myself. As a boy I was not aware that I would one day be able to go to the Himalaya. But this incredible desire for the peaks, to have experiences, and to go out to meet many situations—this desire—made it possible to survive.

I think, when it comes to whatever is happening above 8,500 meters [27,887 feet], or 8,800 meters [28,871 feet], many of the things you do, or Messner does, or I do, you're not thinking about it. It is automatic. You do it.

"Below the summit of Kanchenjunga there is a little chimney, maybe only four or five meters [fifteen feet] high. When I was there, I climbed automatically. The automatic part comes from the training, and the climbing. The more different situations you have gone through before, the more these things are automatic.

"I know Buhl trained very hard for his climbs. He was a truly remarkable, and interesting, person.

"Train hard, go as naked as you can, don't make it too complicated. Go and do it. In the background was a lot of training; even the guiding was training. Often after bringing the group back to the hut, I would do something for my fingers, or do something for my lungs. I was never too lazy in the early days. I trained hard. I did a lot of ski touring too. When I was training, I was enjoying the training. For me it was never an effort. I was never angry about it. I was happy. I saw how I was improving.

"I would tell the young people to get together with good friends who can withstand difficult situations. With Michael Dacher on Nanga Parbat, with Reinhold Messner, some others, it happened that when things got bad, they got stronger. They became calm; they took care of things. These are the best partners.

"Looking back at all the things I was able to do . . . it might be boring, but I would do the same thing again. In every case, Eiger, Matterhorn, Pilier du Freney, Grand Pillar d'Angle, the soloing I did in the Wilder Kaiser, I don't have any idea what I would change.

"I hope there will be real climbers. I hope so. Because now, here, very few people are going to the summits. Everyone now is at the sport climbing areas, in the climbing gyms. The Himalaya will always be a goal for some young climbers, but these young climbers have to climb the smaller mountains too.

"Mountaineering is emotions to me—happiness, joy—and that is still true today. I still get a kick out of the mountains. I like it. I like to be up there."

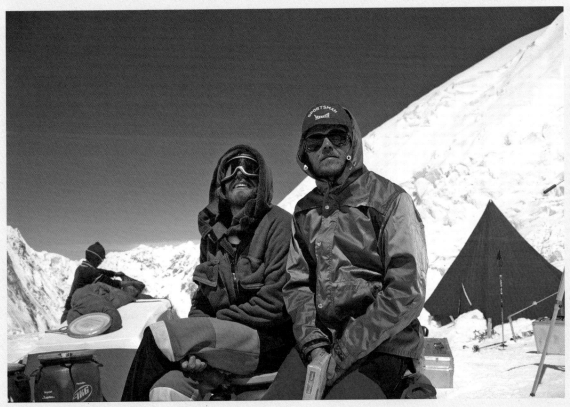

Reinhold Messner and Peter Habeler resting at Camp 2 on Mount Everest a few days before they became the first men to ascend the world's highest peak without supplemental oxygen. *Photo: Peter Habeler collection*

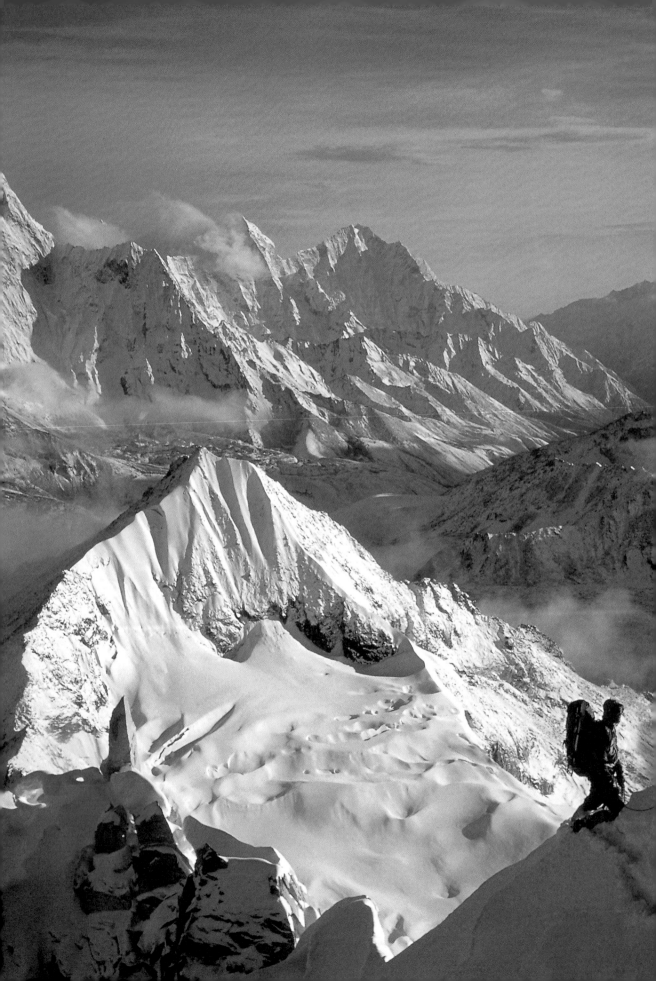

Chapter 12

Altitude: Climbing Higher, Faster

"Every alpinist who climbs 8,000-meter peaks searches for ways to prepare the body so that it will adjust to the variables. The environment at extreme altitudes is as alien as outer space; the dynamics play out in ways that we cannot fully understand. A mountaineer can only hope that a commitment to constant training will prop up his or her ambitions to explore the earth's highest reaches."

— ANATOLI BOUKREEV, *Above the Clouds*

ALTITUDE PHYSIOLOGY BASICS

Let's review a few important facts of altitude climbing and physiology. Perhaps one of the most obvious and least discussed facts of altitude is that we need to provide the same amount of oxygen to our muscles to do a given workload at sea level as we do at 10,000 feet (3,048 meters) and at 26,247 feet (8,000 meters). The VO_2 max of an acclimated climber at 29,028 feet (8,848 meters), the top of Everest, is 20 percent of his VO_2 max at sea level. Recall from chapter 3 that VO_2 max represents the maximal amount of combined aerobic and anaerobic power that

Opposite: Steve House high on Nuptse (25,791', 7,861m) during an acclimatization climb of the 1961 British-Nepalese Route.
Photo: Marko Prezelj

your body is capable of for a few short minutes. This translates directly to how fast you can move. At 29,028 feet (8,848 meters) a climber will be 80 percent slower at any given task, whether it's packing a tent or ascending a snow ridge. Above 26,247 feet (8,000 meters) the volume of ventilation, air in and out, approaches the lungs' mechanical limits, approximately 200 liters per minute. Maximum attainable heart rate and the volume of blood pumped with each heartbeat are reduced at altitude.

The history of mountaineering is full of great ascents by difficult routes of the highest peaks. How is it physically possible to make these climbs? Where is the boundary of possible and impossible? It will soon be abundantly clear that high levels of fitness pay the biggest dividends at the most extreme altitudes.

To climb high mountains you have to adapt to new altitudes, to acclimate. There are two pathways by which your body can acclimate:

- Increasing its ability to deliver oxygen to the muscles.

- Increasing the efficiency with which those muscles use oxygen.

The first happens as your body's natural response to going high. The second can only be affected by the training you've done before you set out on your expedition.

Relationship Between Barometric Pressure and Altitude

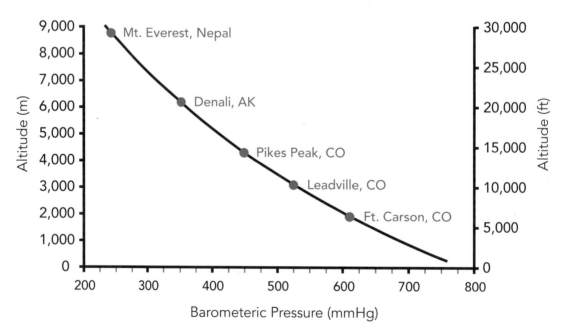

Source: US Army Technical Bulletin, Medical #505

The First Adaptations to Altitude

Within hours of getting to high altitude your bone marrow gets the message to start making new red blood cells, your diaphragm ramps up your respiratory rate, your heart beats faster, and your blood pressure increases. These changes are obvious as you feel yourself get out of breath and your heart beating harder as you ascend.

The new altitude immediately stimulates the release of erythropoietin in your body. Erythropoietin is the hormone that triggers your bone marrow to build more red blood cells. Newly minted red blood cells take seven to ten days to mature. During this time, your plasma volume decreases. (Red blood cell volume plus plasma volume equals your total blood volume.) This drop in blood volume was originally thought to be due to dehydration. The current theory is that the body reduces the plasma in order to effectively increase the concentration of red blood cells. This increased concentration of red blood cells does not mean that more oxygen can be carried to the muscles as the number of oxygen-carrying red blood cells does not increase until the new red blood cells are produced and have time to mature, then total blood volume begins to increase.

Steve House and Vince Anderson heading up for their first acclimatization climb during a 2008 expedition to Makalu (27,825', 8,481m). *Photo: Marko Prezelj*

It is worth stating that doping with synthetic erythropoietin (commonly known as EPO) for purposes of ascending to high altitude would be extremely dangerous. The sudden rise in red blood cells would increase your blood's viscosity and result in a very high risk of stroke. I believe that due to this danger, and the expense, it is unlikely to have ever been attempted in climbing.

One of the most difficult to observe bodily changes is the shift in the pH of your blood to greater alkalinity (increased pH). Once you get to very high altitude, above about 16,000 feet (4,877 meters), blood pH rises because when you breathe more, you hyperventilate, so you are exhaling a greater than normal volume of carbon dioxide.

Mechanisms for Increased O₂ delivery in Response to Altitude

Adaptation	Time for adaptation to begin	Time to end
Increased ventilation rate	Immediate and ongoing	Weeks
Increased heart rate and blood pressure	Immediate	1 week
Blood pH increases	1–3 days, above 16,400 feet/5,000 meters	Several weeks
Decrease in plasma volume (Effectively increases hemoglobin concentration)	1–2 days	1–2 days
Increase in red blood cell mass and increase in hemoglobin concentrations	Within hours	10–14 days
Decrease in the size of muscle cells	Weeks	Months
Increase in capillary density (due to shrinking muscle cell size)	Weeks	Months
Increase the density of mitochondria	Weeks	Months

A decrease in muscle fiber size and an increase in the capillary density has been verified in studies of subjects who spent seventy-five days at 17,225 feet (5,250 meters). This makes sense as an adaptation; it gives the oxygen less distance to travel from the capillary to the mitochondria. Scientists are unclear whether capillary density actually increases during this stage or simply appears to in the face of reduced muscle cell size.

Respiratory Muscles at Altitude

At altitude, the respiratory muscles, primarily the diaphragm muscle, require a greater portion of your cardiac output than the muscles being used for locomotion. Only 5.5 percent of your cardiac output goes to respiration while you are at rest at sea level. But at an altitude of 16,400 feet (5,000 meters), a full 26 percent of your cardiac output must be dedicated to the effort of operating your cardiovascular system while at rest. It is obvious that with only 74 percent of your engine available to supply oxygen to climbing muscles instead of 94.5 percent, you're working at a great disadvantage that increases the higher you go. While exercise physiologists debate whether the muscles' ability to take up and use arterial oxygen or the heart's ability to supply oxygenated blood is the main limiter to exercise at sea level, at altitude cardiac output very much limits exercise.

It follows that we should train the diaphragm muscles to be miserly in their use of oxygen. After reading about the physiology of training endurance, you will know that, like any other muscle, efficient diaphragm muscles are best gained by high volumes of heavy breathing over long periods: lots of long-duration aerobic efforts. The diaphragm and cardiac muscles are almost entirely made up of slow twitch fibers that respond best to long-duration training.

The work done by the diaphragm muscles can be measured as maximum ventilations. The first three examples in the table below were measured during 1960–1961 Silver Hut expedition and the value for 27,230 feet (8,300 meters) was measured by Dr. Chris Pizzo on the 1981 American Mount Everest expedition. Though not ideally executed scientific studies, this is still the best information available. The lower max exercise ventilation at higher altitudes reflects that the diaphragm muscles themselves can do less work at height.

Maximum Exercise Ventilation at High Elevation

Altitude	Max exercise ventilation per minute	Power
19,000 feet (5,800 meters)	173 L/min	1,200 kg-meters/min or 196 Watts
21,000 feet (6,400 meters)	161 L/min	900 kg-meters/min or 147 Watts
24,400 feet (7,440 meters)	122 L/min	600 kg-meters/min or 98 Watts
27,230 feet (8,300 meters)	107 L/min	Not measured

During the test at 27,230 feet (8,300 meters) in 1981 Dr. Pizzo observed his breathing to be extremely shallow and rapid, eighty-six breaths per minute at an average volume of 1.26 liters. At sea level it is not uncommon for an athlete to be able to inhale six liters in one breath. The rapid, shallow breathing seemingly preferred by the body is thought to be indicative of the body's attempt to minimize the work of breathing.

Looking at this chart, notice the drop in the amount of power the climbers could produce. Your body is clearly incapable of achieving anywhere near sea-level rates of work at high altitude. One of the most common mistakes first-time altitude climbers make is expecting their bodies, once acclimated, to feel as strong at height as down low; that never happens.

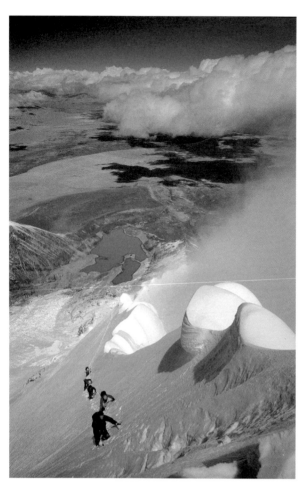

A team of Slovenian climbers acclimates before an ascent of Chomolhari (24,035', 7,326m) in Tibet. *Photo: Marko Prezelj*

Heart Adaptations to Altitude

What happens to the heart at altitude is extremely interesting and sometimes seems contradictory. When you first go to altitude, you feel your heart pounding, leaping out of your chest. But once acclimated your heart rate at rest will drop. Logic seems to indicate that due to less available oxygen your heart rate for climbing at a given pace would be higher than it would be at lower altitude. A higher heart rate for a fit climber should be no problem, right?

Not so fast: In fact your maximum heart rate decreases at altitude. The brain appears to limit your maximum heart rate at altitude. As at sea level, your heart has some regulator on it that keeps its rate below a certain level, presumably to keep it from damaging itself. That level is further reduced as you go to higher elevations. A reduced maximum heart rate reduces the volume of blood pumped by your heart each minute; this is thought to be a major part of the reason for the reduction in cardiac output found at an early stage of altitude exposure. Less blood pumped means less oxygen carried to the muscles, which in turn means less power capacity. The outcome is that you climb more slowly at high altitude and it takes more effort.

Let's review what happens in the first days you ascend.

- Your respiratory rate increases.

- Your resting heart rate increases.

- Erythropoietin (a hormone that stimulates red blood cell production) levels increase.

- Red blood cell production begins.

- Your maximum achievable heart rate is reduced the higher you go.

- Your heart's stroke volume drops.

- For any given workload, your heart must beat more to deliver sufficient oxygen to the working muscles.

- The higher you go, the less oxygen is available to the red blood cells.

- Plasma volume decreases.

- Blood pH shifts to become more alkaline.

All of this information is evidence to further support the value of training our cardiovascular system to do days and days of relatively low-intensity work. Long days of low-to-moderate heart rate and lots of rapid, shallow breathing is the most specific training for altitude.

How Hard Can You Go up High?

Because your maximum heart rate is reduced, the stroke volume of each heartbeat is reduced, and you can breathe less deeply, your VO_2 max drops as you increase altitude. Remember that VO_2 max is the maximum work rate (or power) you can achieve. The figure below shows a clear curvilinear relationship between decreasing VO_2 max and

The Relationship Between Elevation and VO_2 Max

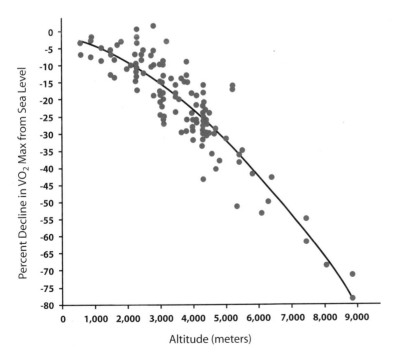

With increasing elevation comes a drop in the amount of oxygen contained in each breath you inhale. The red dots represent the measured VO_2 max of individual climbers the researchers studied. This has the result of dropping your aerobic power output as measured by VO_2 max. A 10–15 percent decline in aerobic power even at submaximal exertion will have a noticeable effect on your climbing speed. By the time you get over 20,000 feet (about 6,100 meters) your will be a mere shadow of your sea level self with only about one half of your aerobic power available. Source: US Army Technical Bulletin, Medical #505

increasing elevation. Notice that reductions in VO$_2$ max are measurable at elevations as low or lower than 2,000 feet (600 meters). It is also interesting to note that studies have found a wide variation in VO$_2$ max decline between individuals at nearly all elevations, especially between 6,560 feet and 18,040 feet (2,000 meters and 5,500 meters). It would be interesting to examine whether or not that variation had any relation to sea-level interpersonal anaerobic threshold variations.

Work capacity progressively decreases with increasing elevation. It has been measured that mountaineers self-select a pace 50–75 percent of their VO$_2$ max at any given altitude up to 19,685 feet (6,000 meters). Higher altitudes have not been studied, but it can be assumed that the same trend would continue.

The end result of an increase in elevation like that shown in this figure is that your perceived exertion increases dramatically.

Consequences of Diminished VO$_2$ Max

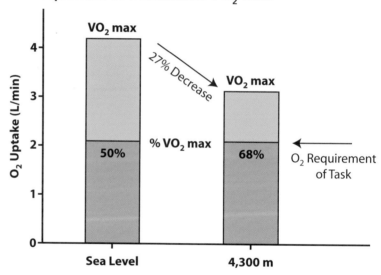

For the same climber, it takes the same amount of oxygen to complete the same amount of work whether the climber is at sea level or 14,000 feet (about 4,300 meters). With the diminished aerobic power due to the lowered amount of oxygen you are breathing, the task of climbing at altitude requires a greater percentage of your maximum aerobic capacity. In this case your VO$_2$ max is reduced by 27 percent but the work rate has stayed the same. The intensity of this same work rate has increased from 50 percent of VO$_2$ max to 68 percent of VO$_2$ max. This is a 36 percent increase in effort.

What Role Do Genetics Play?

You often hear it said that your physical capacity at altitude is largely predetermined by your genetics. It is true that some people simply acclimate more quickly and more thoroughly than others. A good portion of that difference between people may be due to their body size, shape, and aerobic background. As you can see by the data scatter in the figure on the relationship between elevation and VO$_2$ max, there are large differences between how much individuals' work capacities are diminished at altitude. Marko Prezelj acclimates more quickly than anyone Steve has climbed with, although after a few weeks, others tend to catch up with him.

The fact that genetics do play a role in adaptation to altitude was demonstrated clearly by a study published in the *Journal of Applied Physiology* in 1994 by Dr. R. L. Ge of the Qinghai High Altitude Medical Science Institute in China. He studied seventeen Tibetans and fourteen recently migrated Han Chinese, all living at 15,420 feet (4,700 meters) in Tibet. The Han had higher VO$_2$ max levels (36 cubic centimeters per kilogram per minute) than did the Tibetans (30 cubic centimeters per kilogram per minute), but the Tibetans did more work in less time at their maximal levels than the Han (176 versus 150 watts), had higher lactate thresholds as a percent of maximum (84 percent versus 62 percent), and lower blood lactate levels.

The Tibetans had what we referred to in chapter 3 as a high fractional utilization of their VO$_2$ max, which allows them to function at a higher work rate level than the Han despite that the Han are, on paper, fitter. These are remarkable measurements, and in fact it has often been observed that Tibetans, who typically live their entire lives above 15,000 feet (4,600 meters), are superb performers at high altitude.

Then the question becomes: Are these characteristics inborn or adaptive? If they are the latter, then it would be helpful to know the what and the how of the adaptations so we can train efficiently.

Charles Houston, MD, writes in his book *Going Higher*, "Based on what we know today, most of the extreme climbers differ very little from the rest of us. Whether genetically or through exposure, they may have a larger ventilator capacity or a more sensitive hypoxic ventilator response. . . . After having acclimatized many times, their bodies remember how and do so more easily and completely. These are the only differences we recognize today."

Dr. Houston thinks the ability to acclimate is adaptive. Thinking back on our twenty or so Himalayan expeditions, I would concur with him and add a few specific observations. In my experience, those who acclimate best meet several conditions.

■ They have been to altitude before. Experience teaches you when to push and when to rest.

- They are slim of build.

- They are great eaters.

- They are fit and have a high anaerobic threshold. This high fractional utilization of VO_2 max, what gives the Tibetans their edge over the Han, is one of the most trainable qualities we possess.

- They are efficient. Efficiency in specific movement has been studied in Tour de France riders whose continual, specific training leads to marked gains in efficiency of movement. Such gains can also make a climber more efficient. These efficiency differences are clearly visible if you watch a veteran and a beginner ascend an alpine peak side by side. In environments such as extreme altitude, every small advantage in oxygen delivery, or oxygen utilization, will be crucial.

HOW TO ACCLIMATE: TWO STRATEGIES

Strategy One: Climb High, Sleep Low

The phrase, *Climb high, sleep low*, may have first been proposed to mountaineers by Dr. Houston, and it indeed has proven to be invaluable advice for acclimating. Houston's Law is that your average elevation gain of each night's sleeping elevation shouldn't exceed approximately 300 meters or 1,000 feet. That's not much if you're moving fast. A strong climber will be able to ascend 1,000 feet of elevation in an hour below 16,000 feet (4,900 meters) assuming good conditions. Yet, when this 1,000 feet per day is considered as an average over the course of an expedition, it's not far off what is commonly practiced while climbers are prepping for their summit bids.

Strategy Two: The Soviet System— Spend One Night High, Descend Low

Another approach was developed in the Soviet Union, specifically in their mountaineering camps in Kazakhstan, home to the five northernmost peaks above 23,000 feet (7,000 meters). Their methods differ in that when they ascend to a new elevation they carry a light kit to spend the night and then return all the way down to base camp the next morning to rest. Each acclimatization trip takes two to four days, and each rest period is of equal length.

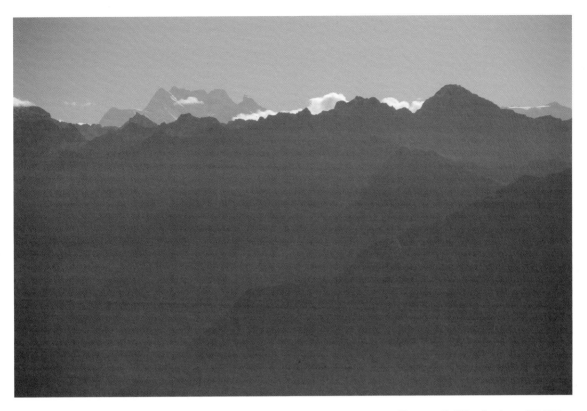

The massif of Kanchenjunga (28,169', 8,586m), the world's third highest peak, viewed from seventy miles away. *Photo: Marko Prezelj*

The Soviet system seems to express something I have also experienced. The body cannot easily do the work of acclimating while remaining up high. The night spent high provides the stress, and the recovery period at base camp allows better recovery and rest, which provides the energy for physiological changes.

In one remarkable expedition, eleven years after the first ascent of any 8,000-meter peak without bottled oxygen (Habeler-Messner, Hidden Peak 1978), and shortly before the Soviet Union collapsed, thirty-two Soviet men and seventeen Sherpa men demonstrated how well they understood high-altitude climbing. During an expedition to Kanchenjunga, the world's third-highest peak, they recorded the following:

■ Eighty-five individual summit successes, most without using supplemental oxygen.

■ Six Soviet members ascended the highest peak twice.

■ The first traverse of all four summits (following the difficult crest) by ten climbers climbing simultaneously in two directions. (Using bottled oxygen.)

■ New route variations.

Comparison of Acclimatization Schedules for Several High Peaks

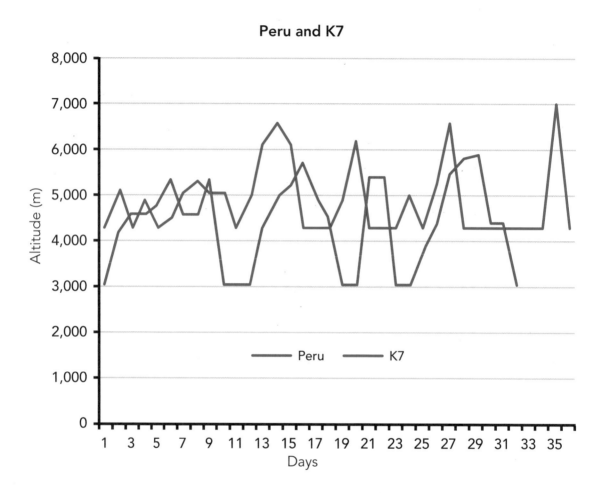

Peru and K7

The blue line shows the acclimatization schedule of Steve House and Marko Prezelj during a thirty-two-day trip to Peru. After a relatively long period, eight nights, at a 15,100 feet (4,600 meters) base camp climbing one-day rock routes up to 17,470 feet (5,320 meters) they gained a solid base of acclimatization. After resting in the town of Huaraz (9,843 feet/3,000 meters) for three days they went on to climb three much bigger (in terms of vertical gain and loss) single and multi-day alpine objectives as none of those summits were more than 3,000 feet (roughly 1,000 meters) higher than the summit they'd been on two times during their first week.

The red line shows Steve's acclimatization for and attempts on K7. You can see that on the fourteenth day of the trip he was acclimated enough to sleep at 19,685 feet (6,000 meters) and climb a 21,500-foot (6,554-meter) summit, Kapura Peak. After a four-day rest he began to attempt his route on K7, eventually succeeding on the fourth try.

What these examples have in common is ten days spent sleeping and climbing between 14,100 feet (4,300 meters) and 17,500 feet (5,335 meters) followed by a succession of quick ascents and descents to elevations up to approximately 23,000 feet (7,000 meters). This strategy works very well for trips to sub-7,000 meter summits. In our experience this amount of acclimatization allows us to move fast and climb technical terrain to 23,000 feet (7,000 meters) within a three-week trip.

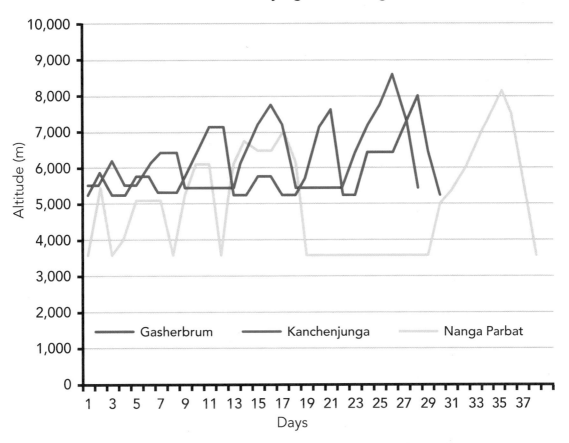

Gasherbrum, Kanchenjunga, and Nanga Parbat

These three expeditions to three different 8,000-meter peaks all show remarkably similar acclimatization schedules despite the differing camp elevations. The valleys and peaks of the three lines show all these teams going up high for one to six days, then returning to base camp to rest. On Steve House and Vince Anderson's Nanga Parbat climb they had a considerable period of bad weather to wait out before starting their climb. They were counting on the further acclimatizing during their six-day ascent followed by a very rapid descent back to base camp. It's also worth noting that in all of these examples the climbers are above 20,000 feet (6,000 meters) in seven to ten days after arriving in base camp. In the case of Denis Urubko's Kanchenjunga expedition, they were above 6,000 meters for multiple days starting on the seventh day of their trip. In the case of Nanga Parbat, very short rests at base camp were utilized because of the extremely low altitude of the Rupal Face base camp (11,750 feet/3,580 meters). The altitude they stayed at during their first two forays up the mountain were lower than the base camps of Gasherbrum I (with Denis Urubko as team leader) or Kanchenjunga.

Comparison of Acclimatization Schedules for Several High Peaks (continued)

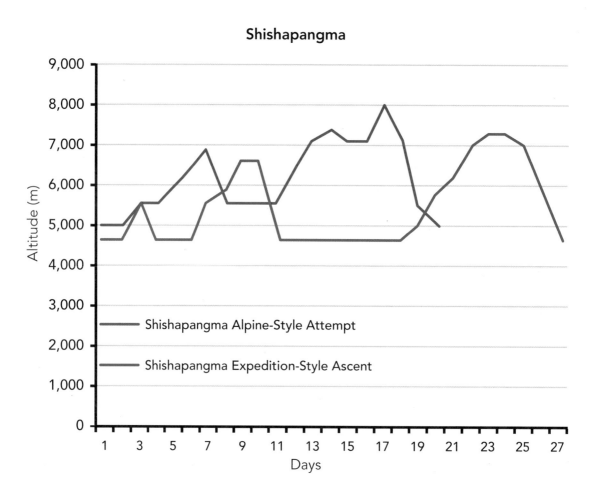

This graph shows the typical difference between traditional expedition-style acclimatization strategy versus alpine-style acclimatization strategy. The red line illustrates the traditional expedition-style strategy with the expedition members staying high for a long time. This is not the strategy favored by these authors, but it has worked many times. The blue line is for a moderately technical route (the south face) and it shows that they made a summit attempt after only one significant acclimatization foray to less than 7,000 meters on the tenth day of their expedition, which was followed by prolonged bad weather. During the attempt their ascent was not overly rapid; they spend four days to arrive at a bivouac at 7,000 meters.

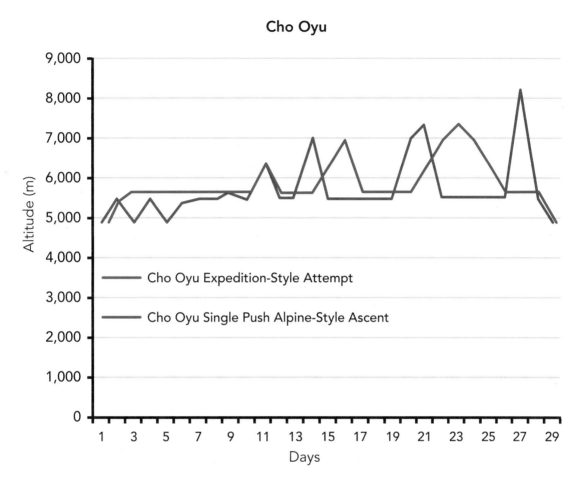

The blue line shows a commercially guided expedition to Cho Oyu and the red line is the alpine-style ascent of that peak by these two authors. One difference is that Scott and Steve spent the first five nights at lower elevations with day trips higher every second day followed by a prolonged rest period at the usual, and very high, Advance Base Camp. Both expeditions climbed above 6,000 meters for the first time on day eleven. After this first foray you will notice quicker ascents and descents by Steve and Scott compared to the commercially guided expedition, which resulted in more rest time and less total time high. Though the maximum altitudes reached at each stage of acclimatization are the same, Steve and Scott didn't climb on Cho Oyu itself until the twentieth day of their expedition. Otherwise the length of the rest intervals were similar.

Altitudes shown represent that day's maximum elevation. All climbs were accomplished without supplemental oxygen.

In terms of the number of people to summit a high mountain, eighty-five, it surely stands as the single most successful expedition of all time. They clearly understood acclimating and climbing to high altitudes.

Unfortunately much of this Soviet experience was scattered with the break-up of the Soviet Union and the 1997 death of Anatoli Boukreev on Annapurna. Today, Russian-born Kazakh Denis Urubko carries on their tradition. Besides having climbed all the 8,000-meter peaks, Denis won the 2006 Elbrus speed climbing competition, climbing at the incredible ascent rate of over 2,600 feet (792 meters) per hour to a finishing altitude of 18,510 feet (5,642 meters). This is 10,663 feet (3,250 meters) of vertical gain in less than four hours! The climbers of the Soviet tradition clearly remain among the strongest high-altitude alpinists in the world.

The Russian Rest

The Soviets conceived the idea that after spending one night at the highest camp, typically within 3,300 feet (1,000 meters) of the summit, they would go very low, preferably below 13,000 feet (4,000 meters) for three nights of total rest. It was Anatoli Boukreev, the highly accomplished altitude climber who stood on 8,000-meter high summits twenty-two times, who popularized with Western climbers what he called the Russian Rest. Today many Himalayan climbers choose to walk to a lower elevation for a thorough rest before embarking on a final summit push. It is not unusual of late for those with the means to helicopter from Everest base camp to Kathmandu for a few days of rest, a few beers, and then heli back in. Must be nice!

How High Do You Need to Go?

Before climbing 26,660-foot (8,126-meter) high Nanga Parbat, Vince Anderson and Steve House had one ascent to 23,000 feet (7,010 meters) and eight nights sleeping at 20,000 feet (6.096 meters) under their belts. They spent about one hour at 23,000 feet before descending back to base camp at 11,750 feet (3,581 meters). There they rested and waited for eleven days before starting their final ascent. They estimated their climb would take six days during which time they'd gain an average of less than 3,000 feet (914 meters) per day, further time to acclimate. This acclimatization regime gave them enough stimuli to begin the adaptation process, but the rest phase at base camp is most probably where the real physiological adaptations happened. As in training, the gains are realized during rest, not activity.

Just how high do you have to go? If you study the figures of various acclimatization schedules you'll notice that in every case the climbers ascended to within approximately 3,300 feet (1,000 meters) of the summit. This seems to work well, building up to a high altitude, then returning low for a rest period, then shooting up high quickly to make the most of typically short weather windows.

Acclimating really is not so different from training. Steve's mantra for acclimating is "Stress the system. Rest the system." You have to climb high, introduce your body to the stress of altitude, and then rest to allow your body to make necessary adaptations. Staying at one elevation acclimates you only to that elevation. Only climbing high acclimates you for climbing high.

HIGH ALTITUDE: YOUR FIRST TIME

Denali is typically a North American alpinist's first taste of a big, high peak. It was Steve's first high-altitude summit, and he spent every season of the next decade climbing and guiding people to its 20,320-foot (6,194-meter) high summit. People understandably approach such a serious peak cautiously, often in big groups and with heavy stores of food and fuel.

The chart below shows two acclimatization schedules: a normal schedule and an alternate (fast) schedule that both authors and many others have used to climb Denali's West Buttress and West Rib routes. The alternate schedule is not unreasonable for a very fit climber and stays mostly within Houston's Law of 1,000 feet (305 meters) per night gain recommendation except at the lower altitudes below 14,000 feet (4,267 meters). The physically hardest day in this accelerated schedule for most people is the move to the 14,200-foot (4,328-meter) camp. This is a big day by any standard considering the heavy packs involved. In our experience, if a climber can successfully make this day then he or she will be able to make the summit from 14,200 feet in a single day with a light pack once acclimated. In the traditional schedule, the move from 14,200 to 17,200 (5,243 meters) is typically more difficult.

To achieve these schedules, and feel good, one must stay within a low exertion level. Conversational pace all the way up; going faster than this is counterproductive in the long run. Scott advised four non-climber Nordic ski racers to a successful Denali summit using the acclimatization plan outlined below; all four were fit but none had been above 10,000 feet (3,048 meters) before nor had any of them stood on a glacier.

My First 8,000er

By Gerlinde Kaltenbrunner

When I was twenty-three years old I started for Broad Peak, my first big expedition. I had no idea about mountains of this height, and before that trip Mont Blanc was the highest mountain I had climbed. I had a lot of experience in rock and ice climbing, but no experience with acclimatizing.

When we hiked into the Karakoram, along the legendary Baltoro Glacier, I moved very slow, trying to give my body enough time to adapt to the lower oxygen pressure. At the same time, a Czech expedition passed us, barreling ahead toward the base camp of Broad Peak. They were very fast and reached base camp earlier than we did.

As I was approaching base camp a group was coming down the glacier toward us. One of the Czech climbers had pulmonary edema and his team was transporting him down to the lower elevation of Concordia. He died before they got there. This was a first tough impression of how serious high-altitude climbing can be.

During this expedition I focused on any advice I could get from the many very experienced high-altitude climbers I met. Once we reached a new camp, I learned to keep moving a little bit instead of resting or sleeping. I collected snow and shoveled, and for hours I melted ice and snow. I always drink a lot, four to five liters per day when possible. I feel very comfortable with that and I believe, because of this big amount of liquid, I never get headaches or have frostbite.

On Broad Peak we did a very nice acclimatization. Many times we moved up and down the mountain, always trying to climb a bit higher than our sleeping elevation. First we climbed up to 5,700 meters (18,701 feet) to establish Camp 1, and that same day we went down to base camp. We rested there for two days before climbing again up to Camp 1. This time we spent one night up there and headed on to 6,300 meters (20,669 feet) to bring up some gear, which we deposited before again going down to base camp.

Afterward we had six days' rest because of bad weather, which for our acclimatization was very good. Again we climbed up to Camp 1 to sleep there, and the next day up to Camp 2 for a night there, and then further up to 7,000 meters (22,966 feet) to deposit gear for Camp 3 and immediately down for four days of rest in base camp.

On our first summit attempt we climbed from base camp to Camp 2, spent one night there, and the next day went directly up to Camp 3 and the next day to 7,600 meters (24,934 feet). We turned back that day when we couldn't feel our toes anymore.

Since that expedition I have spent at least three months a year at high altitude. I've noticed over time that my body adapts more quickly to the altitude than in the years prior. Nowadays, if we have the possibility, we acclimatize on a 6,000-meter (19,685-foot) peak first so we don't need to climb up and down the 8,000ers as much.

Austrian Gerlinde Kaltenbrunner was introduced to the mountains by her priest, who took the local kids hiking every Sunday after mass.

Opposite: Gerlinde Kaltenbrunner standing on the summit of her final 8,000er, K2 (28,251', 8,611m) which she climbed during her seventh expedition to the peak. With this ascent, she became the first woman to climb all fourteen 8,000 meter peaks (without supplemental oxygen). *Photo: Maxut Zhumayev*

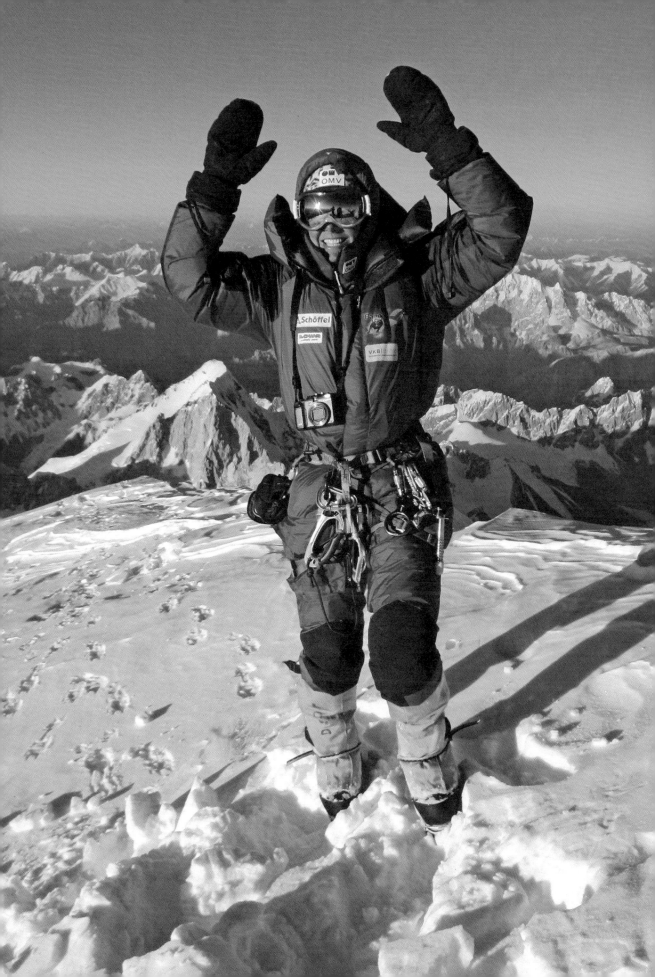

Two Acclimatization Schedules for Denali

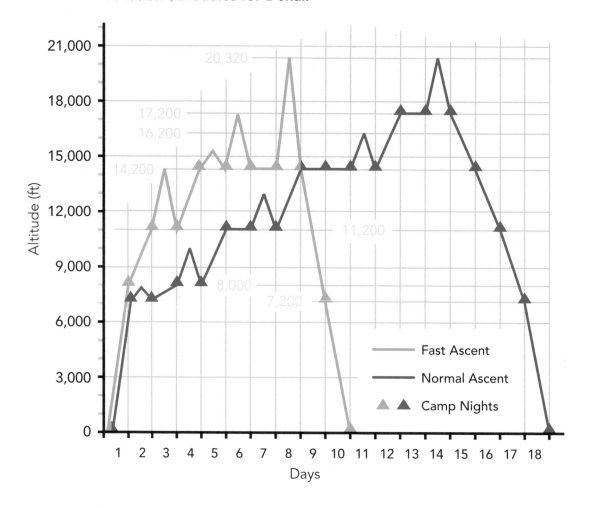

Steve has guided eleven parties carrying sixty- to eighty-pound loads on the arduous climb from the 14,200-foot (4,328-meter) camp to the 17,200-foot (5,243-meter) camp on Denali's West Buttress, often to find that almost everyone is too tired to make the summit when the weather did clear. Unless you are really fit, it is nearly impossible to recover at this altitude because your body has so much to do with managing basic functions, let alone acclimatizing. Aim to be fit enough and go slow enough that you arrive in each camp in a reasonable amount of time, feeling fresh. This is a good time to know what to eat for recovery; consume a good snack as soon as you arrive.

In 1978, Galen Rowell and Ned Gillette climbed from the original base camp site at 10,000 feet (3,048 meters) to the summit in nineteen hours with no prior acclimatization. That's an average ascent rate of 544 feet (166 meters) per hour. Fast by the standards of the

Himalayan giants and considering their utter lack of acclimatization. We have both been to the summit as quickly as day five of a Denali trip from sea level. Fully acclimated, Chad Kellogg went from the current base camp at 7,200 feet (2,195 meters) to the summit in fourteen hours and twenty-two minutes, an average ascent rate 917 feet (280 meters) per hour.

How Long Will My High-Altitude Climb Take?

On the twenty-fourth day of an expedition to Cho Oyu, the world's sixth-highest peak, the authors were faced with the question: How long will it take to climb 8,500 vertical feet (2,591 meters) from base camp to the summit? We might have been wise to ask this before the expedition so we could have done some research. We had to guess, but we've since done that research and have compiled ascent rates from various mountaineers at various altitudes. Ascent rates can vary considerably based on conditions as well as fitness, but the numbers in the chart on the next page provide a basic guideline.

The 14,200-foot (4,330m) camp on Denali (20,320', 6,194m) with view of Mount Foraker (17,402', 5,304m). The climb of Denali by the West Buttress route is most North American's first exposure to high altitude. The cold weather and harsh environment make it a difficult place to learn how to acclimate. *Photo: Marko Prezelj*

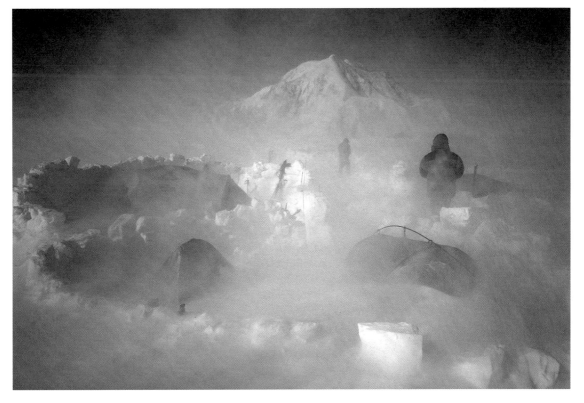

General Ascent Rates for Nontechnical Climbing in Good Conditions.

Altitude	Ascent rates for a fit, acclimated climber	Actual ascent rates will vary considerably
13,123 ft 4,000 m	1,000–2,000 ft per hour 300–600 m per hour	3,300 ft per hour is not unheard of; 2,600 ft per hour of technical climbing has been recorded by soloists.
16,404 ft 5,000 m	1,000 ft per hour 300 m per hour	Infinte Spur: 400 ft per hr Cayesh: 240 ft per hour
19,685 ft 6,000 m	820 ft per hour 250 m per hour	Slovak Direct: 133 ft per hr Rupal Face day 3: 165 ft per hr
22,965 ft 7,000 m	656 ft per hour 200 m per hour	K7 (6,942m): 340 ft per hr
26,246 ft 8,000 m	328 ft per hour 100 m per hour	Rupal Face summit day: 190 ft per hr Cho Oyu 8,201m (from BC): 500 ft/hr
27,887 ft 8,500 m	164 ft per hour 50 m per hour	

*These figures assume no supplemental oxygen.

ACCLIMATIZING: TIPS AND TRICKS

The trickiest part of acclimating is having the right strategy. There are several different approaches, including pre-acclimating at home.

The Scott Method

Doug Scott, one of the godfathers of alpine style, may be the pioneer of the multi-peak expedition. In 1983 he and a number of strong climbers started their season in the Karakoram by making technical ascents on rock towers low on the Baltoro Glacier, then climbed Broad Peak before unsuccessfully attempting K2, all in alpine style.

Marko Prezelj has leveraged this strategy to allow him to climb more new routes in the Himalaya than any one person in history. He routinely ascends three to five routes per expedition and has been known to go on as many as three expeditions per year.

An Experiment on Cho Oyu

The authors combined the Soviet method of acclimating with the Scott/Prezelj approach to ascending multiple peaks when we went to Cho Oyu in 2001. We climbed three 20,000-foot (6,096-meter) peaks and one 23,000-foot (7,010-meter) peak before stepping onto Cho Oyu. There we made one acclimatization trip to Camp 2 at 23,000 feet (7,010 meters), spent a restless night, hiked up to 24,000 feet (7,315 meters) the next morning, and returned to base camp that day. After four days of rest Steve climbed to the summit in seventeen hours, but Scott unfortunately was turned back by intestinal illness at 24,000 feet on the dawn of his forty-seventh birthday.

On the 26,906-foot (8,201-meter) high summit, Steve felt great, drank a liter of water, and ate two energy bars. Our acclimatization strategy coupled with sufficient fitness is clearly a safe way to climb a big mountain. Other climbers, with less fitness, needed six days above base camp to reach the same summit. Scott and Steve spent a total of twenty-seven hours on their final ascent and descent of Cho Oyu, thereby reducing their exposure to the objective hazards inherent to any big mountain.

The Denali Method

This requires access to a relatively easy route. The common practice for people attempting technical routes on Denali's South Face is to first ascend the West Buttress route, usually to the summit if weather allows. Steve did this before two of his new routes on Denali—First Born and Beauty is a Rare Thing—as well as before ascending the Slovak Direct, and on Mount Foraker, the Infinite Spur. After all of these ascents he returned to 7,200-foot (2,195-meter) base camp, in one case even flying out to Talkeetna. These precautions gave him the necessary acclimatization followed by solid rest before taking on high, strenuous climbing.

CAN YOU PRE-ACCLIMATE AT YOUR LOW-ELEVATION HOME?

The short answer to that question is no, almost certainly not. The long answer is more interesting.

Intermittent Hypoxic Exposure, sometimes called altitude training, is living at low elevations and periodically exposing your body to

Climb and Acclimatize

By Marko Prezelj

Adaptation, to new situations and to altitude, is necessary for every high-alpine ascent. This process is most pronounced on expeditions where you must adjust to changes in environment, food, and even the people with whom you will share your experiences. With so much new information, my senses intensely perceive these differences, which triggers strong reactions and impressions—the high of being on an expedition. Spontaneity and relaxation are both essential for all types of adaptation; you need to tune both the body and mind into the new environment.

In 1991, Andrej Štremfelj and I wanted to climb the first ascent of the south pillar of the south summit of Kanchenjunga (27,808 feet/8,476 meters). We were independent members of a larger expedition organized by the Alpine Association of Slovenia. This was a big relief for us because this meant that we didn't have to concern ourselves with expedition logistics. We left home ten days after the majority of the group. At the last herder's pasture before the Yalung Glacier we caught up with the main group. United with our expedition we were able to slow down, settle into the mountain environment, and focus our thoughts on climbing.

After a rainy day and night, we woke to a clear morning. The view from the tent door was the top of the pyramid of Boktoh (20,091 feet/6,142 meters).

"*Should we go climbing?*" was the question at breakfast.

"*When we run out of breath, we can turn around. Come on,*" was the spontaneous answer.

Uroš Rupar joined us. Our line of ascent was not technically difficult, but we did need to use both axes. After six hours, we were on the summit. Of course we felt the air was thinner, but we didn't think about it much. At the time, we did not know we had made the first ascent of the peak.

Several days later, at base camp, we decided to climb the striking Talung (24,110 feet/7349 meters). This time we wanted to get high enough to visually explore and understand the upper reaches of Kanchenjunga South. The first day we ascended to a bivouac in the middle of Talung, the next day a strong wind accompanied us as we climbed separately. Andrej decided to descend 160 feet (49 meters) below the summit. I was able to stand on top. Ten days after Boktoh I was 3,900 feet (1,189 meters) higher. At the time I did not suspect that I had made the second ascent of the peak.

After five days of rest we approached Kanchenjunga by saying that we had to give it a try. Andrej brought his extensive experience and let me ascend in my youthful enthusiasm. On the fifth day we reached the south summit of Kanchenjunga, and we descended, with luck, to the Normal Route where we joined other members of the expedition.

On any climb, I remain chronically curious to explore everything around me. When I'm not deliberately thinking about it, the acclimatization to altitude occurs by itself.

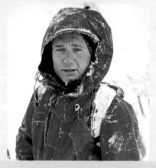

Marko Prezelj in the French Alps.
Photo: Manu Pellissier

Since the late 1980s Slovenian alpinist Marko Prezelj has consistently made successful expeditions to peaks around the world, succeeding in all forms of alpinism. He has climbed many high-altitude summits as well as new routes on demanding summits in the mountains of the Alps, Patagonia, Alaska, Peru, Canada, and Iran.

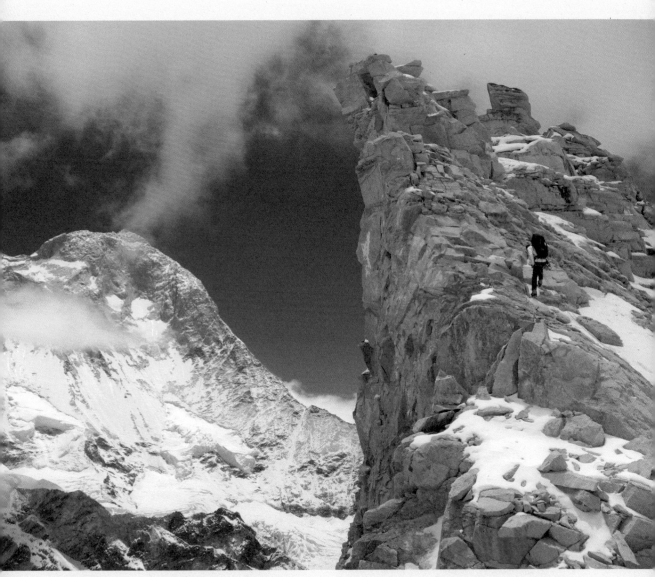

Marko Prezelj descending after making the first ascent of an unnamed, unclimbed 20,000-foot (6,000m) peak while acclimating to attempt Makalu (27,825', 8,481m) in Nepal during a 2011 expedition. *Photo: Steve House*

a simulated or real high altitude. Simulating altitude usually involves sleeping in a tent with a mechanical compressor that pumps low-oxygen air into the tent. This is certainly the most common and most affordable method. Altitude tents are used by triathletes and other endurance competitors to improve sea-level performance.

In some countries it is possible to find special nitrogen houses built for World Cup–level competitive athletes. These houses change the ratio of oxygen to nitrogen in the air to simulate altitude; you can rent time in them like a high-altitude hotel. In a few places in North America, especially in California and Colorado, you may have easy access to 13,000- or 14,000-foot (3,962- or 4,267-meter) peaks. Breathing exercises with masks that restrict airflow have also been studied, and found ineffective. The US military favors the use of unpressurized aircraft flying at high altitudes as their low-pressure environment.

Most of the studies on hypoxic training have been completed without control groups doing the same exercises at normal altitudes. Because of this flaw it is impossible to separate the improvements in performance from the training effect resulting from the ongoing physical exercise and the artificially induced hypoxia. When used under close supervision these modalities return, at most, a 1 percent improvement in VO_2 max. That 1 percent may be the difference between first place and

When planning an expedition try to research routes where you can easily and safely reach a high elevation for acclimatization. Here two climbers ascend an easy snow peak in the Karakoram Range in Pakistan.
Photo: Steve House

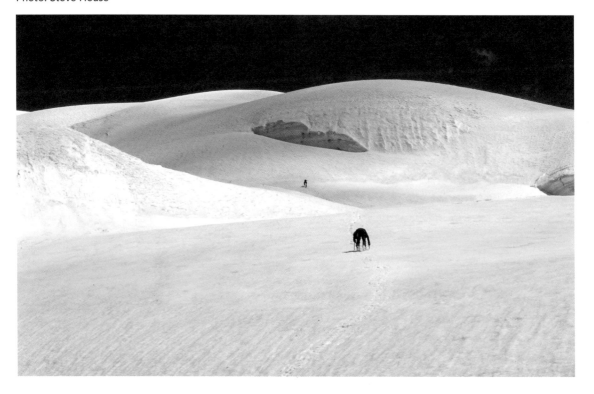

fifteenth place in the Olympic marathon, but for climbing at high altitude, the performance gain does not seem relevant.

Is IHE for Climbers?

The important question for climbers is whether or not this approach could help us to pre-acclimate before a high-altitude expedition. No studies concerning intermittent hypoxia have been made concerning climbers or trekkers ascending to very high altitude, which we would define as above 16,000 feet (4,900 meters). When you speak with altitude experts, most quickly point out that it is unknown if the modality of these tents, which work by pulling oxygen from the air as opposed to lowering the pressure, trigger precisely the same physiologic response as does the decreased pressure that you experience as you ascend. This is one problem. The second big problem for alpinists is that it simply takes a long time to travel from your home to the high mountains.

In 2003, we conducted our own experiment with hypoxic tents. Before traveling to Pakistan, Steve slept in a tent that lowered the oxygen content of the air to the equivalent of 10,000 feet (3,048 meters) for several weeks. It took seven days of travel from Steve's home to reach 10,000 feet again in the Karakoram; he felt no extra acclimatization. The tent rental had been expensive, and it was difficult to sleep with the noisy compressor switching on and off all night. He actually acclimated worse than usual on that expedition, most likely due to a recent illness. We did not repeat the experiment.

The Central Governor Theory

The central governor theory predicts IHE as a pre-acclimatization supplement to altitude will not be useful because, according to this theory, it is the heart that limits exercise performance at altitude, as well as at sea level. The central governor theory leads us to the conclusion that the only altitude training that will be of any value are modalities that contribute to increases in the amount of oxygenated blood reaching the heart muscle itself. Going back to fundamentals, remember that the heart needs the same amount of oxygen to produce one full contraction at sea level as it needs at 8,000 meters. More red blood cells delivering more oxygen to the heart muscle has been identified in studies as a limiting factor for increasing performance at altitude. In testing, no amount of time spent in an altitude tent or nitrogen house resulted in increased red blood cell counts.

Right now there is zero evidence that the body will perform better on a climb at moderate or high altitude after IHE. We would like to see a well-designed study aimed at rapid ascents to moderate altitudes (below 13,000 feet/3,962 meters), as this seems the only likely area for successes for these tools.

Go High, Naturally

The most relevant type of pre-acclimatization is to have access to relatively high mountains all year long. Anatoli Boukreev, who made his home in Kazakhstan, wrote: "To maintain a basic level of adjustment to altitude and to keep up endurance, my routine training includes rapid ascents on 10,000- to 13,000-foot (3,048- to 3,962-meter) high peaks all year." For those lucky enough to live in Colorado, California, Washington, or Western Canada, this is not unreasonable and seems likely to be the best way to help yourself perform at altitude in the long term. Any adaptations must be the result of years of repeated exposure to exercise at these moderately high elevations. This matches our own observations of native altitude dwellers and highly experienced high-altitude mountaineers, and we would hypothesize that this adaptation is long-term and in fact the result of increased capillarization of the heart muscle itself, which allows the heart to beat more strongly and with greater stroke volume at altitude.

PREPARING YOUR BODY TO GO HIGH

Pre-Expedition Weight Gain

There is a persistent idea in expedition climbing that you should gain weight before an expedition because one invariably loses weight at high altitude. This has considerable anecdotal evidence in successful 8,000-meter peak climbers such as Jerzy Kukuczka. However, there are many more examples of climbers—Messner, Habeler, Bonatti, Scott, Prezelj, and Bookreev, to name just a few—who accomplished their greatest climbing in the peak fitness of their lives. A quick look through archival photographs of these climbers will reveal that they were very slim in their primes.

Personally we don't like the "fat down low to be fit up high" philosophy. In fact we believe that it slows acclimatization. Our experience is that extra body mass puts more stress on your circulatory and respiratory systems. The less energy your body has for acclimatization, the less well one acclimates. Marko Prezelj, who concurs with this theory, acclimates better and more rapidly than anyone we've climbed with; his 5'10" frame carries a mere 145 pounds. Boukreev was also tall and thin. Denis Urubko, among the most accomplished alpinists on 8,000-meter peaks in history, is also tall and lean. Five pounds of fat is five pounds of extra tissue to keep oxygenated and fed no matter what it's made of. Remember the piano mover analogy from chapter 3? On your next training mission bring an extra half-gallon of water, or four additional pounds, and see if you don't notice the weight by the end of the day.

Some argue that being overweight gives them valuable energy stores up high. Accessing subcutaneous fat and metabolizing it is more expensive from the physiological standpoint than is accessing intramuscular fat and fat stored around your organs. Recall from the previous chapter that we have enough of the intramuscular and intra-organ fat to fuel many hundreds of miles of running.

Our view is that you want to be as healthy and fit as possible when you depart on your expedition or climb. Your body will have a lot of stress to cope with and the healthier it is, the more easily it will deal

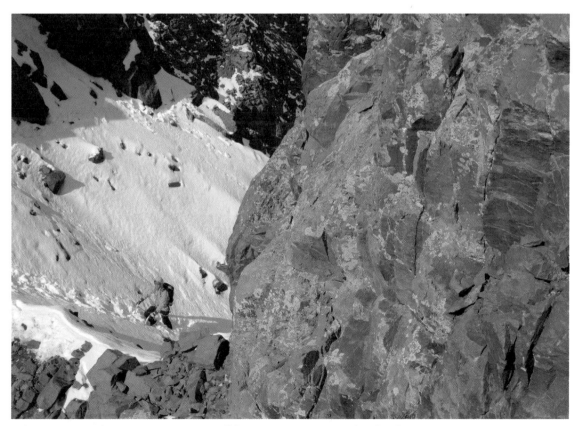

Colin Simon ascending a route on Mount Sneffels (14,157', 4,315m) in Colorado. *Photo: Steve House*

with the challenges to come. Expeditions are stressful, and the final weeks before departure are full of last-minute tasks, spending time with family, and of course making sure you've packed all of your equipment. If you've completed a long-term training program, the drop in intensity and volume of physical work will have the effect of creating a period of super-fitness exactly when you need it most.

Staying Healthy

Staying healthy on long expeditions in developing countries can be one of the biggest challenges to the climber. Paying a bit more money to stay in cleaner hotels and lodges, hiring more experienced base camp staff, and using a reputable trekking agency to help you organize your logistics all pay dividends in staying healthy. A wonderful, but expensive, solution is to bring an expedition doctor. A better alternative for most expeditions is to have a doctor familiar with expedition climbing and developing-world travel help you assemble a solid arsenal of medicine, and be available to consult with you by satellite phone.

Eating at Altitude

We've already discussed nutrition extensively in the previous chapter, but here's the reminder: at altitude, everything is magnified—including your need for eating well. We follow three simple rules:

- Try to eat frequently; every two hours is ideal.

- Eat as much as you can while at base camp.

- Eat lightly and mostly carbohydrates while acclimating and climbing.

Appetite is an excellent indicator of acclimatization, and therefore performance. Exploring why this might be will illuminate some basic truths we've already learned about acclimating.

When you go to a new altitude, and stay there, your appetite is usually weak. In our experience it will be good for the first two to six hours after you arrive, and then it will diminish as your body registers the new altitude. Use this window of time when you're feeling good one of two ways: either get a bit higher to stress the system—1,000 feet (305 meters) higher is highly relevant to furthering your acclimatization—or use the time while you still have an appetite to eat and drink. Eat simple foods that are palatable and easy to digest. Nothing processed. A handful of roasted, unsalted cashews and half a packet

The Khumbu Cough

By Steve House

We crossed the last glacial stream and walked into Makalu Base Camp after seven long, wet days of trekking through the end of the monsoon. It had been a difficult trip to here: cancelled flights, porters stealing some loads and breaking into others, and coaching two friends who had not been to the Himalaya before. I approached the kitchen tent and heard the distinctive, hollow sound of a deep cough.

"Oh, dammit!" I stopped in my tracks, staring at the tent door, suddenly afraid to go in despite my chill and hunger.

Ian looked at me quizzically.

"Our cook is sick. That's not good." I went inside, accepted a cup of tea, made the introductions, and began to inquire about the kitchen's sanitation precautions.

On Himalayan expeditions it is mandatory that the expedition hire a base camp cook to prepare meals and serve the government-assigned liaison officer. The same cook also serves all the base camp meals for all the members, which is a huge benefit, especially when you find a good cook who can prepare diverse and tasty meals. Chest infections are common because the immune system is depressed by the other stresses on the body and the dry, often raw state of mucous membranes in the nose and throat.

Sure enough, within a week I had my own horrible cough. Vince, Marko, and Ian somehow escaped, but I stayed sick for the entire expedition. Vince and Marko climbed a new route on 25,190-foot (7,678-meter) Makalu II while I watched from below. When it came time to attempt Makalu itself, I was dragging far behind.

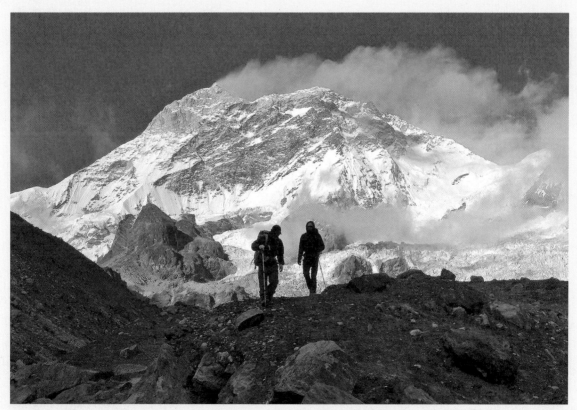

The trek to Makalu takes you up the remote Barun Valley. Here two climbers complete the final leg of the trek to the Hillary Base Camp at 15,750 feet (4,800m) with the south face of Makalu (27,825', 8,481m) looming above. *Photo: Marko Prezelj*

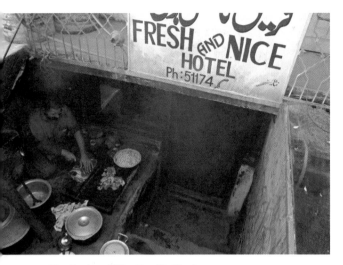

The Fresh and Nice Hotel in Khaplu, northeastern Pakistan. We did not have lunch here. *Photo: Steve House*

of ramen noodle soup without the spice packet is plenty; dehydrated potatoes flavored with melted cheese is a feast. Expecting a diminished appetite, and eating while you can, will help your body get the calories it needs.

Entering a negative energy balance—losing weight—on an alpine climb is normal, whether it's a one-day ascent of Mount Whitney or a sixty-day siege of K2. This is due to a number of factors: eating less, possible altitude illness, diuresis, increased time being physically active, heavier loads being carried, malabsorption of nutrients above 20,000 feet (6,100 meters), and elevated basal metabolic rate when you are living high. Body weight losses of 5 percent are typical and should not affect performance. After climbing Nanga Parbat in 2005 Steve lost seventeen pounds, 11 percent of his body weight. This type of weight loss will affect strength and endurance, and if you've lost that much weight, your expedition is finished, with or without the summit.

It can take months to recover from the stresses imposed on your body that caused the weight loss in the first place. Not to mention regaining the muscle and other vital tissues that were broken down during such an extreme catabolic period. Recall Steve's story in chapter 2 of not allowing enough recovery after his Rupal Face climb before starting back into serious training. The lack of complete recovery came back to haunt him months later when he struggled to regain strength.

The best altitude climbers invariably seem to be smart eaters. Ask someone about time spent on an expedition with Anatoli Boukreev how he would sit, teaspoon in hand, and consume an entire jar of jam for dessert in base camp. It might take him two hours, but he'd do it. While climbing, he would not eat much, preferring light, carbohydrate-rich dinners, sometimes only dried fruit for dinner and hot chocolate or coffee for breakfast. In his 2001 book, *Above the Clouds*, Boukreev wrote: "Appetite at high altitude is an individual thing. For me it is generally best to consume as little as possible (while climbing), and then only those foods that are metabolized quickly."

We concur. As you ascend, eat frequent, small meals with the aim of maintaining your muscle glycogen stores. Eat as if you're on a long training run or hike back home. An energy gel and a handful of nuts may be enough for dinner at a new elevation. This works for a number of reasons: When burdened with the work of acclimating, your body does

Expedition Eating

By Steve Swenson

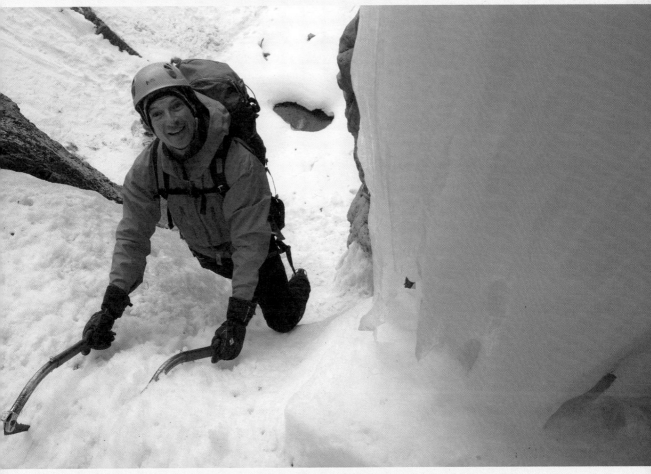

Steve Swenson approaching Whiteman Falls, a classic ice climb in Alberta, Canada. *Photo: Steve House*

At base camp where you are at altitude for extended periods, my one suggestion is to eat as much as you can. You can never eat too much. Your appetite will be naturally depressed, and if you let yourself succumb to that you will become progressively weaker. Force yourself to eat if you need to. If you really can't eat, then you are moving up too quickly and need to go down to an elevation where you can eat more. I don't believe that fancy diets with special foods are necessary—eat what you enjoy so you can get enough down, as long as it is a good mix of fats, proteins, and carbohydrates.

Once you go high on the mountain and are eating your mountain food, weight becomes more of an issue, so it's acceptable to have a more minimalist approach to food as it's only for short periods of time. I can always tell who is strong enough to get up a high mountain by how they eat at base camp.

Past-president of the American Alpine Club, Steve Swenson has been climbing since 1968 and made twenty expeditions to mountains in Asia. He has made ascents of K2 and Everest without supplemental oxygen.

not need the added strain of difficult digestion. It is also important to minimize the weight of food and fuel because you have to carry it all up there. Plus you have little time to devote to the difficult task of melting snow into water and heating enough water to make food. Forcing larger amounts of food at altitude may put you at risk of nausea and vomiting, a sure way to lose loads of fluids and calories that only have to be replaced.

The most common strategy for eating on expeditions is to follow your appetite—and the human appetite at altitude can be a strange thing. Slovenians love to eat raw garlic, six to eight cloves in a sitting, which they believe helps acclimatization. Many Americans, these authors not included, seem to be fixated on Pringles potato chips. We like strawberry jam on chapattis or canned mackerel in a spicy tomato sauce. Instant soups are popular, but from the nutritional standpoint, salty foods are best avoided. Salt is overused in most expedition kitchens. As is the case with too much water, too much sodium can cause trouble at altitude. Bring a supply of low-sodium instant soups and other simple, easily digestible foods from home.

Caffeine: Help or Hindrance?

Many altitude residents are known to drink frequent cups of black tea heavily laden with milk and sugar. Caffeine is commonly thought to be bad at altitude, because of its possible negative effects on sleep and fears of dehydration. In a thorough 2010 review, altitude expert Dr. Peter Hackett concludes: "Fears of dehydration from caffeine are exaggerated. Its effect on ventilation and cerebral circulation and its action as a psychostimulant are likely to be helpful at altitude. Caffeine may also help exercise performance at high altitude. Importantly, habitual caffeine users should not discontinue caffeine because of travel to altitude." You will also remember from our discussion of nutrition that caffeine is known to have a positive effect on fat metabolism.

HYDRATION AT HIGH ALTITUDE

You will hear it frequently repeated that at altitude you must drink six liters of water per day. According to the Wilderness Medicine Newsletter, this is based on dehydration by exhaling 250 cc of water per hour, which computes to six liters per day. We have been unable to find any studies that measured this much dehydration by respiration. On Steve's first expedition to Nanga Parbat in 1990 he and a German climber did drink six liters each on a rest day at 20,000 feet (6,096 meters). It was difficult and time consuming to melt enough snow to get so much fluid, and they both felt nauseous and uncomfortably bloated afterward, so much so that they couldn't eat dinner. In fact too much water can result in problems because the body secretes abnormally large amounts of antidiuretic hormone at altitude, meaning you don't pee off as much as you normally would.

According to the most recent research the best indicator of hydration is the degree of your thirst. You should certainly endeavor to stay hydrated, but do not obsess about hitting six liters or peeing clear; straw-colored urine is ideal. There are in fact many stories of climbers staying out for multiple days above 8,000 meters with nothing to drink. This is not recommended, but a fit climber can survive and climb on much less than you think. It's one paradox of alpine climbing that when you need fluids the most, while climbing hard and high, they are the most difficult to produce.

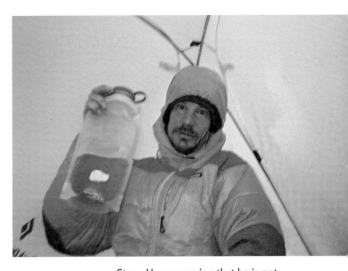

Steve House proving that he is not well hydrated at the third bivouac at 20,000 feet (6,100m) during the the first ascent of the Central Pillar of the Rupal Face of Nanga Parbat (26,660', 8,126m). *Photo: Vince Anderson*

At high altitude there are physiological reasons behind your abnormal thirst. After ten weeks at 20,000 feet (6,096 meters), total body water is 20 percent above normal, plasma volume is 30 percent above normal, and total blood volume is 84 percent above normal. All that fluid starts as liquid you drink. That said, it should never be necessary to spend ten weeks above 20,000 feet. In our experience more than two weeks that high begins to produce diminishing returns of fitness.

On expeditions you should bring a wide variety of herbal teas and drink flavors to keep yourself motivated to drink. Marko Prezelj insists on portering in at least one case of beer per climber to base camp. (You can't put a price on morale!) When climbing, try to avoid cooking in the pot used to melt snow for water. This keeps your water tasting like water, since nothing dispels the urge to drink faster than water that tastes like ramen.

SLEEPING AT ALTITUDE

Sleeping well at altitude is both the most important thing and one of the most elusive. Plan ahead to be as comfortable as possible during an expedition. Your own tent, a wide, warm base camp sleeping bag, extra sleeping pads, pillow, and down booties—whatever it takes. Boukreev wrote: "After years of self-analysis, I know that the ability to fall asleep after hard work is an indication that my body is properly adjusting to the altitude. Difficulty falling asleep indicates that I must reduce the stress on my body and slow my rate of ascent." You will recall that this concurs with the earlier discussion of autonomic nervous system balance between sympathetic and parasympathetic systems. An overstimulation of the sympathetic can leave you feeling wired and restless in bed, even when you're exhausted.

Sleep is made difficult by any number of factors, but the primary culprit is that your respiratory rate naturally drops when you go to sleep, leading to lower oxygen-saturation levels in your blood, which can cause periodic breathing that, if it's bad enough, can wake you up. This breathing pattern, known as Cheynes-Stokes breathing, is exceedingly common during acclimatization. When Steve first gets to any new sleeping altitude above 20,000 feet (6,096 meters), he knows he will not sleep a wink. Headaches, an inability to eat enough, feeling cold, periodic breathing, and general discomfort all will conspire against you. Expect it. Take some aspirin against the headache and keep a large thermos and your pee bottle nearby, put a hot water bottle in your bag, and frequently sip tea to soothe your throat.

HOW FAST DO YOU DE-ACCLIMATE?

In one of the best studies of this question, sixteen-day residents of a 13,287-foot (4,050-meter) altitude were brought to sea level for seven days and then taken back to 14,107 feet (4,300 meters) and tested to assess acclimatization. They were found to retain about 50 percent of their acclimatization. Adaptation to higher altitudes is postulated to take longer to lose than adaptation to moderate altitudes. In Operation Everest III after thirty days in a chamber ascending to the equivalent height of the summit of Everest, the subjects' hemoglobin levels were back to normal values after only four days at sea level. The previous hypothesis seems to conflict with this data, but we find that studies on altitude done in laboratories more often than not do not correlate to what we've experienced in the field. When we examine our own experience, look at the historical record of high-altitude climbing, and ask others, we find that the most common rule of thumb is that you lose your adaptation to altitude at about the same rate as you gain it.

ALTITUDE ILLNESSES AND THEIR CAUSES

As you ascend, your brain swells inside the rigid container of your skull. Picture a bag of potato chips at high altitude. This swelling of your most important organ can lead to acute mountain sickness (AMS) and high altitude cerebral edema (HACE). You may also encounter high altitude pulmonary edema (HAPE), the leaking of fluid into your lungs due to excessive blood pressure in the pulmonary capillaries. A full review of altitude illnesses is beyond the scope of this book and indeed there are many good books devoted solely to this subject. The most compact, simple, and concise book is Dr. Peter Hackett's *Mountain Sickness*. Dr. Charles Houston's book *Going Higher* is the classic in the field and delivers much rich history written by one of the pioneers of altitude medicine. Mike Farris' *The Altitude Experience* is a comprehensive and up-to-date treatment of the full spectrum of altitude issues and covers the science as well as a number of specific recommendations for climbers.

Bruce Miller and Steve House at a bivouac at 23,620 feet (7,200m) with typical symptoms of altitude illness, including lassitude and edema of the face and extremities.
Photo: Bruce Miller

Field Treatment for Altitude Illnesses

All altitude illnesses have, to use Dr. Hackett's popular dictum, three cures: descent, descent, and descent. Failing descent, medical doctors have studied a number of drugs, some of which will help to buy you time so that you can descend.

Altitude Drugs

Climbing at altitude seems to bring out the drug users. In no other area of climbing do people take so many medicines to try to help themselves adapt. I want to discuss drugs used at altitude from the perspective of training and performance. The previously mentioned books will discuss in much more detail how these drugs actually work and when they are contraindicated. As always, a medical doctor must be consulted before ingesting any of these medicines.

Most of the properly designed clinical studies related to altitude medicine are conducted at altitudes below 13,000 feet (3,962 meters), which is not really high altitude in the sense of mountaineering, so right away most of these studies should be viewed skeptically if your goal is to climb high.

Aspirin

Aspirin is perhaps the most common, and one of the most helpful medicines to have on an expedition. It has long been the practice of

Disclaimer

The following descriptions of prescription drugs, over-the-counter medicines, vitamins, and nutritional supplements are for informational purposes only. You should consult with your physician concerning the proper use of any of these items. If you find that you are suffering from the symptoms of any physical or medical condition, you should consult with your physician or other qualified health care provider immediately. Do not avoid or disregard professional medical advice or delay in seeking it because of something you have read in this book.

many high-altitude mountaineers to take a children's aspirin daily to help thin the blood; remember that your plasma volume drops as you ascend. Buffered aspirin can be nice in the event you want to take it on an upset stomach while at altitude. We found no studies that show any effects, positive or negative, of taking aspirin at altitude.

Acetaminophen

Acetaminophen, or Tylenol, is a great drug to have on an expedition for its fever-reducing capacity and as a headache medicine at altitude. Tylenol PM is popular at many base camps because it contains acetaminophen as well as diphenhydramine, which is the active ingredient in Benadryl and causes drowsiness as well as being a cough suppressant. It is a very mild respiratory depressant, so should be used very sparingly at altitude and not at all above base camp.

Non-Steroidal Anti-Inflammatories (NSAIDs)

NSAIDs, such as ibuprofen (Advil) and naproxen (Aleve), may be the most used medicines at altitude. These medicines are effective at helping with altitude headaches, a common cause of sleeplessness. We suspect that the same anti-inflammatory effect they have on the muscles acts on the brain and the brain swelling that is the root cause of AMS (acute mountain sickness) and HACE (High Altitude Cerebral Edema).

A 2012 study found that 600 mg of ibuprofen three times a day starting six hours before ascent resulted in a 26 percent reduction in symptoms of Acute Mountain Sickness versus the placebo group. How this works and whether or not ibuprofen will replace acetazolamide as the altitude drug of choice remains to be learned.

The downside of NSAIDs is that because they take a lot of water to process in your kidneys, they dry your throat, make you thirsty, and therefore tend to exacerbate any dry-air or altitude cough you might have.

Acetazolamide (Diamox)

Acetazolamide is a well-understood and frequently used medication for prevention and treatment of Acute Mountain Sickness by North Americans. We find that Europeans use this drug much less frequently.

There are good studies that show it works to both prevent and treat AMS. As with any medication, there are responders and nonresponders. We've personally climbed with and without it at elevations of up to 26,000 feet (7,925 meters). It does help us to sleep, though we find ¼ tablet (62mg) before bedtime to be enough to affect improved sleep without the annoying side effects of having to pee all the time (it's a diuretic). The tingling of fingers and toes that is a usual side effect is distracting during technical climbing.

In our experience Diamox is not the altitude wonder drug people want it to be. We have concluded that it is only marginally effective in relieving AMS symptoms, and the side effects are annoying. We haven't used it in about ten years.

Need another reason to skip the Diamox? Acetazolamide has been found in studies to worsen performance of high-intensity tasks that involve prolonged whole-body effort or rapidly repeated local muscular effort.

Dexamethasone

Dexamethasone is a steroidal anti-inflammatory used in the treatment of High Altitude Cerebral Edema (HACE) and sometimes High Altitude Pulmonary Edema (HAPE). In North America this must be prescribed and administered by a physician and is available as a tablet or as an intramuscular injection.

We've heard, but not observed, that it is becoming common to use "Dex" in an attempt to prevent symptoms brought on by insufficient acclimatization, effectively as a performance aid. It seems unlikely to have significant benefits in this way and there is little science to back up this type of use. The best study showed an almost immeasurable preservation of individual VO_2 max at altitude; this test was conducted at only 14,750 feet/4,559 meters.

Tadalafil and Sildenafil

Tadalafil (Cialis) and sildenafil (Viagra) came onto the altitude-medicine scene with quite a lot of buzz. We have not known anyone who has taken sildenafil or tadalafil prophylactically against the effects of altitude. In some well-designed studies it has been shown to prevent HAPE and significantly increase an athlete's abilities to exercise at altitude. As is often the case with these studies, the modalities and altitudes don't strongly correlate to what we're interested in as alpine climbers. The best study used a 10-kilometer time trial on a road bike at 3,874 meters, quite different than the intensity and the task faced by a mountaineer.

While these drugs have been hailed as a major advance in the field treatment of HAPE, in our one experience we have been unimpressed.

Phenergan

Phenergan is an anti-nausea medication that climbers have used successfully at altitude to help reduce the nausea and vomiting often inherent in climbing to very high elevations. As does aspirin for a headache, this drug has the advantage of making the symptom tolerable without completely masking it. This is important because if your nausea (or headache) gets worse you may have Acute Mountain Sickness—and that needs to be treated with immediate descent.

Ginkgo Biloba

Ginkgo biloba became the focus of a lot of attention after a 1996 French study caught the eye of Dr. Peter Hackett. Hackett designed further studies carried out at Pikes Peak in Colorado, and they do show that Ginkgo biloba reduces the incidence of AMS, though not as well as acetazolamide, which was used as a control. The latest review states that the primary challenge to investigating whether Ginkgo biloba is effective for preventing or ameliorating AMS symptoms is the lack of standardization in the Ginkgo biloba preparations themselves.

Ginger and Garlic

Ginger and garlic are two common foods that many high-altitude climbers swear by. There is no scientific evidence to support their efficacy as an acclimatization aid, but these foods have never been studied.

Iron

Hypoxia (low blood oxygen) is known to increase the demand for iron in athletes training at altitude and many, especially women, may prove to be iron deficient. Again, few altitude studies have been conducted, but differences in iron status was proposed as an explanation of differences in individual hematological response, meaning differing abilities to generate new red blood cells at altitude.

Hemoglobin, the iron-containing protein in our red blood cells, is an important determinant of oxygen transport, but iron is only one factor in the complex biochemistry of oxygen transport. If you're not sure if you are iron deficient, get tested, as recommended in the previous chapter. You want to make sure your iron levels are within normal range before embarking on an expedition to altitude.

Having above-normal levels of iron is unhealthy and so supplementation must be done intelligently, if at all.

Supplemental Oxygen

Supplemental oxygen is by far the most effective drug at altitude. A three-liter bottle holds about 720 liters of compressed oxygen. Typical flow rates are one to four liters per minute for climbing and one

Alone with HAPE

By Steve House

I n 2009 I was alone at 21,000 feet (6,401 meters) on the west face of Makalu when an unexpected storm began. I decided to wait out the bad weather since I had a tent and plenty of food and fuel. The second night of the storm I noticed a funny noise in my lungs and realized I had high altitude pulmonary edema (HAPE). I immediately took sildenafil as well as nifedipine, the more traditional drug indicated for HAPE. At first light I began to fight my way down 3,300 feet (1,006 meters) of exposed down climbing and rappelling in a raging storm. I had real difficulty breathing and was scared. My pulmonary edema continued to get a lot worse, even after I got to base camp at 13,800 feet (4,206 meters). My symptoms weren't relieved until I walked down below 11,000 feet (3,353 meters) the next morning.

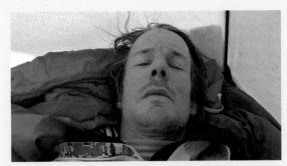

Steve House, very weak and very sick, prepares to leave the tent at first light. His HAPE continued to worsen over the next twenty-four hours. *Photo: Steve House*

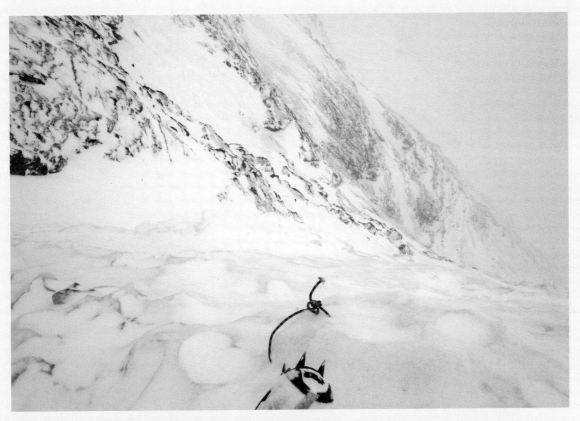

The first rappel anchor at the top of a long descent. Since Steve did not take drugs prophylactically to aid his acclimatization, starting the medicine may have bought him enough time to be able to extricate himself from a very dangerous situation. *Photo: Steve House*

liter per minute for sleeping. So it follows that you have 180 minutes to 720 minutes of climbing or rescue oxygen in one full three-liter bottle. Above four liters per minute is too much, and at higher flow rates it becomes toxic. Guided parties on Everest reportedly carry three to five bottles per client on a summit day. Small, privately funded expeditions can rarely afford to have bottled oxygen as a base-camp emergency drug due to its high up-front cost and the expense of transporting it.

Steve House tries to catch his breath just a few feet below the summit of Nanga Parbat (26,660', 8,126m). *Photo: Vince Anderson*

Using oxygen to ascend lowers the altitude of the peak you're climbing. Supplementing with a flow-rate of two liters per minute effectively reduces the summit of Everest by 3,300 feet or 1,000 meters. This classifies it as a performance-enhancing drug in our book. Some argue that supplemental oxygen is a tool, like an ice ax or a rope. However, a tool is an inert object. Supplemental oxygen is a gas that you inhale to endow yourself with physical capacities you otherwise wouldn't have. Administering drugs to an athlete, whether by injection, pill, or gas, to enhance physical performance is the definition of doping.

Everest was very nearly ascended without supplemental oxygen during the British expedition in the 1920s and again in 1952, the year before the first ascent. In 1939 German-American climber Fritz Wiessner climbed within 660 feet (201 meters) of the summit of K2 without supplemental oxygen. One wonders how different the history of climbing would be had they succeeded.

We believe that the use of supplemental oxygen is ethical to facilitate emergency descent, to keep someone alive while awaiting improved weather that would allow an emergency descent, or by rescue personnel trying to reach a patient.

BE TOUGH AND SMART

Acclimatization turns out to be a fine microcosm of alpinism, embodying so much of what makes climbing mountains compelling and interesting. It takes years of apprenticeship in the various acts of climbing rock and ice to gain the efficiencies you need before beginning to climb really big mountains. Having a healthy and strong heart and robust diaphragm muscles are exceedingly important and can only be developed by years of climbing and training. Arriving at the start of an expedition to high altitude in prime fitness and extraordinary health is as important as clear skies on summit day. What you eat and how much you can eat becomes critical. Arriving at a new altitude, your body will react differently than others. Your own body will feel a bit differently each time you go high.

In all of these ways, climbing at high altitude becomes a goal and a specialty in and of itself. The only way to improve is to do it often. Boukreev, who we've mentioned frequently, once summited four 8,000-meter peaks in a span of four months. Based on these types of experiences he was able to climb 26,906-foot (8,201-meter) high Cho Oyu in five days with no prior acclimatization. Of course he had summited 8,000-meter peaks without supplemental oxygen five times in the previous twelve months, including Everest twice. Cho Oyu in five days was only possible in his mind and body after he had spent countless weeks living and climbing above 8,000 meters and even more months living and climbing above 16,404 feet (5,000 meters).

After studying this chapter, you will be familiar with the basic science of acclimatization. To learn the art of acclimatization, you must climb high yourself. We feel compelled to warn people embarking on high-altitude climbing for the first time: It is uncomfortable, painful, and often sickening. There is, as is so often the case with climbing mountains, a fine line between being tough and being smart. You have to be both. Successful high-altitude mountaineers are survivors who look to the long-term success and not the short term of a single day, a single summit, or even a single expedition. Listen to your body and what you are feeling. Listen carefully. Each experience going high is a lesson. Make frequent adjustments to your expectations based on the changing realities of your body's performance, weather, conditions, and partners. It will get easier the more you climb.

> "You get these high-powered people who want to climb Mount Everest, they spend $85,000 . . . there is a Sherpa in the front pulling, a Sherpa in the back pushing, carrying extra oxygen bottles so you can cheat the altitude. You haven't climbed Everest. The purpose of climbing something like that is to affect some kind of spiritual or physical change. When you compromise the process, you're an asshole when you start out, and you're an asshole when you get back."
>
> – YVON CHOUINARD, founder of Patagonia

Altitude: A Sufferfest

After winning the grueling Mount Elbrus running race Kevin Cooney was invited to join a 1991 Soviet expedition to Everest. There he partnered with the second-place finisher on Elbrus, Anatoli Boukreev, in a speed attempt during which they used Adidas javelin spikes with super gaiters up to Camp 2 in the Western Cwm. The expedition was an eye-opening experience in the Soviet climber's toughness and created a strong friendship between Cooney and Boukreev. A few years later Kevin remarked to author Scott Johnston while the pair was at 22,966 feet (7,000 meters) on K2 that high-altitude climbing is like having the flu all the time: "If I felt this shitty at home I'd call in sick at work." Yet, far from being able to pull the covers up and have another bowl of chicken soup, they were trying climb the world's second-highest mountain.

The Art of Suffering

By Voytek Kurtyka

*Originally printed in *Mountain Magazine*, #121, May/June 1988. Reprinted by permission of Voytek Kurtyka.

It's hard to believe, but the tongue-in-cheek speculation in the pub in the '70s has become a Himalayan reality of the '80s. We once joked about climbing naked at night (the ultimate lightweight), and it's now happening! During the past few years a new Franco-Swiss generation have made a number of ascents at night, and given the circumstances, they might well be considered naked. But no perverse sense of humor drove them to choose such outrageous tactics, rather a spirit of adventure and sporting calculation.

There was once much truth in the saying "alpinism is the art of suffering." The masters of this art ruled and shaped Himalayan climbing. Neither age nor lack of ability deterred the masters of suffering from achieving their aims. To survive intense cold, starve for days on end at high altitude, and still be able to wade through deep snow, a man requires a peculiar and stolid brand of passion and determination. A prerequisite for Himalayan climbing was an ability to accept pain. It was considered a sort of psychological triumph of mind over matter.

Only a few appreciated the psychological costs, yet it is true that inner strength is sometimes mirrored by an outward callousness. Physical dangers and the distress of partners may be blotted out. Hard work and suppressed fear, when combined with competitive determination, tend to narrow the field of vision. I am sadly convinced that egocentricity and a kind of inner deafness are common personality blemishes in our climbing community, more so than many care to admit.

Am I merely being sarcastic? I may be, but not without reason. Too often heroic performances are achieved at

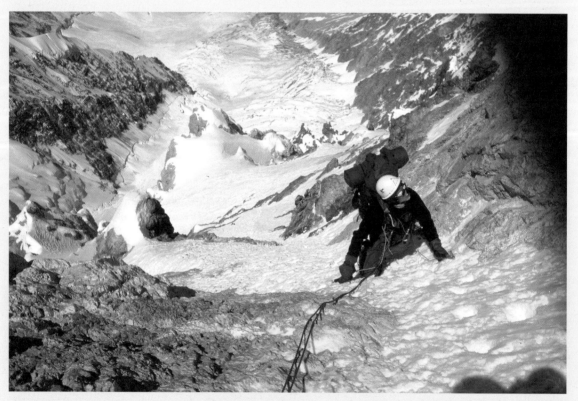

Voytek Kurtyka during the ascent the 10,000-foot (3,000m) west face of Gasherbrum IV (26,001', 7,925m) which he and Robert Schauer climbed in alpine style to the North Summit in 1985. *Photo: Robert Schauer*

the expense of partners. *"He's tired, well so am I. Some-one's coughing behind? There's always someone cough-ing behind . . ."*

This attitude is not an inevitable consequence of Hima-layan climbing. The choice of a partner in the Himalaya is increasingly important to the successful lightweight group. If there is a strong bond, stronger than just companionship, an individual is less likely to miss possible fatal signs of distress in a partner.

I believe that the latest trends exhibit different quali-ties than those of the traditional *masters of suffering*. They are successes both in sporting and human terms. Extreme lightness, the ease of action, and the natural relation-ship with the mountain environment characterize these ascents. Mind and body seem to listen to a new voice, follow a different rhythm. Suffering has been replaced by composure as the long hours of the night are paced away. In two of the following ascents, it is astonishing that the climbers seem not only to have deceived the human psyche, but also the human body since acclimatization was minimal. Possibly the speed of the ascents, with only short spells at altitude, prevented deterioration. Erhard Loretan for one is convinced that by depriving the body of sleep, stagnation is inhibited and the chance of edema and altitude sickness is reduced.

The first ascent I will relate was a relatively cautious affair on the Abruzzi Spur of K2 climbed in July 1985. The team members, Loretan, Eric Escoffier, Yves Morand, and Jean Troillet, acclimatized traditionally, spending one night at 8,000 meters (26,247 feet). At midnight on July 3, they left base camp at 5,000 meters (16,4040 feet) and by 10 a.m. were at Camp 2 at 6,800 meters (22,310 feet). Here they stayed until 7 a.m. the following morning. Previous ascents from this point had taken at least three days, but the plan now called for a single push. At 11 a.m. they reached Camp 3 at 7,300 meters (23,950 feet), where the lads fancied a "picnic" and waited for dusk. Leav-ing behind bivy gear and even the stove, they climbed through the night and reached the summit at 2 p.m. on July 6, having climbed 1,800 meters (5,906 feet) without sleep. They descended to Camp 3 before nightfall and down to base camp the next day.

Next, the east face of Dhaulagiri, which Alex MacIntyre, René Ghilini, and I had first climbed in 1981. The Swiss team consisted of Loretan, Steincr, and Troillet, and this time they chose winter for their night-naked tactics.

The team spent little time acclimatizing, spending one night at 5,700 meters (18,700 feet) and climbing to 6,500 meters (21,325 feet) on the NE Ridge as a warm-up. At midnight on December 5, they left base camp and climbed to the camp at 5,700 meters. Here they rested in a snow hole, departing at midnight on the 2,500-meter (8.200 feet), 50-degree ice face. This time they were not only naked, but cheeky: no ropes, hardware, sleeping bags, or bivy tent; just their one-piece suits, one stove, and a

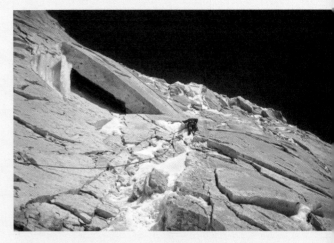

Voytek Kurtyka leading on the eighth day of the first ascent of the south face of Changabang (22,520', 6,864m) in September 1978. At this point they had climbed the crux of the route, but did not know what lay ahead.
Photo: John Porter

chocolate bar each. Winter in the Himalaya is character-ized by continuous hurricane winds and –forty degrees C, but the lads guessed the weather right. They climbed continuously for nineteen hours through the night and the following day, emerging on the summit ridge at 7,700 meters (25,262 feet) at 7 p.m. Here they sat out the night, huddled together, brewing drinks during twelve hours of what Loretan described as "convulsive shivering." At first light the desire for the summit was still with them and at 8 a.m. they set off again, reaching the summit six hours later. They descended immediately and at 2 a.m. reached their snow cave at 5,700 meters (18,700 feet).

This incredibly bold and cold feat is to me more inspi-rational and revelatory than frenzied 8,000er collecting. These three had discovered a new secret, proved the possibilities of extremely lightweight winter ascents, and suffered successfully together. Peak bagging is a form of emotional consumption, a sign of a mountaineer over-whelmed by a desire to collect. If there is such a thing as spiritual materialism, it is displayed in the urge to possess the mountains rather than to unravel and accept their mysteries. Adventure is thus replaced by a regimen of routine actions and emotions.

The collectors make clever use of the magic of numbers such as 8,000 and 14 x 8,000. These figures were once symbols of extremes in Himalayan achievement, but now have been skillfully turned into commercial measures of mountaineering fame. Numbers are simple and under-standable, even by those who have never had cold fingers. The demand for numbers is unlimited. The number eaters gulp them greedily, for they confirm the illusion of posses-sion and soothe the nerves of the consumers.

It is difficult to imagine a sport without numbers, and many now classify mountaineering as sport. No doubt, there is excellent sport to be found in the hills, but is it merely sport? How do we excuse the common and horrifying presence of death in the mountains? Do we really accept it as part of a funny game and competition? I believe that the inner response that drives us onto the precipices and into danger has nothing to do with competition. As an activity, it expresses the classical opposition of the urge for self-preservation and the need to test mortality. To feel in control of one's fate spontaneously frees the spirit from mortal skin. While sensing these frontiers, a mountaineer experiences his greatest joy. How much of this is expressed in collecting numbers? To me, the Swiss ascent of Dhaulagiri, gambling with their nakedness at night, was a return to the essence and good taste in mountaineering.

In 1986, there were two superb night-naked-style ascents on Everest and K2. The first, an ascent of Everest's fine Japanese/Hornbein Couloir Direct, was made by Loretan and Troillet. With them was Beghin, but he rebelled after the first night, when instead of sleep the team climbed a mère 2,000 meters (6,560 feet). The total ascent time from the base of the wall to the summit was forty hours!

Almost as incredible was the time of descent. Finding the snow in condition, the pair made a sitting glissade (in Polish this is literally translated as "arse sliding") down the majority of the route and reached Advanced Base Camp in only four hours. As a Pole, I find it difficult to stay cool knowing that the Swiss have beaten us at one of our national sports! I don't mind hangliding or parapenting from 8000ers, but I am boiling with rage to know that these two Swiss have experienced the greatest arse slide in the world! This very rapid ascent was preceded by a five-week stay during the monsoon in a base camp at 5,500 meters (18,045 feet). Acclimatization above base camp, however, was minimal. They spent one night in Advanced Base Camp (ABC) at 5,850 meters (19,029 feet) and ascended two 6,500-meter (21,325-foot) neighboring peaks.

That was enough; all other energy was saved for the face. They left ABC at 10 p.m. on August 28 carrying no more than had been used on Dhaulagiri. The first 2,000 meters (6,560 feet) took thirteen hours. At 11 a.m., the team had reached 7,800 meters (25,590 feet), where they spent the rest of the day continuously brewing up. At 9 p.m., Loretan and Troillet continued without Beghin. Sometime after midnight, at about 8,400 meters (27,560 feet), the intense cold and pitch darkness forced them

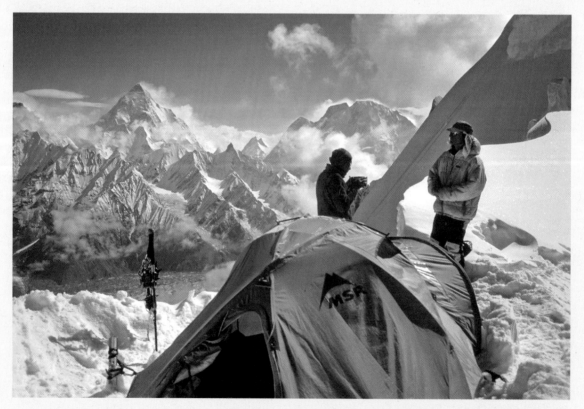

Marko Prezelj and Matic Jost relax during a climb of Biarachedi (22,247', 6,781m). K2 (28,251', 8,611m) on the left and Broad Peak (26,414', 8,051m) are both visibile behind them. Both peaks have seen several history-making ascents. The Abuzzi Spur, the most frequently ascended route on K2, is visible as the right skyline. *Photo: Steve House*

to a halt. They huddled close together and waited for the cruelest hours to slip past. Around 4 a.m. when the first glimmer of dawn had crept into the couloir, they set off and at 1 p.m. they reached the summit. They lounged on top of the world for one hour. By 7 p.m., and hopefully a little sore in the hind parts, they were 3,000 meters lower.

The one night and day ascent of the Abruzzi Spur of K2 by Benoit Chamoux is the simplest story to tell. He set out from base camp at 5 p.m. on July 4 and at 4 p.m. the next day he stood on the summit. Clearly, he had no time to sleep. A few days earlier he had made a sixteen-hour ascent of Broad Peak.

When I met Loretan and Troillet in Kathmandu two summers ago, my curiosity provoked a few questions aimed at Loretan.

"Do you train for climbs?"

"No, the best training's here," tapping his forehead.

"Do you smoke or drink?"

"No to the first, yes to the second."

"Any medications taken?"

"Only mild sleeping pills, never anything to improve blood supply."

"What do you want most in high-altitude mountaineering?"

"As difficult, high, and quick as possible; alpine style of course."

"What advice would you give to aspiring Himalayan climbers?"

"Try to listen to and to understand your body systems."

Although the four climbs described here are athletic feats, their appeal is not that of sport, but lies in the style in which they were done. Traditional methods were abandoned in favor of a new approach.

Whenever a climber leaves the known paths, he enters an area without rules or routines to rely on. The only advice comes from deep inside the self, and hopefully the motivation is true. At such moments, the mountaineer is creative, not merely a participant in sport. This creativity manifests itself in styles of climbing or in exploration of unknown areas. It is impossible to cram mountaineering into a sport framework. To me there are as many ways to experience the mountains as there are real and passionate emotional bonds with the mountains. If you allow my earlier sarcasm, permit me a momentary contact with the mystical. I conclude that mystery is essential to mountaineering. What is unveiled to the individual when involved with creative mountaineering forms part of a new bond with the mountain experience.

One needs to recall only a few figures such as Bill Tilman, Naomi Uemura, or Gary Hemming. It is in forging true bonds rather than the collection of numbers or establishment of records that unveils a bit of mystery. But mystery remains a mystery and sport is sport.

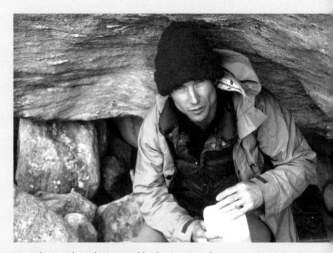

Voytek Kurtyka relaxing and hydrating near base camp before the ascent of the west face of Gasherbrum IV. *Photo: Robert Schauer*

Polish climber Wojciech (Voytek) Kurtyka, born in 1947, was one of the most influential and important practitioners of alpine-style climbing in the Himalaya. He climbed many important new routes, always in small teams, expeditioning with many of the most important alpinists of the twentieth century: Alex MacIntyre, Jerzy Kukuczka, Doug Scott, Erhard Loretan, Reinhold Messner, and Yasushi Yamanoi, to name a few. In 1985 with Robert Schauer, he climbed the west face of Gasherbrum IV in alpine style to the summit ridge, an ascent considered by many to be one of the finest climbs of all time. Writing about that ascent in 2003 he said, "Strangely enough, the climbing community accepted the ascent as a finished work. That's an obvious hint that alpinism is an art rather than a sport. Only in art does a missing piece contribute to the meaning of the piece."

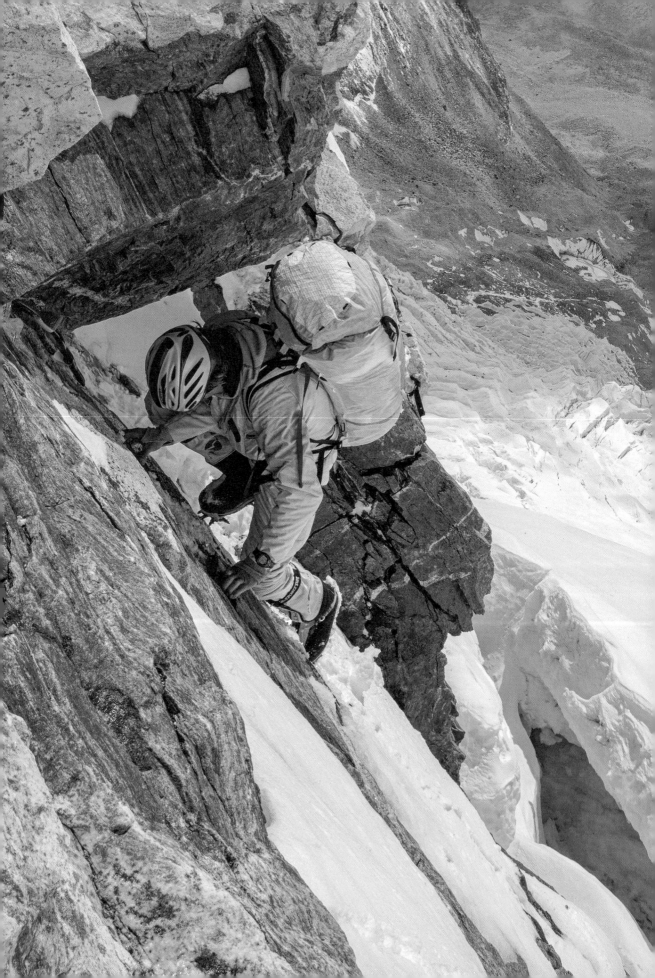

Chapter 13

Mental Fitness: The Most Difficult 80 Percent

"There are a dozen reasons for climbing, some bad, and I've used most of them myself. The worst are fame and money. Commonly people cite exploration or discovery, but that's rarely relevant in today's world. The only good reason to climb is to improve yourself."

— YVON CHOUINARD

THE MENTAL/PHYSICAL BALANCE

To proffer this book on training without addressing the mental aspects of climbing is tempting; the subject itself is ill defined and the evidence anecdotal. As such this chapter makes controversial assumptions, unlike the rest of this book, which is based on scientific inquiry, empirical testing, and peer review. We feel compelled to include this chapter although many of you already know that in climbing, the mind is primary.

Opposite: Steve House soloing across a short, dangerous section of rock at 21,000 feet (6,400m), carrying a pack with food, fuel, shelter, and clothing for a planned seven-day ascent of Makalu (27,825', 8,481m) in 2011. *Photo: Marko Prezelj*

YOUR IDEAL MENTAL STATE FOR CLIMBING?

What is the ideal mental state for entering the mountain arena? A good goal for each of us is to find an answer to this question. The fact is, the answer is ephemeral; it may change from day to day and place to place. This is a process of self-discovery, unique to each of us. In an attempt to create some order out of a complex subject we will divide the mental aspects of alpinism into what we feel are the major components: motivation, emotion, fear, fulfillment, concentration, flow, confidence, and transcendence.

MOTIVATION

> "You can't coach desire."
>
> — SCOTT JOHNSTON

All actions start and end with motivation. Motivation directs and energizes our every behavior. The motivation to climb seems odd considering the fact that alpinism contains significant deadly risks to yourself and your partners. When we've climbed we've experience pain throughout our whole bodies. Feet, hands, and nostrils freeze. Muscles burn with fatigue. Bodies shiver from exhaustion as well as cold. Physical suffering is a profound fact of alpine climbing.

Climbing is often viewed by outside observers as a selfish pursuit providing no visible benefits, and indeed frequent injury or death to the climbers themselves. These points are rendered moot if you take the position that the person who has not known him- or herself in a deep way has little to offer family, friends, or society in the first place. Motivation to do something lacking outside approval is intrinsically rooted in the question of why we climb; a deceptively simple query that has no easy answer.

Each and every one of us who climbs has our own unique blend of motivating factors. Motivation is one of the most important forces in life. To examine some of the various motivations climbers feel in hopes of better understanding ourselves, we've created an incomplete list of some common motivations we've observed in ourselves and others.

Feeling good: The movement of climbing can feel good and be enjoyable. Many people get into climbing this way, and many enjoy a wide variety of sports in addition to climbing.

Eighty Percent

By Steve House

Pulling onto the ledge I grabbed a mess of old slings hanging off of the anchor next to Ljubo. Tugging on my rope, he lifted me to standing. *"Alpinism,"* he said, nodding at my exhaustion, *"is 80 percent mental and 20 percent physical."* I inhaled briskly and clipped myself in as he already had me off belay. We finished our route to the saddle, rock slabs graded an easy 5.5 in summer, but slow and difficult when blanketed in cold, powder snow.

We started rappelling at sunset and later that night as we wound down the tired Yugoslavian road, I questioned him. *"Ljubo, how can climbing be only 20 percent*

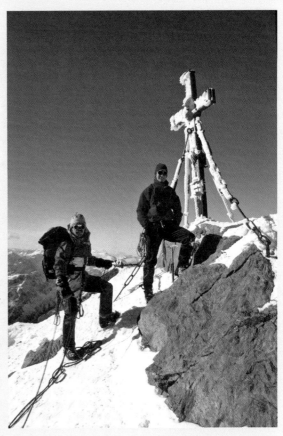

Steve House and Branko Starič on the summit of Austria's highest peak, Grossglockner (12,461', 3,798m) in December 1988. *Photo: Steve House collection*

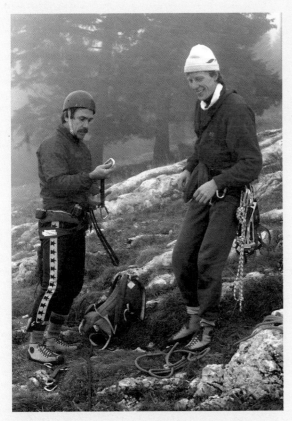

Slovenian alpinists Ljubo Hansel and Branko Starič were two of Steve's earliest climbing mentors. During a year-long student exchange (1988-1989) Steve climbed frequently with these two. Here they prepare to rock climb as a light drizzle comes down. They only went rock climbing if the weather was too bad to climb in the mountains of Slovenia or Austria. *Photo: Steve House*

physical? Isn't it all physical? Or at least the other way around; 20 percent mental?"

"Stef," he said simply, *"you will see. After, you will decide."*

Since that night in 1989, I've often considered Ljubo's law and whether or not he was correct. In my younger years I thought that my initial feeling had been right, that he had the numbers flip-flopped. But as I gained in years and experience, watching myself as well as others, I have slowly migrated toward his version of 80/20 mental/physical ratio. Today I believe that Ljubo's estimate is largely accurate—that, above all else, alpinism is a mental practice.

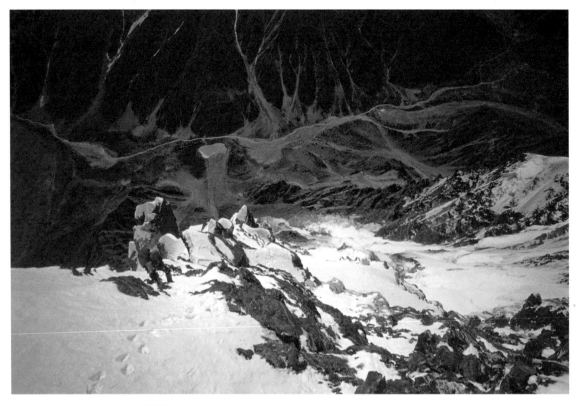

Vince Anderson looks down 13,000
vertical feet (4,000m) to base camp
on day five of the ascent of the
Central Pillar of the Rupal Face of
Nanga Parbat (26,660', 8,126m).
Photo: Steve House

Simplicity: Some are attracted to the monastic lifestyle that a mastery
of climbing asks.

Explorers: This is the adventurer who is always looking around the
next corner.

Collectors: Collectors enjoy checking their lists: all the fourteeners, all
the 8,000ers, all the seven summits, etc.

Humanists: The ones who care largely *who* they are climbing with.
These people are intensely interested in the cultures they travel through
and the partners with whom they share the journey.

Anger: Anger, angst, and rejection of society's values are common
themes in many climbing stories. Climbing channels and processes such
emotions in an exquisite way that has to be experienced to be appreciated.

Self-Loathing: Like anger, climbing processes deep-rooted, post-
modern anxieties like few other activities.

Performer: One who generally prefers competitions or forms of climbing where easy comparisons can be made. These people often come from a conventional sports background or enjoy competition as a motivation.

Insecure: These people are inherently unsure that they are worthy of others' love and will go to great ends of accomplishment to assure themselves and others that they are worthy.

Narcissists: Driven by ego, these personalities overlap in many ways with the insecure and the performers. The key difference is that these people are driven to prove that they are better than everyone else.

Think about what you first felt about climbing. To discover your motivations, it may help to trace your inspirations. What got you into it? Was it a book? The scenery? Your friends? What your parents wanted you to do or what they didn't want you to do? Consider setting a timer for ten minutes and write nonstop about why you got into climbing; retell yourself the story of how you started and write deeply into your memories.

It can be important to know your DNA as a climber. Are you really a sport climber, or a big-wall guy, or a Himalayist? Why is this important? Motivation is connected to inspiration. The ancient Greek maxim, "know thyself" is very relevant in climbing. Knowing yourself allows you to know what you should and should not be doing.

Steve long ago dreamt of climbing new routes on all of what have been called the king walls of the Canadian Rockies. Over fifteen years, he has succeeded on Alberta, Fay, Robson, and North Twin. He still has a lot of work to do: Temple, Geike, and Assiniboine to name just a few, but knowing that these mountains motivate him allows him to make time and space in his life to repeatedly go climbing there.

Likewise, when Steve was nineteen years old he stared up at the world's biggest wall, the Rupal Face. He couldn't imagine how to climb it at the time. Yet fifteen years later he did just that, by a new route and with one partner. Many long approaches and hard days were fueled by the desire to one day be good enough to attempt that wall.

Most people function best, especially in a training environment, if they have something to think about and work toward. Start by asking yourself what the spine of your dreams is. By *spine* we mean, what is the general shape of what you would most like to do? Is it high-altitude alpinism? Is it the Canadian Rockies' classic routes? Is it high traverses in the Sierra? Start with the spine, then build the

The Unbreakable Will

By Stephan Siegrist

When a mountain attracts me not only with its beauty and aesthetics, but it touches me emotionally, then I know that I can apply the appropriate mental motivation. Then I have something really important: a clearly defined goal that will motivate me to work hard during the training phase. The unbreakable will is crucial for success. Only then are hard workouts fun. As soon as you recognize the first success, the happiness is great.

Make these little milestones of success part of the overall experience. Discipline, being hard on yourself, is truly important. The excitement of preparing for a big climb should never disappear behind the shadow of unregulated ambition.

I print a photo of the mountain, if possible from different perspectives. I draw the planned route with a visible color. I mark possible bivouac spots, and potential pitfalls are highlighted with an exclamation point. And very important: On the top is a stick figure with a smiley face and arms held high—the joy my partner and I will feel upon reaching the summit. Although I am physically still in the valley, mentally I've already reached the summit.

This photo of the mountain sits on my nightstand for about thirty days before I leave for an expedition. Each night before I go to sleep, I climb the route in my head. Then I go through it as a team; I imagine standing happily on the summit and climbing down safely as a team. I take the time to imagine I can feel the experiences of the upcoming climb. I imagine I feel the cold, the thin air, and the effort. This way I mentally prepare myself for as many different situations on the mountain as possible.

Of course, those mental climbs are not the ideal activity before going to bed and not the top priority of my wife. She understands, though, how how important this mental preparation for me is. Good teamwork starts at home.

Swiss alpinist Stephan Siegrist is best known for establishing very difficult modern routes on the north face of the Eiger. A professional climber, he has climbed new routes in Patagonia, the Himalaya, and Antarctica.

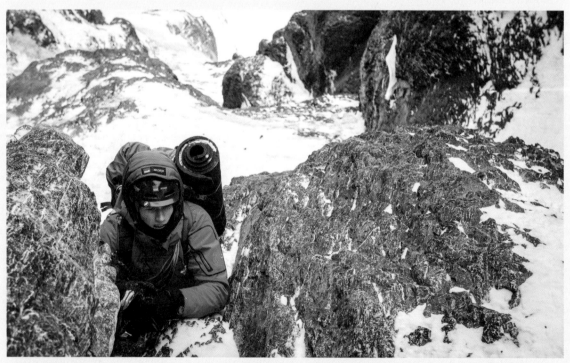

Stephan Siegrist making a winter ascent of the 1938 Route on the Eiger (13,025', 3,970m). He first climbed this route when he was twenty years old. *Photo: Thomas Senf*

skeleton. Let's say you want to climb the classic peaks in the Canadian Rockies. What are the routes you'd like to climb? What is the season for each? Which is the easiest, the most difficult, the most dangerous, the most aesthetically pleasing? Which one are you going to attempt next season and with whom? If the idea is the spine, the answers to these specific questions are the bones that form the skeleton of your goal.

Motivation is will, and will has two parts: *power* and *purpose*. Without power, your purpose cannot be realized. Without purpose, your power will be diffused and will become impotent.

Money Is Not the Limiting Factor

When Steve was in his twenties he heard a rumor that a top climber was paid a salary many times greater than the $10,000 a year he was living on. He daydreamed about all the expeditions he could do with such an allowance. Looking back now, he is glad no one handed him that much money when he was twenty-five. Financial limitations focused his climbing on Alaska, where he could travel for free as part of his work as a mountain guide. A solid decade of expeditions there paid off in practicing skills he would come to rely on when he eventually managed to get to the Himalaya.

Money is rarely, if ever, the ultimate limiting factor in any creative pursuit. There is no way to be more invested in your own success than to finance your own road trip or expedition yourself. The storied Polish Himalayan climbers painted bridges and smokestacks to pay for their expeditions in the 1980s. The Slovenes would drive overland to Pakistan in their own trucks. Steve sold his only belonging of value, a motorcycle, to go on his first expedition. It's no wonder so many underfunded expeditions are successful; they have too much invested *not* to try their hardest.

Traits That Deliver Success

In 2008 an article was published in the *Harvard Business Review* in which the author reported studies of commonalities between Olympic medalists and successful businesspeople. The author, Graham Jones, a former sports psychologist turned executive coach, delineated the following characteristics and common motivations that contributed to the successes of his subjects:

- Self-directed

- Very confident of their abilities

- Focused on excellence

- Internally rather than externally focused

- Not distracted by others

- The ability to psychologically manage pressure

- Meticulous attention to goals

- Careful planning of short-term goals

- A relentless focus on the long-term attainment of goals

- An ability to shrug off their own failures

- Masters of compartmentalization in their lives

- Celebrate their wins

- Analyze the reasons for success

- Reinvent themselves following a success

- An unstoppable striving for success

Let's contrast the above list with a list of attributes that we think make a great alpinist:

- A good all-around technical climber, but most importantly skilled in ice and mixed climbing

- Very good cardiovascular fitness

- Patience

- Perseverance

- Discipline

- A high tolerance for suffering

- An ability to form partnerships and contribute to a small team

- An ability to plan for medium- and long-term goals

- Good mountain-sense: knowledge of weather, avalanche hazards, geology, glaciology

- Good route-finding skills

- A solid base of outdoor skills: navigation, survival, cooking, camping, etc.

- A good learner

- Comfortable with travel, other cultures, and other languages

- An outlook that blends optimism and pragmatism

- Clear intentions

These lists mention personality traits as well as skill sets; all are somehow related. What are the most successful internal motivators? What ignites the fire of your ambition? Your chances for success will increase dramatically when you search intently for reasons to go up instead of inventing reasons to go down.

EMOTION

In August 2004 Bruce Miller and Steve House climbed to 24,800 feet (7,559 meters) on Nanga Parbat's Rupal Face before Bruce decided they had to descend because he thought Steve was dangerously pushing himself too far. Steve's emotional state during that climb was introverted and fatalistic. His awareness of risk and his reaction to discomfort, hard work, danger, and cold were numbed. Some might argue this is a necessary state for that type of climbing. His friends worried; Barry Blanchard wrote to him that he had "become a creature of the wall" and advised that he back off for a while. Scott Johnston took him aside to warn him that he was treading a thin line between hubris and destruction.

Steve recalls in 2004 visualizing every detail of imagined climbs and their possible outcomes, both successful and tragic, such as the one on the Rupal Face. These visualizations, coupled by deep self-doubts and profound feelings of unworthiness, created a steely, heavy sensation in his stomach that he can recall even today. Those sensations were tightly tied to resolve and determination. He would not do anything at the time that might negatively impact his goals, to the point where he'd avoid relationships that he might become attached to.

Emotion provides a component to motivation that can be either positive or negative. Motivation colored by satisfaction is more positive than motivation driven by anger, contempt, or inadequacy. In climbing, this is a worthwhile distinction, especially considering the inherent risks.

Emotion is the most powerful human motivator. Hate and love play an oversize role in the actions of humanity. A desire to bring glory to the crown launched early British expeditions to the Himalaya. Walter Bonatti famously opened his route on the north face of the Matterhorn to spite his critics. In climbing, as in art, being pissed off is an emotional state that can be exploited. As rock singer Zack de la Rocha put it: "Anger is a gift." Alpine climbing hurts, and nothing dissipates pain like anger, which may be why we get mad when we hit our thumb with a hammer, or conversely punch a wall when we're mad. Anger and its variations are not likely to be sustainable as fuel for motivation, though that is where many start.

The Subconscious Roots of Our Emotions

What you are telling yourself, thinking about, or being told, often on the edge of your own awareness, is what builds up or degrades your sense of well-being and self-efficacy. Consider how well the marketing industry has mastered this concept. Do a self-test: Observe your emotional state as you watch a slate of television commercials. Good ads make you feel something. As you later encounter those advertised products in daily life (in the supermarket, for example), what feeling is evoked?

Imagine one of those long, miserable uphill slogs, and you're telling yourself, "This is hard," "I feel so tired," over and over again. This wears you down more than the actual physical exertion. Thoughts create emotions, which in turn create sensations in your body, in this case, tiredness. If you still doubt us, meditate on the last time someone wronged you and tell yourself how unfair it was. How did your emotional state just change?

Emotions run the show far more often than we'd like to admit—in climbing, and in life. This is a powerful lesson that most of us have to learn the hard way. The less you are aware of this, the more you need to try to understand it. Most of us would like to believe that our dispassionate and reasoned thinking selves make the decisions but this is simply not the case. As Nietzsche tells us, "One ought to hold on to one's heart; for if one lets it go, one soon loses control of the head too."

This is particularly true of our childhood through the mid-twenties when the brain of the human male completes its development. (This happens earlier for women.) The oftentimes subconscious, or barely audible, signs, words, and feedback we get from those around us—parents, friends, classmates, teachers, coaches—go a very long way in forming our opinions of ourselves and establishing our baseline emotional state.

Emotions and Risk

Climbers are risk managers. In business, good risk management begins with a balanced, unemotional assessment of what the risk is. One then asks what the potential consequences of that risk are, and how well a business can survive a bad-case or worst-case scenario. When the physical safety of you and your partner is immediately on the line, it is very hard to isolate emotion from your decision-making. In climbing, no one in their right mind is willing to accept a worst-case scenario (i.e., death).

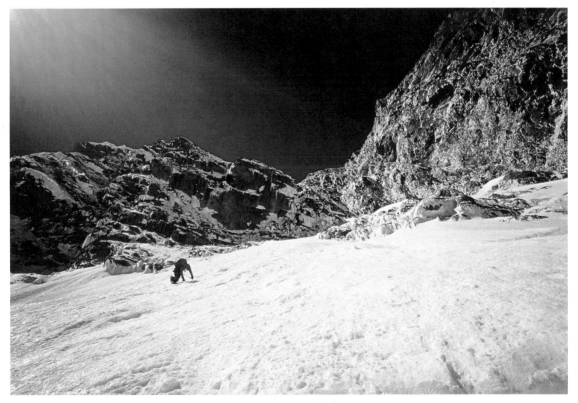

Vince Anderson soloing easy terrain on day four of the climb of the Central Pillar of the Rupal Face. We had no idea how difficult the climbing immediately above him would be despite studying numerous photographs and probing the wall with a small telescope. We were somehow confident that we could climb whatever we found up there. We had to, because we did not have enough equipment to safely descend from this point. This confidence, and the calm emotional state that accompanied it, allowed us to commit ourselves fully to the climb and therefore succeed. *Photo: Steve House*

Increasing your emotional intelligence—your ability to identify, assess, and control your emotions—is not easy. But you can, and most people do, develop emotional intelligence over time. Experience and self-awareness guide that process. We have observed that raw, transformative journeys, development of a personal philosophy, and ability to manage risk can be great accelerators to this process.

The business model approach to risk management can be boiled down to three questions you can ask yourself in the field:

1) What are the chances of me falling (or getting avalanched, stormed in, etc.) here?

2) What would be the consequences of that fall/avalanche/action?

3) How honestly have I answered questions one and two?

It takes emotional maturity and equanimity to answer these questions correctly time and time again. Excitement to do a long-dreamed-of route is an emotion that can easily get you into trouble: The dreaded summit fever. Group dynamics, such as the anxiety created by multiple parties rushing toward a coveted climbing objective, also clouds judgment.

Our emotional lives have two important roles in our climbing. And while emotions fire our motivation, emotions can also warp our judgment and get us into trouble. Reflecting upon climbs that we've completed, and lessons learned from failed attempts that we've survived, can teach us lot about ourselves.

Steve has seen this process play out on his three expeditions to Makalu's West Face. Each time he felt the balance between his motivation and his ability to make good decisions in high-pressure, dangerous situations was not correct. Each time he walked away with a clear understanding that he was not yet emotionally prepared for the objective. A younger Steve would have been full of angst and negative self-talk after each of these three failures. For a small team to raise the money, organize, acclimate, and attempt such a route is a huge undertaking, and failure can be a difficult pill to swallow.

In an age where expeditions often reach out to sponsors for funding, this can be especially volatile. Before asking for money, consider the price of your freedom and the price of a free conscience if you decide not to do a climb you don't feel right about. Consider the worst-case scenario, and whether or not you can turn around without making the video your sponsor wanted. Can you return home without news, without even a story? If the answer is no, that is something to meditate deeply upon.

The best approach to failure, if we rely on the model of the successful habits of the Olympic competitors and business leaders, is to use it as motivation to improve—not quit. In the emotional balance between success and failure, life and, possibly, death, you must get it right.

These self-explorations may seem abstract, but we believe they bring you closer to being capable of an ascent that would be personally groundbreaking. We must each realize that our ideal emotional state for a given objective will evolve over time. You can, and should, come back to an objective you were not ready for in the past. Returning to a dreamt-of climb can be one of the climbing life's most rewarding experiences. In doing so, you are able to revisit previous mental states by returning to the same physical places. There you can learn, and understand, just how dramatically your emotional state changes with time.

No one is capable of reliably finding the ideal emotional state before a climb. There is no perfect; good enough is good enough. Over the course of two lifetimes of climbing the authors have learned to recognize if we're emotionally in the right ballpark—or not. Being able to recognize, achieve, and maintain a good-enough emotional state is a highly valuable attribute as an alpinist; it's crucial.

Best Mental State Enhancers

Listening to or creating music is a big mental boost for several of Steve's partners. For others, it's painting or taking pictures. Steve reaches for his diary. Writing slows him down and puts him in a more centered state. Writing makes ideas concrete. Painting turns emotion into color and, sometimes, form. Any of these activities help you to process things that might be bothering you, help you to understand your current state, which is the first step to affecting and directing your emotional state in a way that helps you realize your goal.

Meditation, to be discussed later, is also a powerful tool. But so is the ritual of packing, or approaching a climb in the dark. Bad weather can also be a powerful motivator. When storms have derailed our climbing plans, it makes us a bit angry, and we try harder.

Nutrition and food are important components of a normal mental state. If you start doubting yourself, mentally or physically, check your fuel and fluid levels. Sugar, glycogen, is the fuel your brain needs. If you have an important decision to make, consider eating a snack first.

Finding Your Ideal Mental State

Write down one climbing goal and postulate what your ideal emotional state is for that goal, a state that would give you both the motivation to succeed and the balance to make good judgments in dangerous circumstances. Now list what you might do to encourage and achieve that state. What thoughts could you have to encourage those feelings?

My ideal emotional state for climbing is an optimistic, slightly anxious, and slightly agitated or frustrated state. My climbing used to thrive on self-loathing. Having found that to be a dead end, I now focus on helping other climbers, as well as myself, who are passionate about climbing mountains, to improve.

— Steve House

Prepare Yourself to Suffer

By Jean Troillet

For me, the most important thing I find in preparing for an expedition is to prepare psychologically, mentally. Voytek Kurtyka described this well in his article titled "The Art of Suffering." We know that when we go into the high mountains, on expeditions, that we are going to suffer. Climbing big mountains is not easy. Nothing is easy there.

So prepare yourself mentally that something bad might happen. And when it happens, you will survive. If you aren't ready, you may not survive. Say you are at 7,000 meters (22,966 feet), for example, and you have a small break in the weather, but you don't feel strong at the moment. If you know yourself, if you are prepared for this moment of suffering, of hardship, you can say to yourself, "OK, keep going slow." In those moments your success, even your survival, can be decided.

Experience is key: If it is your first time at 7,000 meters and you take a break, and you say, "Oh-la-la, I don't feel good, and it will surely be worse at 8,000 meters (26,247 feet). I shouldn't go farther." And then you turn around. You fail to climb the mountain because you didn't have the experience. If you know that if you keep going step after step, slowly, when you get to 8,000 meters you might think to yourself, "Oh, I feel better now." Then it's OK, you recovered. Experience is the only way to learn this about yourself.

Attitude is important. In 1995, I went to Kanchenjunga (8,586 meters/28,169 feet) with Erhard Loretan, and I was not climbing much before the expedition because I did some guiding, some canyoneering, some scuba diving, and some sailing. I climbed Mont Blanc once before we left for the expedition. When I was on Mont Blanc I noticed in myself that I was really enjoying the mountain, really enjoying climbing. Then I went to the expedition, and in the beginning I suffered to acclimate, which is normal. After that, I was in the same condition as Loretan, because I accepted the suffering and I really enjoyed being on the mountain with him.

You need to have your goal fixed firmly in your mind, and you must be prepared to suffer for that goal.

Otherwise you climb until you say to yourself, "Oh man, I've had enough of this snow and these crampons." When I go on an expedition, I go for the full experience of climbing the mountain.

When I was young, to prepare myself for a winter climb here in the Alps, I slept outside on the balcony. I needed to do that because I needed to know myself, to know if I could accept the suffering of sleeping outside in the cold and storm.

When people ask me if they should climb an 8,000-meter peak, I say to them: "If you want to go to an 8,000er, you should go. But prepare yourself to suffer. Don't push too hard, and go slowly from the beginning to the top."

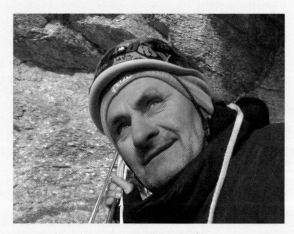

Jean Troillet *Photo: Jean Troillet collection*

Jean Troillet has climbed ten of the 8,000-meter peaks in alpine style and without supplemental oxygen. Troillet, along with Erhard Loretan, Voytek Kurtyka, and others, pioneered new routes on 8,000-meter peaks in a "night-naked," bivouac-less style.

If you feel under-motivated, or tired, especially upon waking, drink a glass of water. Dehydration presents as fatigue; tiredness sows the seeds of doubt. The one phrase of negative self-talk, "Maybe I'm not ready for this today," will rob all your motivation. Don't allow it. Instead try a phrase like "Today I will set aside any doubt and I will try to climb as best I can, come what may."

FEAR

Fear warrants its own special treatment here because it can so easily undermine all of what we are striving for. A sense that you are risking your own death or injury is a powerful message to your mind and body that is impossible, indeed, wrong to ignore. Secondarily, fear of failure is powerful in its own right.

"Focus on the task at hand, break that task down into attainable parts, get yourself from one point of safety to the next." This is what you hear Steve say when someone asks him how he handles fear. Easy to say, hard to do.

Let's begin with fear of failure, which is a good place to begin addressing fear. These are the situations where you are totally safe while failing, let's say falling off of a steep sport route. There is no danger to your person, but your ego or self-image may be in jeopardy. Especially if there is an audience.

The first step is to reject the negative association of not succeeding. When we set goals, when we strive for growth and improvement, we are going to fail along the way. A sport climber may spend weeks or months projecting a route, trying many times knowing that they are getting better and (hopefully) stronger with each attempt, and eventually the hard work will allow them to send the route. This type of failure is necessary and good provided that you are not failing 100 percent of the time.

To overcome this fear, we recommend that you fail in private, and where it's most safe. It's easier to fall at a secluded crag with a couple of nonjudgmental friends than at a popular crag on a busy Saturday. The more you can try in this safe situation, the less likely you are to fail. Because less of your attention is occupied by fear, more of your attention will be on climbing well.

Jerome Robbins, the film director and dance choreographer, observed that creative people do their best work after their biggest creative failures. Probably because after a big embarrassment, they are free to try their hardest. We like to think that climbing is no different. To be able to *fail well*, it is vital to shake off the sting of disappointment and retain, indeed focus on, the lessons from your efforts. This vital exercise requires intention and consistency. If you can experience humiliation as not being bad, then you're free to try harder than ever before.

Types of Failure

Colorado climber Michael Gilbert originated the saying that there are only three reasons people fail to climb a route: "Not strong enough, not brave enough, or not good enough." All of the following could fit into one of these categories.

- A failure of skill. This can apply to just about every climbing situation; even the most skilled of us can find a wall so blank we can't climb it. Internal voice says, "I'm not good enough."

- A failure of fitness. If you can't hold on, or can't hike uphill fast enough, you can't get to the top because you're tired.

- A failure of confidence. This is ultimately an indication you did not yet spend enough time developing your climbing skills and/or fitness in relation to the route you're attempting. Your internal voice says, "I can't do it" (which is different from "Can I do it?") before you start. Different people develop confidence at different speeds.

- A failure of judgment. This is perhaps the most common reason, especially in the case of accidents. You should have known better, or you didn't have the right experience or knowledge to guide you.

- Strategic failure. The route could have been climbed in a thirty-hour push, but you packed bivy gear and got stormed off after three days. Your inner voice says (after the fact), "We should have . . . "

- A failure of nerve, or letting fear make your decision for you. Your inner voice says, "I could have . . . "

- A failure of repetition. We include this because we think that over-frequenting the alpine environment can lead to complacency, overconfidence, and rushing that leads to a drop in attention. Ask any assembly-line worker. Inner voice says, "Merde . . . "

- A failure of resources. This is not so much a failure as a choice, and not necessarily a poor choice. Legion are those who might have the skill and stamina to climb great mountains, or ride the Tour de

Practicing Failing

By Scott Johnston

Famed alpinist and all-arounder Charlie Fowler and I frequently partnered for challenging winter routes in Rocky Mountain Park outside of Boulder, Colorado, in the 1970s and '80s, inventing tools and techniques suited to our purpose. Charlie was well known for backing off of climbs (both with and without partners) if he didn't feel that all the stars were aligned properly. He was often heard bragging about bailing off such and such route, or how many difficult winter routes he had failed on that month. He was fond of saying that he liked to practice failing, or that backing off allowed him to live to climb another day.

Of course when Charlie was on his game he was nearly unstoppable and was a bit like having a secret weapon on dangerous pitches. So, this bit of self-effacement was never taken too seriously by anyone as any indication of weakness. In retrospect it seems that this was his way of easing the pain of failure by putting it front and center in his and others' minds. No equivocation, no excuses—he'd just say he was not up to the task and immediately remove any sense of guilt or shame. His practice of this skill removed any stigma of failure from his mind, which was where it could potentially do the most damage.

Charlie once told me (and others in the tightly knit Boulder climbing community of the '70s) that I was the strongest worst climber he knew. His honesty could be brutal, but like his own self-deprecation, I used this to remove the stigma of being a second-tier climber and adopted the habit of bragging about my shortcomings as a climber. It kept us both from taking ourselves too seriously. Besides, our shortcomings never stood in the way of the two of us having some amazing climbing days.

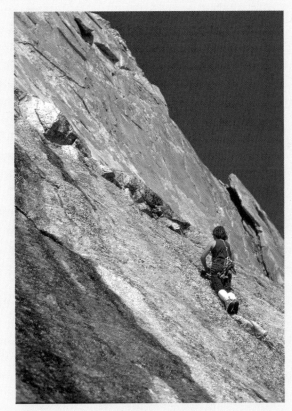

Charlie Fowler climbing Sykes Sickle on Spearhead Peak, Rocky Mountain National Park, circa 1979. *Photo: Scott Johnston*

France, but make other things priorities in their lives, and so they never fully develop one specialized area of skill and stamina. That's normal and OK. Eighty percent of being good at any skill is showing up to work every day. Either devote more time to climbing or lower your expectations. Inner voice says, "I can't afford the time or money to do this."

- A failure of will. This is the most common, but the least commonly admitted. Inner voice says, "I can't because x-y-z circumstances are against me." You are really saying, "I don't want to try that hard." No one worth knowing is going to judge you negatively for truthfully acknowledging what you are or aren't willing to do.

Use Fear as a Trigger for Concentration

To control fear is not to let go of it or ignore it, but rather the opposite. Samurai warriors famously meditated daily on all the ways they might die. Own your fears. As with emotions, fears must be acknowledged and examined before they can be managed. As Danika Gilbert eloquently describes, they can be touched and played with.

In climbing we find that it is invaluable to use fear as a trigger for concentrating on action. To take the next steps, you must have already eliminated all the negative associations that fear is bad. Fear is healthy.

Detach from Fear

To put this into practice, you must cultivate a sense of detachment from your fear. Our goal is enough detachment and enough awareness that you notice the first moment you begin to sense fear. When it comes up, in your brain or more often in your gut, repeat to yourself that fear is information, and that you don't let fear control your emotional state. You can try to widen your awareness, as Danika does by naming the objects around her.

It is quite reasonable to be scared when cramponing down a narrow ice ridge after a summit. Especially if you are tired, the partner who you are roped to is clumsy, or the wind is gusty. Acknowledge that this fear is telling you that it's important to focus on standing well and placing your crampons in the best spots. Take control of your body and make those movements deliberately and precisely. Stay alert and in communication with your partner. Notice options for other strategies so that if your fear continues to build, you will

On Fear

By Danika Gilbert

Fear is a very real part of alpine climbing. I try to meet my fears head-on, which can be uncomfortable. I believe you can work with fear and as a result improve your climbing and your inner well-being.

As I experience it, fear is generally of two types: one keeps me alive in the face of real-life threats, the other keeps me from doing something I am indeed capable of doing without dying. It can be difficult to tell these two apart. When scared enough, we go into fight or flight mode: our vision narrows, our heart races, other senses dull while those keeping track of the fear sharpen. This can be both good and bad. When we need to get the hell out of the way of a fast-falling ice chunk, this response is good. The muscles run without thinking. When we need to think rationally and move cautiously and calmly, this response is bad; it leads to hasty movements and rash decisions.

I watch for the fear that creeps up on me gradually—that pit-in-my-stomach feeling. Once I recognize this fear rising, I see if I can keep climbing with it. Some days it may be too much, and it is time to turn around and try the climb another day. Some days I can safely touch and play with that fear. If that's the case I start by noticing my vision; if it has narrowed, can I force it to widen a bit? I look around and note five things I can see, what color are they? What can I smell? I try to note four things. What can I feel? I touch three different things and notice their texture. What can I hear? I pause and note two sounds around me. This process brings me into a calmer space where I can breathe. With a few additional deep breaths, I can usually focus and begin to make good judgment calls. With practice, I have learned to do this automatically, quickly, and quietly. Then I can evaluate my situation a bit more clearly and calmly—and decide if I can continue or need to retreat.

Be respectful of fear and choose when you can and cannot work with it. While climbing, and at home, reflect on the process of fear. This is where we can each look into ourselves and sometimes uncover clues as to what drives us and what holds us back from our greatest potential.

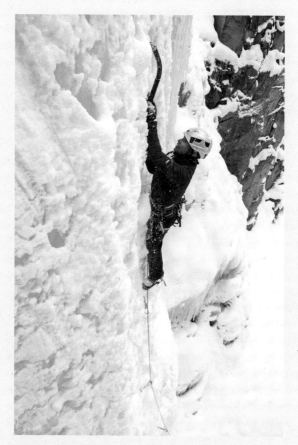

Danika Gilbert climbing ice near Ouray, Colorado.
Photo: Kennan Harvey

Danika Gilbert has been on climbing expeditions throughout the world. She is a botanist and a climbing and ski guide making her home in the San Juan Mountains of her native Colorado.

have a plan for where to belay, or how to alter your climbing tactics to gain more security. Fear is often simply the messenger who says, "Hey, you need to really concentrate on doing this well, or you need to change something." Solving the problem at hand, concentrating on the bits you can control such as placing your crampons well, placing an anchor and belaying, these are things that are possible once you detach from the fear enough to respond to it rather than feel controlled by it.

Know What Risk You Can Handle

Both Scott and Steve love motorcycles. When Steve was nine years old his great-grandfather, a machinist by trade, installed a lawnmower engine in a homemade steel frame with two wheels and gave it to him. The brake was a pedal that pushed against the rear tire. The first and only fast street bike he owned, he sold after one year. The reason? He'd had three close calls in the previous nine months, laying it down once. After that third close call he understood that he was not mature enough to ride a fast motorcycle safely.

In climbing, accept the level of risk you are able to handle. If you can feel solid and steady on difficult free-solos, more power to you. If exposed scrambling is terrifying for you, you'd better know that about yourself.

There is a training adaptation to fear: The more you increase your exposure to fear, the more exposure you can handle. Climbers who take this to extremes will have to consciously set limits in order to live to an old age, as risk always contains some degree of randomness. Steve has enjoyed his solo climbing, but knew he would stop when he got married. Though he still craves the solo experience at times, he has set that limit on his risk.

Frequent visitation to a high-risk environment can make it hard to re-adapt to normal life. Frying eggs for your kids may seem a little mundane after eating a gel for breakfast on a chair-sized shelf of ice thousands of feet above a glacier. As you must acclimate to fear, so too must you de-acclimate. A high degree of experience and self-knowledge is needed to handle fear, in both increasing and decreasing doses.

Let's work backward to re-examine the relationship between fear, risk, self-awareness, and climbing. The key to handling fear in life-threatening situations is to possess a well-developed ability to channel fear, without panic, into deliberate actions that result in survival. In other words you must constantly be anticipating risks and making plans, often on a subconscious level, so that if the bad or worst-case scenario arises suddenly, you will be able to react with life-saving decisiveness. At the root of this ability is a level of self-knowledge of how your emotional reaction to fear affects you that is so ingrained as to be automatic.

Effectively managing fear while climbing requires self-awareness. Without self-awareness, you cannot control yourself well in daily life, let alone in a dangerous situation. Climbing—especially alpine climbing—as well as training for climbing, enforces self-discipline; the first form of self-mastery. You must develop self-mastery, be open to and aware of the power of the transformative experience. Climbing and training are potential vehicles for both self-mastery and transformation. The mountains will take care of the rest.

FULFILLMENT

"The struggle itself . . . is enough to fill a man's heart. One must imagine Sisyphus happy."

— ALBERT CAMUS, "The Myth of Sisyphus"

In his essay "The Myth of Sisyphus," Albert Camus explores the fate of a man who repeatedly struggles to push a rock up a steep hill, only to have it slip from his grasp at the last moment, rolling back down to the bottom of the hill, as a metaphor for modern lives spent working jobs in factories and offices. One can imagine climbing's zero-sum gain of ascent and descent subbing in for Sisyphus in Camus' essay. Is it true, at least for some of us, that fulfillment, even transformation, can be found only though struggle, sometimes on the edge of disaster? Doug Scott pejoratively argued that enlightenment is not found on a full belly.

Many people want to believe that life is perpetually difficult, that we will always lose, or that by only doing things involving toil and sacrifice will they achieve peace and happiness. How is this possible? And why?

Many of us self-identify as climbers, it's who we are. We advertise this fact through the people we befriend, the clothes we wear, the places we live, and the types of cars we drive. With so much of ourselves invested in being climbers, it is not surprising when we judge ourselves harshly for falling at a crux, or not making a summit. The allure is not the pain and work itself, but in the aforementioned mastery, attainable only by way of an all-consuming concentration.

CONCENTRATION

"To be completely concentrated on what you do,
that is simplicity."

— SHUNRYU SUZUKI, author of *Zen Mind, Beginner's Mind*

Feeling concentrated is a good indicator that you're in your ideal mental state for climbing. Concentration is something everyone thinks they have but, when you challenge them, very few people can truly focus and remain concentrated for long. Climbing at a high level requires you to be concentrated for an extended period. It is not unheard of for difficult leads to take between two and three hours. That's the nature of hard climbing, especially when falling would be lethal. So it makes sense that the more one can remain truly focused on the climbing at hand, the better.

During Steve's final year at university he had the opportunity to take a course that included a ten-day meditation retreat. During the silent retreat, hosted by the Northwest Vipassana Association, he sat in meditation for fourteen hours per day, ate one vegetarian meal per day, and had no contact with other students. The first three days were spent sharpening the concentration by meditating on one's own breath. The following seven days the students were taught further concentration in part by moving their awareness through their bodies. It is well beyond the scope of this book, or our expertise, to teach meditation techniques. But Steve insists that his experience with meditation had a profound effect on his climbing.

After the Vipassana retreat, with its 140 hours of practice, Steve found that he was able to apply new awareness and concentration to his climbing. Instead of meditating while sitting, he did it while climbing. Try it. Put as much awareness as you can into your big toe and push up on a small hold. Notice the sensations. Move the toe, stay with the sensations in your toe. Do the same with your fingertips, your hips, with the points of your ice tools. When the ice gets thin, rather than get panicked, increase your focus on where and how the

Steve House concentrates on a difficult mixed pitch at 22,000 feet (6,700m) on the south face of Kunyang Chish East (24,278', 7,400m). *Photo: Vince Anderson*

ice is bonded. Tap it with the side of your tool, listen to it. When you swing into it, swing into the best possible point. We're not talking about the best area; we're talking about the best possible one square millimeter with precisely the right amount of force. Awareness is in fact concentration.

A good analogy to this is hitting a golf ball; you're aiming with your awareness, controlling direction and distance more by feeling than by conscious aiming. Back to climbing and concentrating on the ice in front of you: do not forget your feet, don't get lazy on your crampons, you cannot afford to place 100 percent of your focus on the icicle, so how much? That's for you to learn.

Most meditation classes start with breathwork. Yoga is another practice that emphasizes the alignment of breath with movement, which also has many parallels with climbing.

The next time you are climbing close to your limit, try to observe yourself and remember how you react, how you behave, in extremis. By all means continue to climb, but assign a sliver of your consciousness to observe yourself, your technique and surroundings, as if from the outside. With this you are already heading in the right direction. The more you practice, the bigger the sliver of awareness will become. This acute awareness is one of the best parts of climbing. Never have snow crystals seemed so perfect, or a sunset so vivid as when we've been intensely focused for one or more days. Consciousness, awareness, and concentration *can* be expanded.

One Thing at a Time

A lesson Steve learned from Alex Lowe was to concentrate on finding and placing good gear, and then worry about the climbing. To say it another way: Once you have good gear to protect you, forget about the gear. Maintain your focus on one thing at a time—on protection, then on ascending. This is similar in many ways to our discussion of fear, but concentration is a crucial piece of that equation.

Studies have shown that once your heart rate exceeds roughly 145 beats per minute (145 was the mean found in the study; for a highly fit individual this may be as high as 170 bpm), people have a very hard time focusing on anything but moving their limbs enough to maintain that level of exertion. Think of sprinting full-out and what that mental experience is like. You aren't contemplating what you'll do after the sprint, you're entirely focused on continuing to run as hard as you can. The climbing analogy to this is being completely pumped, and when you do manage to grab a cam off your rack, it's probably the wrong size.

Know where this point, this level of heart rate or lactic acid burn, lies for you. When you start to feel this coming on, allow it to trigger your focus on the immediate task. Find a rest spot. Place some gear. Bring your heart rate down. If you let it go too far, most people tense up, try to place gear in a panic, grab the gear, or down climb. If you're climbing well you've already calculated where your gear is and where the best holds are, and you've already placed good gear below you. Stay with your plan and climb through the crux to the next rest, the next gear placement.

Breath is a wonderful trigger for focusing and is directly adapted from meditation techniques. Breathing through the nose is usually impossible when leading a hard pitch, so breathe through pursed lips to trigger your brain to go into a meditative, focused state. It is a powerful nonverbal reminder to yourself to be fully present in the climbing.

This is a very powerful tool once you're good at it. It does require work to maintain or regain this ability. Steve finds it useful to practice the sitting meditation to relearn and hone this ability. For him, climbing alone is not enough. He brushes up when he expects to be climbing a lot, such as before or during an expedition or an extended trip to the Canadian Rockies. With practice you can train yourself to use any number of triggers to snap into a flow state with a high level of concentration.

FLOW

Yoga is very similar to meditation, though it incorporates breath, movement, and body awareness in a different way. It is perhaps the oldest and most structured method of achieving what Mihaly Csikszentmihalyi famously coined as *flow* in his now-classic book, *Flow: The Psychology of Optimal Experience*. Csikszentmihalyi references the original basic text of yoga, compiled approximately 1,500 years ago, which describes eight stages of increasing skill. The first two stages are strictly concerned with the mind and are aimed at making attention and concentration easier to control. Exactly what we're trying to accomplish in climbing.

Csikszentmihalyi goes on to cite five requirements for achieving flow—a state where you use less energy on attention, which thereby creates a refreshed feeling afterward:

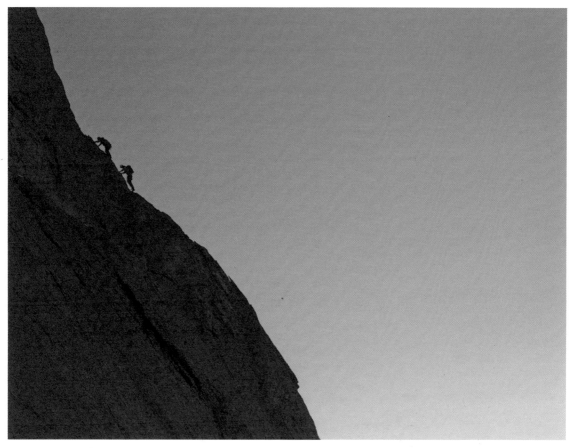

Climbers high on the ultra-classic north ridge of Piz Badile (10,853', 3,308m), Switzerland. *Photo: Steve House*

Clarity: You must know what to expect.

Centering: Attention to the present is required.

Choice: You must have a variety of options that you control.

Commitment: You set aside your defenses and become unselfconsciously involved.

Challenge: You experience an appropriate level of complexity relative to your skill and experience.

Climbing in all its forms can fit every one of these conditions. It helps that climbing is distinct from the realities of everyday existence. Climbers, as is common to other flow activities, dress in specific uniforms and have unique clubs, jargon, and networks to set ourselves apart. While climbing we cease to act in terms of outside

Subtractions

I have some guidelines I've adopted that help me stay close to achieving concentration. I call them the subtractions. These rules help me to create the bubble in which I find my ideal emotional state for climbing and flow.

- No movies, no television, no gaming. This is a hard-and-fast rule for me. Movies easily burn themselves into my consciousness. I first subtracted movies because I was addicted to *Star Trek* in college and found the clips replaying in my head while I was trying to climb. Now that I have a bit more self-mastery I find I can watch an occasional film without affecting my ability to concentrate.

- Reduce music. I limit this as well. I never was that aurally inclined, so this isn't difficult for me. Many people successfully use music to positively modify their emotional state. I find it distracting, again because I hear the tune or the lyrics while trying to focus on the climbing. I enjoy music in a social setting, but when working, training, and climbing I prefer the native sounds around me.

- Reduce Internet and e-mail. This became a problem when I got a smartphone. If you want to disrupt your flow, check your e-mail at the crag or while training. I try to schedule my access to the Internet and e-mail to one time during my day; I get online, do what I need to do, and log off.

- Avoid drama and dramatic people. Cynicism may be entertaining, but negativity is ultimately detrimental when trying to do and be your best. Seek out people who approach problems, training, risk, and life in a proactive, positive way.

– Steve House

common sense and concentrate instead on the peculiar realities of the ascent.

When extrinsic goals—such as fame or money—gain importance, there is a danger that the climbing can become a means to those ends. Someone once said that famous climbers do their best climbing before they become famous. You can find examples of that in many sports, not just climbing. To us, the larger concern is that external goals can and often do interfere with achieving flow, as well as put climbers at risk of injury.

Self-Reliance

> "The power which resides in him is new in nature, and none but he knows what this is which he can do, nor does he know until he has tried."
>
> — RALPH WALDO EMERSON, *Self-Reliance*

There is a long American tradition of giving things up to foster self-reliance and mental toughness in the name of creativity and achieving high levels of flow, and ultimately a transformative experience. Think of Ralph Waldo Emerson or Henry David Thoreau. Within climbing we have the same ideas: expeditions, road trips, bivouacs. These traditions are a form of ritual in that you sacrifice something to partake in them. Building up a tolerance for solitude, or at least being in very small groups, opens channels of concentration. Self-reliance is an important attribute of every alpine climber.

Road tripping in the American West today—or living in communist Poland in the '80s—is conducive to building mental toughness, a requisite for alpine climbing. The Slovenes who drove their vehicles across Iran to Pakistan to climb describe the countless hours on the road as a way of clearing their minds. This surely helped them achieve a state of flow, and they established some amazing climbs on some of the world's biggest peaks. It is worth considering this in light of today's instant-Internet world, with connectivity available even in the most remote places.

The beginning of every climbing day offers a chance to initiate flow. While you are approaching a climb, place your feet very carefully on the trail. Notice your body, how it feels, where it's tight, loose, sore. When you're climbing your first pitch of the day studiously place your crampon points, or boot toes, precisely where you want them to be. Awaken yourself to precise, efficient movement. We find this precision and awareness carrying over to our climbing for the rest of the day without being conscious of it.

Training itself is a great facilitator of flow. Building the hours needed to complete an annual training program is going to give you plenty of time to think, time to calm your mind and ultimately time to hone your ability to concentrate without the effort of searching for concentration.

One of the primary reasons that we believe in training is those hours spent training are crucial to your mental ability to manage fear, risks, and ultimately climb well once you do get to the mountains. Training the body trains the mind.

CONFIDENCE

"I fear not the man who has practiced 10,000 kicks once, I fear the man who has practiced one kick 10,000 times."

— BRUCE LEE, martial artist

When you watch a great climber climbing, you are always impressed by their sense of confidence. When they step on a foothold, no matter how small, they stand on it knowing full well that it is going to bear their weight.

Confidence is born of skill—and skill, of experience. Without having practiced, you cannot expect to have skill. Without skill you will have no confidence. A lack of confidence is not something you can fake your way through. Confidence is earned in the most basic sense of the word. Each of us knows precisely how well we have prepared. Think back to your school days, remember an exam you went into after having studied until you knew the material inside and out. You were confident because you were proficient. Now remember how you felt before, during, and after an exam you didn't prep for.

Now recall a climb where you felt confident. Why were you confident? Because you were prepared or even overprepared, though not in exactly the same sense as with the school exam. Your body, especially your nervous system, remembers every workout you've done, every pitch you've climbed. This explains why, once someone has climbed a hard route, it is easier for them to climb at the same level of difficulty in the future. Our minds and bodies remember previous efforts and this gives us confidence that we can make a certain move. This reveals a big reason why climbing standards increase gradually over time.

The Climb of the Future: 5.13c in 1978

By Tony Yaniro

In 1978, a friend of mine took me to Sugarloaf, California, to show me the "climb of the future." Arriving at the base I was awestruck by a forty-foot (twelve-meter) long finger crack, with one smooth hand-jam rest a third of the way up.

Around this time, several top climbers were, quite controversially, proposing the hangdog method of practicing climbs. I decided to apply hangdogging to this climb, incorporating this new strategy with specific strength training.

This roof demands repeated moves in a very specific position with decent finger locks, but with most of the body weight on two fingers per hand. At first I could barely do two moves in a row. To add to the problem, the rest of the body was in a constant state of tension trying to scrape and stick to a horizontal, open dihedral.

I decided not to visit the climb for half a year and train specifically for this route. I found an open outdoor stairwell and made some wooden finger jam replicates that would not hurt my joints and skin too much. I then trained my strength and muscular endurance in this stairwell for half a year. The first return to the climb proved that the training was effective; I nearly sent the route the first weekend.

I returned home, taking two weeks away from the rock, and trained carefully. I did the climb on the next trip and named it Grand Illusion. [It is now graded 5.13b/c, and since this climb was done before sticky-rubber climbing shoes, it was surely 5.13c for Tony.] We thought it was the hardest pitch of free climbing in the world at the time.

It was certainly many times more difficult than anything I had heard of. Physical training helped make it possible.

The other thing that helped greatly was the mind-set that was involved. It started right from my friend Craig Britton's statement that this was "the climb of the future." Each generation of climbers pushes the edge of the limit, but if you think a generation back, what was then cutting edge is now commonplace. Why were climbers stopped there? What created that limit? As a species we did not evolve physically during that time, so it must be a mind-set. Why not set our mind into the future now?

I decided that someday someone would find this climb not too challenging. I pretended that the cutting edge was already way beyond this route. I tried to imagine what climbers of the future would be doing to prepare for this route. I learned much from that process: Train for what you need. Be creative. Pay attention to the details. Find what works for you and believe it! Think of how, and do it now.

Tony's ascent of Grand Illusion, accomplished when he was only seventeen years old, helped start a revolution in climbing and training for climbing—a revolution that has been universally embraced and led to the proliferation of indoor climbing walls, campus boards (another Yaniro invention), finger boards, and the subsequent general elevation of rock climbing standards.

Opposite: Hidetaka Suzuki on the second ascent of Grand Illusion in 1980. *Photo: Greg Epperson*

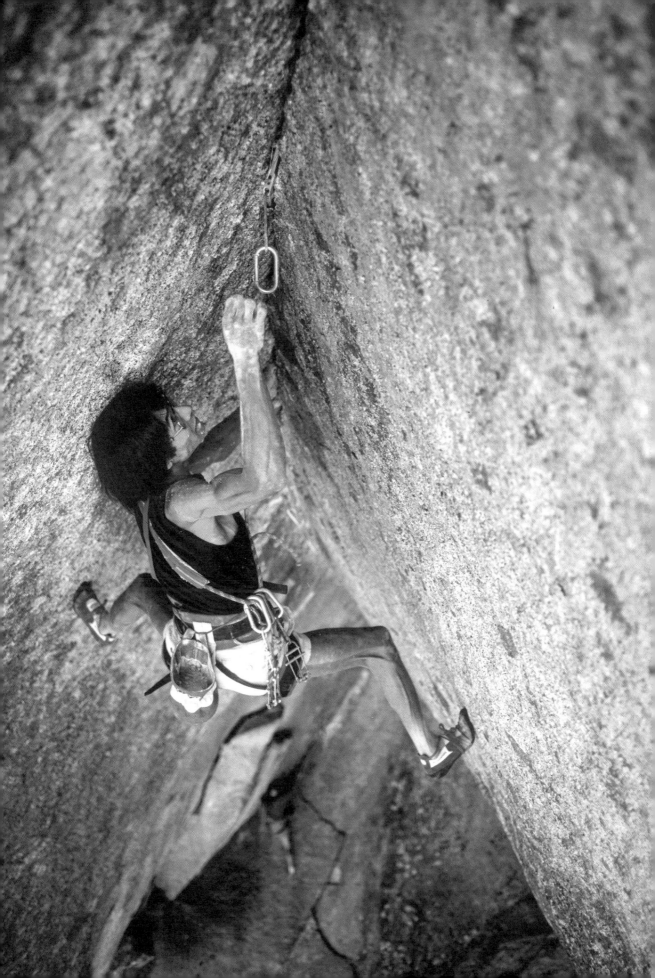

Each of us is born with a predisposition to a certain degree of confidence. What we start with is either fostered or ground away in the course of growing up. Finding the right balance of confidence to fear in the alpine environment is important; the cost of upsetting this balance can be one's life.

Judgment

Confidence is a prerequisite to building judgment: the balancing of ambition, ability, and risk. Judgment itself is a complex set of thoughts, feelings, and sensations that inform us from moment to moment about our safety and security. How this differs between climbers can be illustrated by recognizing that one person may safely solo a difficult route, which for another, even roped, might be life threatening.

Judgment is programmed by experience. The soloist learned judgment—incrementally and imperceptibly—over thousands of hours of climbing. There is no other way. Consider that to confidently solo you must be continually reevaluating your security as you are moving, sometimes from moment to moment. It's so much information that it could never be processed consciously, most of it happens at a subconscious level.

Buster Jesik and Marrianne van der Steen descending Mount Andromeda (11,319', 3,450m) in Alberta, Canada, after climbing the not-so-easy Practice Gully, Grade 3, during an Alpine Mentors climbing trip.
Photo: Steve House

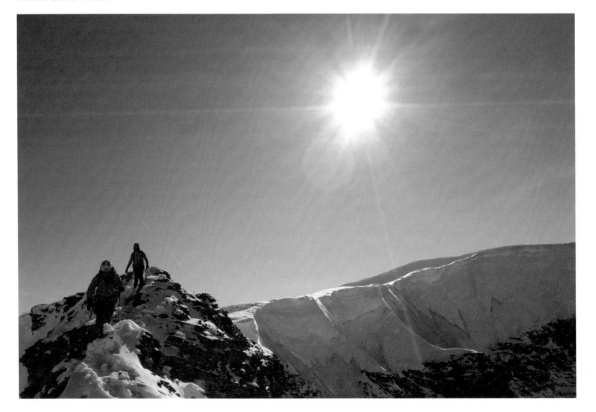

Trusting your own judgment is a big part of confidence. But can you improve your climbing judgment? Or confidence? Psychologists have studied this question. The most effective way climbers can improve themselves is to spend time with people who are better than they are. We can all benefit from the supervision of more-experienced climbers to help us fine-tune our awareness and judgment. Our training recommendations put a lot of emphasis on climbing a very high-volume of moderate (for you) routes, an ideal scenario for enriching your judgment skills. Judgment is earned—and shared—by experience.

Goal Setting and Confidence

Goal setting is an important tool for boosting confidence. Overcoming difficulty and failure with follow-up successes is the only thing that truly builds confidence. Set goals that are attainable and incremental. Be patient. Do not expect to reach the pinnacle of the sport in a few years. Mastery at anything worth doing takes a lifetime. Coaches commonly estimate that it takes five years of focused training to start to approach one's physical potential in any sport. Work in the currency of attainable goals, and your long-term payoff will be much greater.

Mentors

Mentors are invaluable sounding boards for your goals and ambitions. If someone knows your climbing and understands your ambitions, it is easier to have realistic, constructive discussions of your climbing goals. Finding mentors is never easy. We tend to gravitate to people of the same age and experience level. In some countries, mentorship is facilitated by climbing clubs, as was Steve's early experience in Slovenia. This does exist somewhat within clubs like the American Alpine Club, Mazamas, Seattle Mountaineers, and the Colorado Mountain Club. These all foster a mentor-based culture but, in our experience to date, the mentors themselves are often not experienced with climbing outside of the club structure. We don't mean to condemn all climbing clubs, but our personal experience has found their culture of climbing largely at odds with the climbing we know, which relies on a light, fast, low-impact style that rewards skill, confidence, and determination.

The high number of good climbers and alpinists coming from Slovenia, a country with a population less than that of Houston, is due in significant part to a healthy and well-run club structure that

Alpine Mentors

I feel so passionately about the value of climbing mentors that in 2012 my friends and I launched a recurring, two-year mentoring program for twenty-one- to thirty-year-old climbers. During our first cycle four young climbers, as of this writing, have climbed in Colorado and the Canadian Rockies with Vince Anderson, Bryan Gilmore, Steve Swenson, Rob Owens, Raphael Slawinski, Scott Backes, and myself. In 2013 we attained federal 501(c)3 nonprofit status and began raising money to support the program. It is our long-term goal to establish regional chapters of Alpine Mentors throughout North America. The mission of Alpine Mentors is to "promote alpinism by encouraging, coaching, and climbing with technically proficient young alpinists who aspire to climb the world's greatest mountains in a lightweight, low-impact style." Check out what we're up to at www.alpinementors.org.

–Steve House

incubates climbers' ambitions at every level from the beginner to the most advanced.

Moderate experience can foster a lethal type of confidence, one based on ignorance. Think of someone stopping for a lunch break under a dangerous serac. If you are lacking in experience, you may not know you're eating under a possible death threat. If you don't have experience to attempt a climb bigger, harder, or more complex than one you've done previously, be honest about it and find ways to connect with those who are more experienced. Mountain guides are of course the ideal answer. Though costly, guides offer almost every level of instruction and some guide very difficult ascents in addition to easier routes.

Developing Skills

Experienced alpinists must constantly hone their skills. I like the analogy to writing: A great short-story writer can always improve his or her skills by venturing into longer-form literature. Hemingway worked as a journalist, which honed his skills for writing fiction. Likewise, use the seasons to your advantage. Alpinists need to be good at all forms of climbing, so vary your climbing throughout the year. Fall is for rock climbing, winter for ice/mixed climbing, spring is for long routes or big ski tours, and summer is for alpinism. I don't think it's healthy or wise to try to alpine climb year-round—even if you could afford it. Rotating through the skills keeps you on the road of improvement.

Goals Build Confidence, Confidence Begets Skill

The more skilled you are as a climber, the more of the healthy confidence based on experience you will have. Both authors were alpine climbing for a long time before we came by a solid self-assurance that we knew how to keep ourselves safe on an alpine route, objective danger notwithstanding. To wit, Steve wasn't at all scared before he climbed the Rupal Face in 2005. Of course he knew there were dangers on such a wall, and he had a normal level of fear about those, but he also had immense confidence that he and Vince could do the climb safely. Their combined skills and fitness had been building over fifteen years; a lot of experience backed up his confidence.

Rock-solid confidence, refined judgment, deep experience, healthy ambition, good teachers, and past successes are all-important ingredients for a successful mental starting point. But that may not be enough. As we discussed earlier, focusing on past failures creates a negative emotional state in you, the opposite of what you are trying to be. Allowing free rein to demeaning self-talk or dwelling on the risks will deflate your self-confidence and sow the seeds of failure. Consciously narrow your thoughts to things that fortify and build toward the path you want to follow—the path to a transcendent experience in climbing.

TRANSCENDENCE

"All that we are is the result of what we have thought. The mind is everything. What we think, we become."

— BUDDHA

The search for transcendence, a feeling of confidence, mastery, and flow in the face of uncertainty, may be at the core of our quest for improvement in climbing. To us, transcendence is the culmination and the balancing of motivation, emotion, fear, ego, fulfillment, concentration, flow, self-reliance, confidence, and judgment all funneled into the sublime act of climbing. We've discussed each of these points because each represents a rich vein of development you can mine to find your own best performance as a climber.

Each of these components shifts with time, with age, with life. Transcendence is like a mirage in the desert. You see it on the horizon, you approach it, and it recedes. Trust that every step, no matter how small, sometimes even backward, is progress in your quest.

Here is a summary of what we personally found to be most fruitful:

- Meditation. Practicing meditation makes a state of concentration easier to attain and maintain.

- Don't let confidence, or the lack thereof, run the show. Being frozen by a lack of confidence indicates that your expectations are unrealistic; set new goals that you can attain and build up. Don't expect yourself to be climbing new routes on 8,000-meter peaks until you're climbing new routes on 7,000-meter peaks. Set attainable goals that you can achieve with hard work.

- Emotional awareness typically grows in fits and starts throughout one's lifetime, and for many of us it may not begin until middle age.

The Necessity of Cycles

By Andreas Fransson

When I was younger I used to try to follow my passion with 100 percent focus every day, all year. On my biggest seasons, after I had quit school, I averaged around 300 to 340 ski days per year, travelling between the seasons in the Alps, the north of Sweden, and Australia; ski bumming, training skiing skills, guiding heli-skiing and ski touring, as well as coaching clients and instructors. I love skiing, but back then I think it was more like an obsession.

I learned a lot about myself, ski technique, and the mountains, but I got to pay with hitting the wall, a hospital résumé longer than most people I know, and a body aging way faster than normal.

Then I turned to the real mountains, and instead of focusing on ski technique I plunged into the technique, strategy, and philosophy of adventures in the snow, ice, and rock. I started living for the next day's adventure, and for every day I learned something new and also increased the level step-by-step. I was on the same path as before, and my body, mind, injuries, and accidents followed in the same way as before.

The legendary Slovenian alpinist Tomo Cesen once said that after every great challenge he has accomplished he would always pause, draw back, and rest his mind for some time before he took on a new task. He did this so that he wouldn't get carried away by success and lose the fear and respect that comes with a worthy challenge. When you have accomplished a task, you normally want more of that task. You get confident and probably remember that which was hard as being easy, and then you risk pushing it too far.

In steep skiing (and mountain activity in general) it's alarmingly easy to get used to and lose the respect for exposure. If you are skiing the steeps every day you will sooner than later start feeling that extreme slopes are not much harder than walking on a sidewalk. It is worth noting that my hardest beating I have gotten this year was taking a fall on a sidewalk in Stockholm on an ice patch covered by a bit of fresh snow.

You need to be confident to be able to perform according to your potential, but you also need respect and fear as your companions to be around to enjoy the mountains in the years to come.

Cycles help us keep the balance between these opposites and are a key to survival in the mountain environment. Cycles, of course, also help us keep the balance between rest and training—and keep our egos in check.

On the grand scale of the game, cycles serve us with the contrasts that are life defining. Without darkness we wouldn't see light, without a pause from what we love, we wouldn't acknowledge how much we love the things we do.

For me, allowing, accepting, and recognizing this dance of doing and not doing is one of the most important things in a mountain life, if not in life in general.

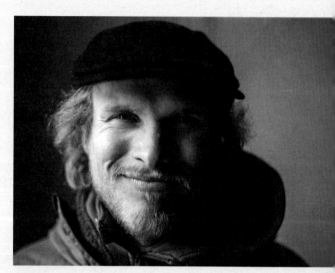

Andreas Fransson. *Photo: Tero Repo*

Andreas Fransson is one of the best big-mountain skiers in the world today. He lives in Chamonix and has made many incredible first descents, most impressively skiing the south face of Denali in 2011.

Opposite: Andreas Fransson beginning the descent of the north face of the Aiguille du Plan (12,051', 3,673m) near Chamonix, France. *Photo: Tero Repo*

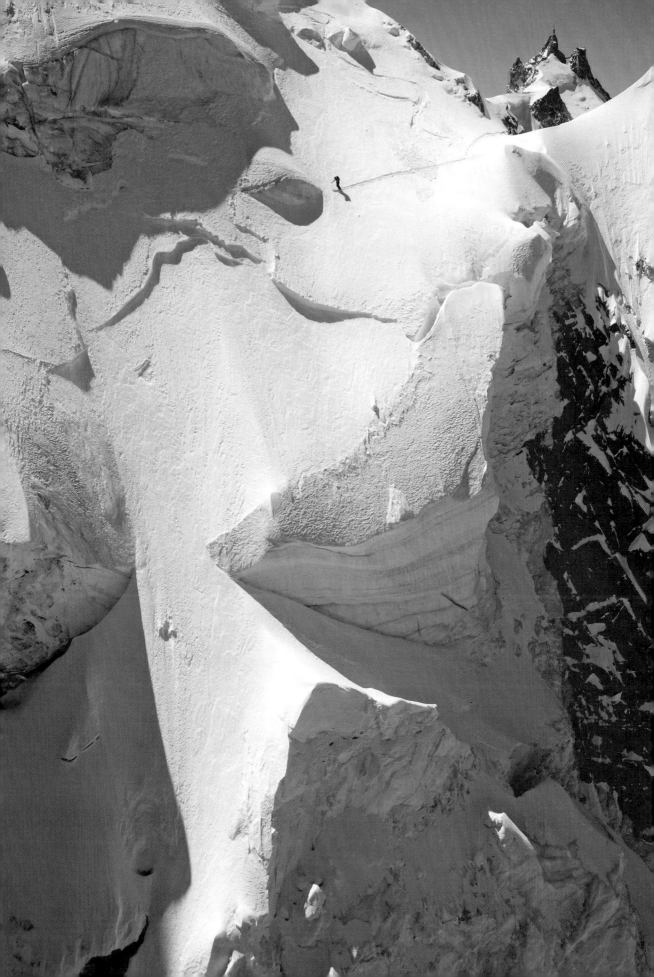

Some people grow up faster than others, but climbers as a group, from our observations, seem to grow up slowly.

- This is for the young readers of this book, those of you who live and breathe climbing: Do not allow motivation to run unchecked. You can visit the edge—and we can vouch for its allure—but you cannot live there full time.

- When you reflect on every big climb you've been on, there will always be a moment at which you knew you would finish the route, or not. Doubts are normal, even healthy. But when the positive aspects of continuing clearly outweigh the benefits of descending, you're on the road to success. Don't stop climbing until something stops you.

- Judgment, knowing when to back off, is imperfect. Accept your decisions without destructive second-guessing. No matter how much you want to go on, accept the occasionally inevitable decision to turn around as part of the practice of alpinism. Accept, learn, move on.

- Grow your awareness of how emotions affect decisions by assigning a sliver of your consciousness to observing your emotional state while climbing.

- Accept your fear and use it to focus your concentration. Turn fear into a catalyst for positive action.

- Any pursuit involving struggle or sacrifice can become a facile escape from broader inadequacies. The constant need for life-threatening affirmation is not a viable long-term solution for obtaining insight. Nevertheless, dysfunction is powerful fuel for hard alpine climbing. But know when to say when.

- Whether to go up or down is a decision to be made before you get scared. You will always be disappointed if you decide to retreat while you are choked by fear. Being unable to find protection, bad snow conditions, loose rock—these are reasons to retreat. Three rules of thumb: Don't retreat or make any important decision (1) in the dark, (2) with your heart rate over one hundred, or (3) on an empty stomach.

- Preparing for your climb may have started years earlier when you identified the goal, and the process of understanding the lessons gained will continue well past the day you return home from your expedition.

■ Learn what you need to do to find a productive, positive mental state for your climbing. Educate your family and your partners about it, and respect that process.

> "Physical or spiritual progress is simple: you must want who, or what, you might become more than who you are, or what you have, right now."
>
> — MARK TWIGHT

NON-LAZINESS AND PRACTICE

There is a story of a spiritual aspirant who was looking for a guru all over India. One day, he saw a guru meditating near a lake. He walked over and sat beside the teacher and waited. Finally the guru opened his eyes and said, "What can I do for you?" The student answered, "I would like to achieve illumination in a very short period of time." The guru said, "Very good, my son." Then he took the head of the student and held it in the water. Finally, when the student was almost drowned, he pulled him up. He asked the gasping student, "What did you desire most when you were drowning?" "Air!" replied the student. To this the teacher said, "If you can desire illumination as much as you desired air, you will have it quickly."

We assume that everyone reading this book wants to improve as a climber. Some of you have already been training. Some of you will train this evening. Maybe you will decide to read the newspaper before going to the gym. Or maybe you will decide to watch TV, check your Facebook page, or call a friend. After this, you might feel tired and decide to go to sleep. Tomorrow comes and you go through the same thing. This can go on for months or years.

You have to decide that you want to climb and train. Nobody can force you. Climb and train only when you really want to, not because others are training or climbing. When you have decided to train, make a schedule and follow it. You need to be true to your goals with your actions. Sticking to your plan to train fundamentally respects yourself. Practice following through constantly and consistently. Constancy of aim and effort, and not being lazy, is the key to developing as a climber.

Climbing starts with the idea, the ambition, and the motivation. Self-mastery and discipline may sound facile. And in fact you may easily attain a settled, focused mind from time to time. But getting what is between the ears to stay on track all the time is a basic, though incredibly difficult skill. One's successes are manifestations of completed growth and development as a climber. When you are internally strong, focused, and in control of lesser emotions, such as greed and envy, you will be much more likely to succeed. Physical training has the power to reinforce your mental focus. The mental focus is the difficult 80 percent: the most difficult perhaps, and the most important.

Experience comes from doing. Judgment develops from experience. Mentors are needed to help guide the process of recognizing your current abilities and setting your next goals. Skill is a manifestation of good judgment combined with practice. Confidence is born from this process, opening you up to the possibility of transcendence.

Observe the masters of climbing and you will agree that they are universally humble people. This is because confidence must be earned honestly and refreshed constantly. Experiencing an earned sense of transcendence brings the knowledge that climbing is both an art and a practice. The masters master the fundamentals and practice them over and over again. So should you.

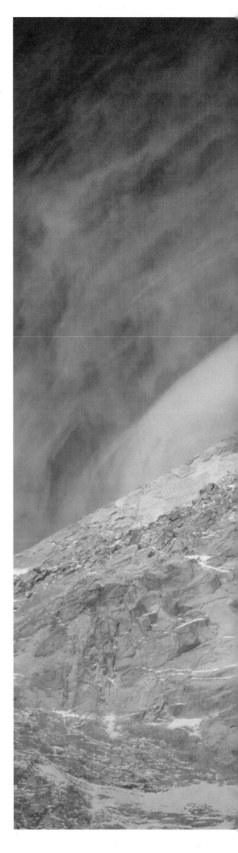

The ascent of the central part of the west face of Makalu (27,825', 8,481m) is destined to inspire future generations of alpinists to train intelligently with the goal to complete this climb of the future. *Photo: Steve House*

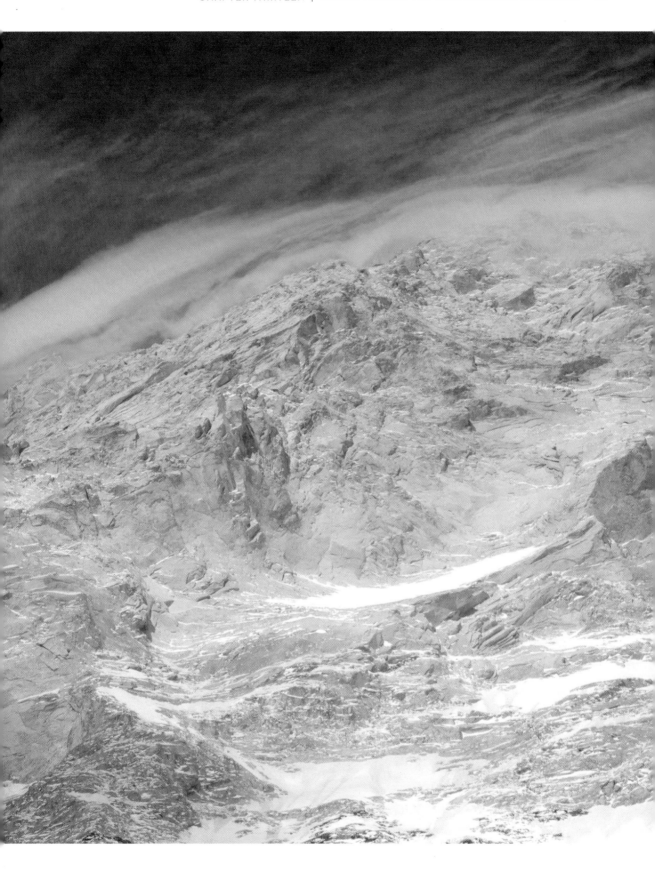

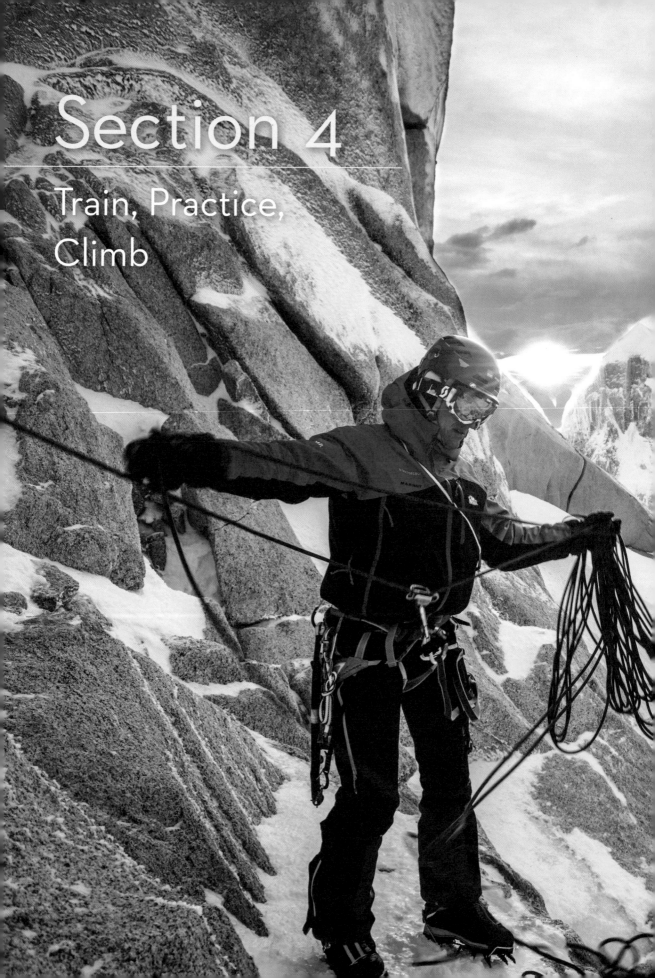

Section 4

Train, Practice, Climb

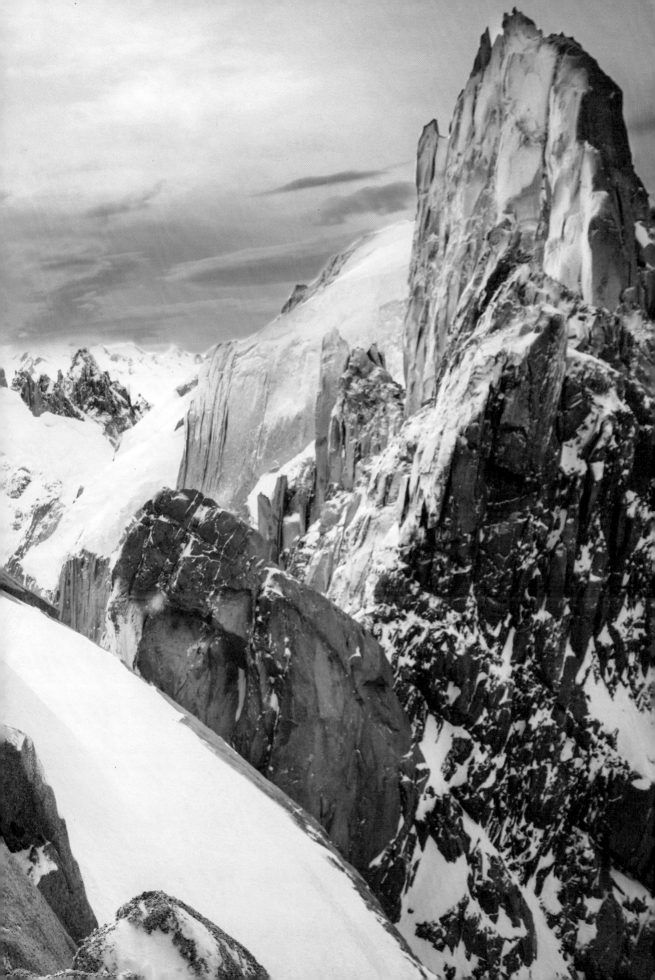

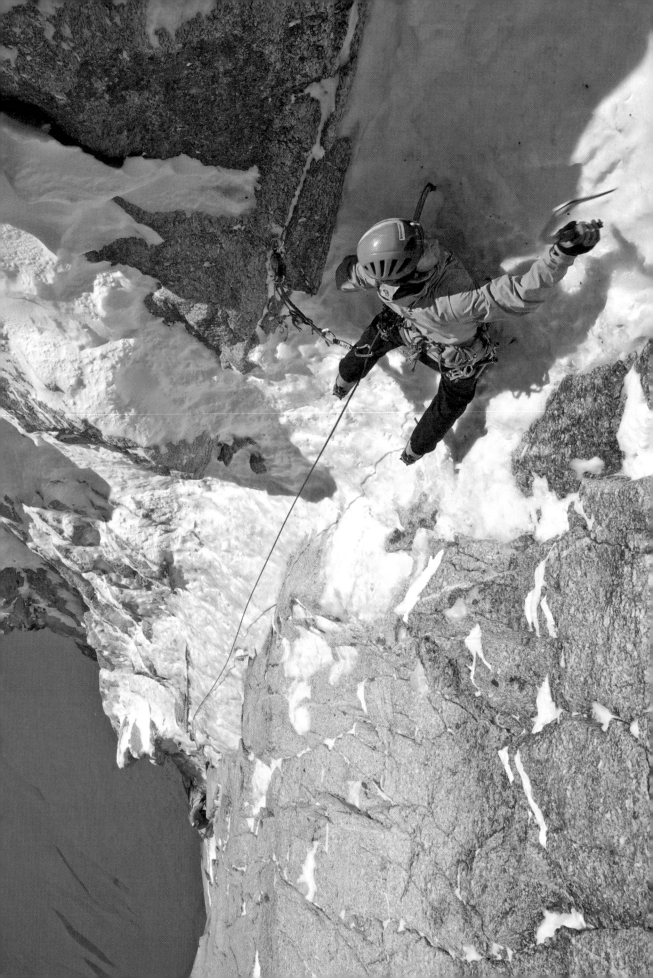

Chapter 14

Training by Climbing

"The world breaks everyone, and afterwards, some are strong at the broken places."

— ERNEST HEMINGWAY

GOING CLIMBING VERSUS TRAINING FOR CLIMBING

Lots of climbers talk about training by climbing. Many will tell you it's the only way to train. When you go climbing all the time, you feel fitter and stronger after a few months or a few years of consistent climbing. The problem with this approach is that it is random and sporadic. If it's not organized and progressive, it's practice, not training; it is just going climbing. The improvements in your abilities are most likely attributable to improvements in technique, efficiency, and specific muscular endurance. While these improvements are crucial to climbing well, many climbers, including both of us, have experienced a plateau or even regression in climbing fitness due to constant climbing.

Training by climbing implies something completely different. Training by climbing means applying the concepts of continuity, gradualness, and modulation to an annual climbing plan. It implies doing a good Transition Period, building a solid Base Period, and incorporating

Opposite: Ueli Steck climbs the Supercouloir on Mont Blanc du Tacul (13,937', 4,248m) in the French Alps. *Photo: Jonathan Griffith*

Previous spread: Stephan Siegrist rappeling down after a long day of climbing in Patagonia in winter. *Photo: Thomas Senf*

Max Strength training as well as Muscular Endurance training within the frequent practice of climbing.

Training by climbing has the advantage of specificity. There is never any need to convert nonspecific fitness gained on trails or in a gym to the mountains. It's all specific. That being said, it is important to recognize that the nonspecific conditioning proposed throughout this book is still a necessary, foundational component of any training plan. What we propose in this chapter is another way for those of you with the most time and motivation and easy access to cliffs, icefalls, and mountains to structure your training. The more technical your climbing goals, the more likely you are to benefit from using climbing as your primary training modality. This chapter will show you how to plan a climbing year through the lens of a training progression.

Defining Goals

First you need to set some goals for yourself. This can be a climb you want to do next year, or it can be more general. Your training will be most successful if you know what you're training for. Around 1990 Steve, at age 20, wrote down the following general goals for his climbing.

- Be able to lead, onsight, any 5.11 rock pitch, of any style, quickly and safely.

- Be able to lead any grade-6 ice pitch quickly and safely.

- To match or better Messner's 1,000-meter-per-half-hour (3,281-feet-per-half-hour) uphill running time.

- Be able to easily ascend 1,000 feet (305 meters) per hour in the mountains with a thirty-pound climbing pack in good conditions (below 16,400 feet/5,000 meters).

- Be able to climb technical pitches in bad conditions, snow-covered rock, rotten ice, wet rock, loose rock, etc.

- To understand and have good mountain skills. Become an expert on avalanche forecasting and safety, navigation, weather forecasting in the field, and to know every rope trick that might be needed.

What is useful about Steve's list is the fact that he broke out the different skill components of alpine climbing and set standards to aspire to in all the component parts of alpine climbing. These standards became goals that would lead him to round out his skills as well as his fitness. To reach these goals Steve focused intently on the components listed

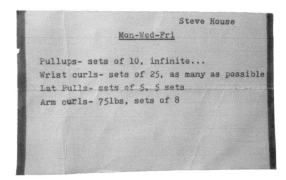

Steve House
Mon-Wed-Fri

Pullups- sets of 10, infinite...
Wrist curls- sets of 25, as many as possible
Lat Pulls- sets of 5, 5 sets
Arm curls- 75lbs, sets of 8

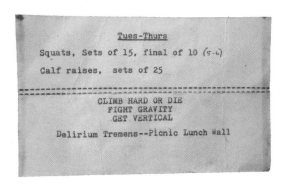

Tues-Thurs

Squats, Sets of 15, final of 10 (5-6)

Calf raises, sets of 25

CLIMB HARD OR DIE
FIGHT GRAVITY
GET VERTICAL

Delirium Tremens--Picnic Lunch Wall

Steve's self-authored training plan circa 1985: He climbed the route Delerium Tremens, but has yet to make the ascent of Picnic Lunch Wall.

above and began to pursue them on an individual basis. Besides the fitness training, he pursued harder technical standards on rock and ice. He took mountain weather and avalanche courses and eventually became the chief avalanche forecaster for North Cascades Heli-Skiing. This systematic approach took years but he was able to accumulate a huge knowledge and skills base, all of which helped in his long-range goals on big alpine walls. Without any formal understanding of training, Steve had an intuitive sense of these fundamental qualities that make up the complexities of alpine climbing and where he needed to start his training progression. In this book we are seeking to formalize this approach and remove some of the trial and error for the reader.

General Mountaineering

If your goal is climbing the Colorado fourteeners or ascending Mount Rainier, there is little point in going sport rock climbing, other than enjoyment. As you know, the less technical your climbing goals, the greater the relative importance of basic cardiovascular fitness. Moreover, mountain skills such as field weather forecasting and navigation will also gain in relative importance. Your ability to route-find out of a whiteout may be just as important as your fitness to your survival.

Technical Climbing

If your technical climbing skill already meets or exceeds the technical level of your climbing goals you will be best served by improving your base fitness as outlined throughout this book. This will also apply if you are constrained by your schedule or geography.

The more technically difficult your climbing goals are, the greater the number of years it will take to gain those climbing skills plus all the other knowledge needed for high-level alpine climbing. The conventional wisdom is that if you want to climb a certain grade and aren't there yet, then go climbing a lot.

This is true: Climbing must be experienced to be learned. Most breakthroughs in technique are attributed to body position and footwork. It is our experience that the more important shift is in perception; that standing on a small rock edge is secure, that the one-inch edge you hold onto becomes a rest, not a crux. As Ljubo warned Steve in 1989, it's more mental than physical. But what causes these shifts? More often than not it's the fitness to do what was previously difficult. If you can do ten pull-ups on your ice tools and hang on to a one-quarter-inch edge without a pump, you'll be much more confident in your climbing than if you don't have these strengths.

Your climbing skills training will progress most quickly if it is related to your goals. Climbing overhanging bolt-protected routes is not going to make you faster on loose 5.8. Maybe you need to be able to do both, maybe not. In our estimation an alpinist needs to be able to climb snow, ice, and rock, in all conditions. To be able to climb snow-covered rock slabs in the mountains you will want to go outside and climb rock routes in winter conditions wearing crampons. Not only will you be faced with the climb, but also dealing with wet ropes, finding solid partners, learning how to stay warm, and what to eat on a sub-zero day.

If you want to improve as quickly as possible, there are better models than the climbing-only model. As you improve your ability to climb technical rock, ice, and mixed terrain well, you will also need to start combining strength and endurance training with your climbing to speed and enhance your technical development.

Cardiovascular Fitness

As we have repeatedly pointed out, aerobic fitness is the cornerstone of alpine climbing. How you acquire that fitness can vary but its importance can never be ignored. If you do a lot of alpine climbing you will be building that base of fitness by virtue of the approach hikes. If you can crank hard moves, but a two-hour approach to a climb is the longest endurance workout you've done all year, then you need to focus on your cardiovascular fitness.

The simplest way to get better at walking uphill is to do it. Most climbers dislike hiking, but if it kicks your butt, choose some routes in your area with long approaches and start to target climbs that are farther and farther from the road. Alternatively, you could start with chapter 6 and assess your fitness and begin to design a mountaineering training program for yourself that would concentrate on boosting your speed and endurance going uphill.

YOUR BEST DAYS CLIMBING

Lots of climbers we see and talk to have reached a certain level of competency and stagnated there, often for years. There is a misguided assumption that you should be improving as you did during the first several years of climbing—the glory days when you went from leading easy, to moderate, to difficult routes in only a few years.

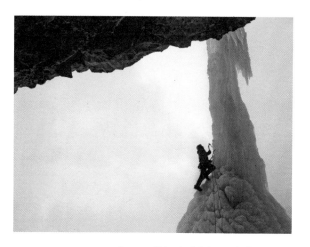

Accomplished alpinist and all-arounder Nick Bullock tunes up his ice climbing near Kandersteg, Switzerland. *Photo: Steve House*

In many cases, climbers plateau because they are trying to climb their best all the time, and wrongly expect continual improvement. Peaks are part of performance. Distance runners know from thousands of races in the history of the marathon that an individual athlete can peak a maximum of five to ten times over a career. In the entire history of the marathon only one individual runner has set the world record more than twice.

Climbing, while difficult, is not of the same intensity as running a fast marathon. There is more of a window of opportunity for alpine climbers to achieve great climbs over a career spanning decades. As climbers we can expect to peak once a year, and after several years of strong peaks we will have to acknowledge the fact that the rest of our lives we will be less strong physically. We will all be well served by understanding where our climbing is along the peaking continuum.

PLANNING A YEAR'S CLIMBING AS TRAINING

As with any training plan, the start of the process is to sketch a plan. For the as-much-of-the-time-as-humanly-possible climber, this will be vastly different from the goals of someone with a day job. For this chapter, we're going to assume that time is not an issue; that you can climb all day, every day, as much as you want.

On the following spread is a sample climb-to-train plan based on Steve's climbing over a twelve-month period.

At first glance, Steve's goals column seems random. But if you look at the period column you see that the goals mimic the structure of conventional periodization. In effect, he has designed his climbing year as a training plan. This is what we mean by viewing a year's climbing through the lens of training.

The approach we've outlined is not identical for someone focused only on difficult, shorter routes; such as hard sport climbing or single-pitch, hard mixed climbs. That is not the focus of this book. However, with a good understanding of the science we've shared here, it would not be a big stretch to design such a program.

PLANNING THE INDIVIDUAL PERIODS
Transition Period

As you've learned from the previous planning chapters, the first eight weeks are a transition back to training and climbing full time. This is an important period for everyone, no matter how long you've been climbing. The Transition Period starts by climbing lots of pitches below your maximum level and adding general strength training twice a week.

Let's talk about volume and difficulty in climbing. As we mentioned in chapter 7, the biggest issue to avoid in this period where you are re-entering a training cycle is coming out of the gate too hard. You will no doubt be highly motivated and energetic after a break from climbing and training. It is very easy to crank up the volume and intensity too quickly when starting out. As a motivated climber it is hard not to try to climb your hardest every time you're out. Sport climbing makes it so easy to quickly and safely get on routes that are close to your limit on any given day. And the peer pressure to do so is omnipresent. Most climbers' routine when they go sport climbing is to warm up on two or three easier routes and start trying harder routes that they can't complete. This is the wrong approach for this period. This is what you will do once you're well into in the Base Period, after you've built up a high level of endurance and general strength.

Not allowing your body to build a solid foundation each year is one of the main reasons most climbers don't progress from year to year. When viewed through the lens of climbing to train, you will see that this approach conflicts with the three tenets of continuity, gradualness, and modulation that you now know to be the basis of training.

During the Transition Period is when athletes address their strengths and weakness and target the low-hanging fruit. By focusing on improving the weakest qualities and bringing them to an equal level with your strengths, you will elevate your entire alpine climbing package. Spending the bulk of your allotted training time on your strengths is fun, and this is most likely why those particular qualities are your strengths, because you enjoy them. But it is not the way to make long-term progress. Remember what the great coach Eddie Borysewicz said to his cyclists: Train your weakness, race your strengths.

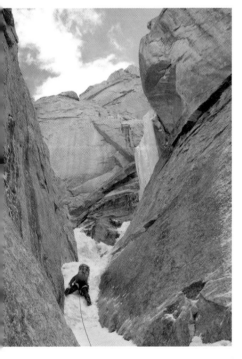

Marko Prezelj uses climbing and guiding exclusively as his training. Here he climbs an ice-choked couloir on the way to the first ascent of K7 West (22,500', 6,858m).
Photo: Steve House

Steve's Climb-to-Train Schedule

Climbs	Goals	Period
Summer 2012: Guiding and climbing in Alps. Focus on length not difficulty. Lots of hiking/approaches. 2 days of easy sport climbing per week, maximize number of pitches, not difficulty. 2 days per week of strength training in the gym.	The goal is to climb consistently, get used to daily, weekly, consistent climbing. Record volume and adjust intelligently.	Transition Period. Transition Period strength training.
Fall 2012: SW Colorado and the Black Canyon. Climbing long routes, 3–4 consecutive days on. 1–2 long easy runs per week for aerobic as approaches generally are short. These will be high volume weeks. First 8 weeks: Max Strength training plus core strength either in the gym or via bouldering 2x per week.	Climbing in the Black Canyon is great mental training due to the nature of the routes. As winter starts, switch to specific Muscular Endurance focus: Mixed climbing and/or rock climbing. Redpointing rock and mixed routes at my limit will ensure good core and upper-body strength. Record volume and adjust intelligently.	Base Period including a Max Strength phase for 8 weeks. Then begin specific Muscular Endurance phase.
Winter 2012/2013: Winter climbing, guiding, and completing some new route projects. Ski touring and Muscular Endurance strength training in the gym.	Guiding will give me the hours at low intensity and lots of pitches that are below my maximum ability. My winter climbing projects will push my skills and improve my climbing-specific muscular endurance. Ski touring is an excellent and most enjoyable endurance builder that can be both base building and lower-body muscular endurance if I go hard. Record volume and adjust intelligently.	Continued Base Period with specific Muscular Endurance workouts.
Spring 2013: March will be in the Canadian Rockies with Alpine Mentors program. Focus on length *and* difficulty. April is prime season to try some harder routes in the Black Canyon. In May I will be guiding the Moonflower Buttress on Mount Hunter.	Spring alpine season is a classic conversion period and brings mental skills into focus. Attempting long, hard rock climbs in the Black Canyon and big alpine routes in Canada will consolidate both muscular endurance and technical skills. Record volume and adjust intelligently.	Conversion Period. The majority of the climbing done here will be on long routes close to max ability.
Summer 2013: Expedition		Peak

Building Up Mileage

Let's suppose that you can climb any day of the week you want. During the Transition Period you will climb long, easy routes two to four days a week. Multi-pitch routes, preferably with sizeable approaches, are best for the alpine climber since they include the aerobic effort of the approach and descent.

The overall goal during this Transition Period is to do lots of pitches that are relatively easy for you; the more the better. The thing to make sure of is that you recover fully from each day's climbing with a single night's rest. There are several reasons for this strategy that should sound familiar. The first is that you are preparing your body for the Base Period, which will entail lots of climbing. As you'll remember, the Transition Period sets you up to start the real training. If you exhaust yourself in this early period then you will not be able to progress in the next periods. You will probably have to hold yourself back. As we discussed in chapter 3, many important adaptations happen during the Transition Period and if you skip or shorten this time frame you will not be able to absorb as much climbing volume during the Base Period, and that will limit how hard you will be able to climb later on.

Trust the process. There are fifty years of physiology and research and practice backing up that theory; this is how professional and Olympic athletes train for all other sports.

The first week of a Transition Period for an experienced climber who has reasonable fitness would start by climbing four to five pitches in a day, two days a week. Add to this two low-intensity endurance workouts a week, each two to eight hours long, which would ideally be long, easy climbs. This can be third- or fourth-class scrambles or easy fifth-class (belayed) climbing. It can also be a hike or a ski tour.

Each week add 5 percent more climbing time and 5 percent more easy climbing, scrambling, ski touring, hiking, or running time to your routine. For climbing, this is typically one additional pitch per week, sometimes two if they're short. It doesn't sound like much, until the eighth week when you're climbing fifteen pitches per day that are approximately one number grade below your best redpoint. During this time, if you want to get on a project, a climb you can't do without working on it, don't, not yet. Remind yourself that your long-term gains will be greater if you wait to tackle a new project until you've finished your Transition Period and begun your Base Period.

A major goal of this training-by-climbing is to practice your craft, to climb as well as you can. During the Transition Period think about solidifying your technical skills. Climb slowly and carefully on routes that are easy for you. If that's too boring, climb in boots instead of rock shoes. Try to eke out efficiency, relax on the climbs, see how lightly you can hold onto a crimp without falling, find out exactly how much pressure that hand jam needs to stay put. Let your speed come from being efficient and smooth, rather than forced or rushed.

A good tool to help with this is to wear a heart-rate monitor and challenge yourself to do pitches while keeping your heart rate as low as possible. As this period reaches its midpoint, try to purposely climb a little faster on routes you know well. You want to move surely, solidly, quickly, and with flow. Your goal is alpine climbing, and the important attributes of an alpinist are climbing smoothly and efficiently, and not falling. If the routes feel too easy, that's much preferable to them feeling too hard. Be patient, store motivation for the harder climbing that is to come. Guard against doing too much too soon. This is why coaches carry a whistle: to tell a motivated athlete when to stop—even when you want to do more.

General Strength

The second goal of this Transition Period should be to complete a period of strength training. As we've said before, there are countless studies that show that a general strength training period will be highly beneficial to developing more sport-specific strength later on. Your strength workouts start immediately, twice a week, and continue throughout the Transition Period. Use the general and core strength workouts introduced in chapter 7.

For general strength conditioning we recommend spending two days a week cragging, and on that same day do a general-strength workout in the gym. Overhanging climbing can also be good to get your core engaged, but for most people steep routes are not easy enough for this period. For now, stay off any routes you can't climb on the first try. Steve prefers a crag with long pitches and as close to vertical as possible since this most closely mimics alpine terrain.

Another good option for strength training during the Transition Period can be bouldering mixed with weight training. As bouldering is climbing, it's prefered by most people. But remember, this is a period for easy (for you) climbing. Don't do boulder problems you can't complete on the first or second try. And because the focus of our training is on alpine climbing, we recommend bouldering on close-to-vertical terrain because overhanging movements have relatively little application in the alpine climbing realm. Search out problems that are moderately overhanging and balancey, require lots of core tension, and minimize the climbing on very overhanging terrain.

Cold and Hungry

By Scott Semple

Will broke up the cheese into chunks while Kevin stirred the instant noodles.

"*Ah, shit*," I said.

We had just failed on our first attempt on what would later become Howse of Cards on Howse Peak in the Canadian Rockies. We'd spent an hour digging a snow cave and getting ready to eat. As I watched the salty, fatty goodness in the pot, I realized that I'd forgotten a bowl and spoon.

I was new to alpine climbing, so it wasn't surprising, and I was later proud of my innocent mistake. My problem was quickly solved, but I wasn't so lucky with a similar rookie mistake a few years later.

My friend Eamonn and I had spent ten hours climbing four demanding mixed pitches on a winter attempt at Snowpatch Spire in the Bugaboos. The ice was thin and the gear was bad—there was no such thing as a #20 Camalot, so the only protection for the third-pitch squeeze chimney was the belay.

Faced with fading light, we looked around at our bleak bivy options. The first option was a twelve-inch horizontal crack that we probably could have crawled into, but claustrophobia made us cringe at the thought. Our second choice was what looked like a big enough snow drift twenty feet (six meters) to the right on a down-sloping slab.

I belayed Eamonn as he traversed to the snowy slab, and then he put in an anchor so we could tram our gear across. I clipped the stuff sack that held both of our sleeping bags to the tram line and then gave it a shove. It bounced off the wall—*click*—the carabiner opened, and we both yelled, "*NO!*" as we watched our sleeping bags fall into space.

I climbed over to Eamonn, and we started digging a snow cave, but the snow was sugary and bondless. The exposed side of the cave quickly collapsed, leaving us with a semi-covered porch. "*Tonight is gonna suck,*" I thought.

In retrospect, we could've rapped off and gone back to the hut a half-hour ski away, but the thought of coming back to jug the pitches below us was distasteful, and giving up those hard-won leads even more so. We had climbed together enough that we didn't need to discuss it: We'd stay there and suffer.

We spent the night doing hundreds of push-ups, squats, windmills, and spooning to keep warm. The warmest position we found was me as the blanket, and Eamonn as the mattress—he's a lot bigger than I am.

It's important to make survivable mistakes. They say that good judgment comes from bad experience, and the hubris that comes with being a twenty-something alpine climber pretty much guarantees such an education.

Going hungry or freezing your ass off for silly errors is necessary and invaluable, primarily because after a lesson has been emphasized with suffering, you're guaranteed to never make that mistake again.

Scott Semple lives in Canmore, Alberta, and splits his time between his computer, his kids, and climbing (preferably with sleeping bags on hand).

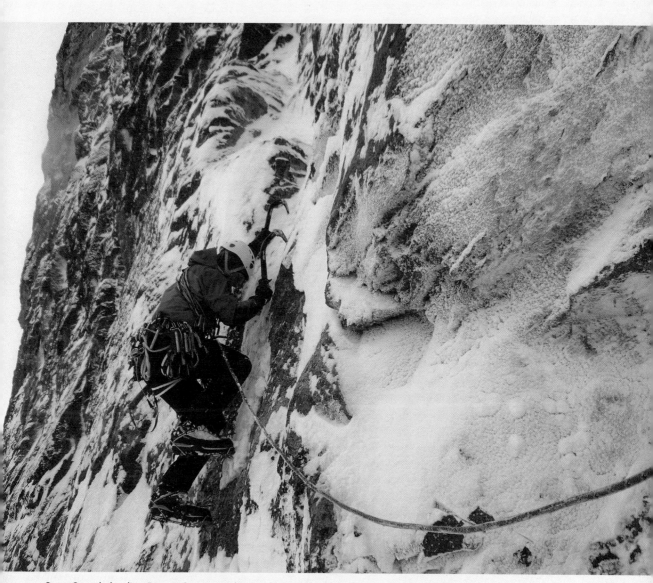

Scott Semple leading Drama Queen on the Stanley Glacier Headwall near Banff, Canada. *Photo: Steve House*

Bouldering during the Transition Period has to be done very carefully if you are to gain the most benefit. It is very easy to overdo it. You are also at risk for a climbing-specific injury. We personally know of a lot of people who have sustained all kinds of fairly serious injuries while bouldering, especially indoors. Most highly motivated climbers are at risk of climbing and bouldering too much or too hard during this period. A gym-based strength workout will be preferable for you if you know you're that type.

The weight room will almost certainly be a necessity; there is no better way to strength train your legs and lower body. We recommend you pick four lower-body exercises from the General Strength Routine that you feel you need to improve on and do these twice a week in the weight room. One-legged movements should make up at least two of these four exercises. If you don't want to go into a gym, or don't have one nearby, use the four exercises as inspiration and create your own, similar exercises that utilize whatever materials are at hand.

The Transition Period is fun and entails lots of climbing. You will see steady gains in strength that will give you confidence that you're making positive progress toward achieving your goals.

A BASE PERIOD OF CLIMBING

As we've said repeatedly, the Base Period is the longest phase of the training year, and it is also the most important. The goal during this period is to develop a resistance to fatigue and accustom your body to doing lots of work. Volume takes precedence over intensity of effort. When climbing-as-training, this is the time you will do lots of climbing at a technical level that is relatively easy compared to the hardest climbing you've ever done. Do not get on routes that you pump out on and fall off of. Climb pitches, pitches, and more pitches. As for approaches, feel free to queue up those remote routes you've always been too lazy to cross off your list. Approaches should be purposefully long to get your aerobic training. Improving your climbing-specific muscular endurance at this stage is a good by-product of all this climbing, but be careful not to overdo it in the early weeks of the base development.

The First Eight Weeks of the Climb-to-Train Base Period

During this time frame, you should be modulating your week-to-week climbing load by feel. Make sure you gradually increase the overall volume from week to week, and take a full, easy week out of every three or four. This is best done with a coach who can simply tell you when to lay off and do some recovery workouts. Assuming that you will be your own coach you must closely monitor your own body, plus use some of the self-test methods discussed in chapter 2. The aim is not to plan recovery weeks per se, but to feel when you're starting to fatigue, and act on that by taking rest as it's needed. That being said, you should take a recovery week after three to four weeks of buildup. Otherwise you are likely to crash in week six or seven when the steady increase in training and climbing volume catches up with you. This requires that you exercise your awareness and discipline to know when to back off and when to start climbing again.

Calculate a Starting Volume

To calculate how much climbing you should do, refer to our previous discussion about training hours in chapter 6. If you count up the time you are climbing and approaching, then you should be able to come up with a starting volume and modulate your volume appropriately each week.

Max Strength: Bouldering

During these first eight weeks of this Base Period, plan two short climbing sessions a week at a bouldering area or crag where you can do short climbs close to your limit. These sessions should last an (action-packed) hour at the most. Essentially, two days a week you want to do a Max Strength workout by climbing. Recall that Max Strength workouts are typically four reps and last six sets and do not result in muscular failure. Rest for three to five minutes between attempts—long enough to attempt a full effort. A couple of different eight-move boulder problems that you can do every time, but not too easily, would be perfect. Remember that going to muscular failure causes hypertrophy, muscle-mass gains, something you don't usually want unless you are especially weak.

Max Strength for Your Legs

This is great time to integrate some of the hill sprint or truck-push training we covered in chapter 8. These exercises will help you develop powerful legs and can easily be added to an intensive climbing program like the one we're describing here.

Climb for Pace

Another two or three days of the week you'll do long climbing routes plus approaches to complete the number of hours you need to top up your weekly volume. If you do not have long climbs nearby, but do have access

Mileage on the Real Thing

By Colin Haley

Most modern climbers make sure to live somewhere with close access to crag climbing or at least a climbing gym, so training for hard pitches is not a problem. The availability of high-quality cardiovascular training, whether in the form of running, Nordic skiing, or biking, is present almost anywhere. What I think is often neglected in the modern climber's training regime is mileage on easy to moderate alpine terrain. I think that spending a lot of time and covering a lot of distance on genuine alpine terrain is useful both physically and mentally.

A benefit of a lot of time on easy alpine terrain is that your base of fitness will improve. More importantly, your movements will become more efficient the more time you spend climbing, down climbing, and traversing on moderate alpine terrain. I have seen plenty of people who can climb WI6 but are very slow on an exposed, sixty-degree snow traverse—they have to think about every movement, rather than just let their arms and legs do it from memory. The benefits are mental as well:

The moderate terrain on an alpine route is usually much more poorly protected than the hard pitches, and often not protected at all. With a lot of experience on fifty- to sixty-degree slopes, you will feel surprisingly confident soloing around on them.

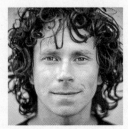

Colin Haley *Photo: Mikey Schaefer*

Colin Haley, a native of the Pacific Northwest, focuses his climbing on the mountains of Patagonia and Alaska, where he is drawn to the steepest alpine faces.

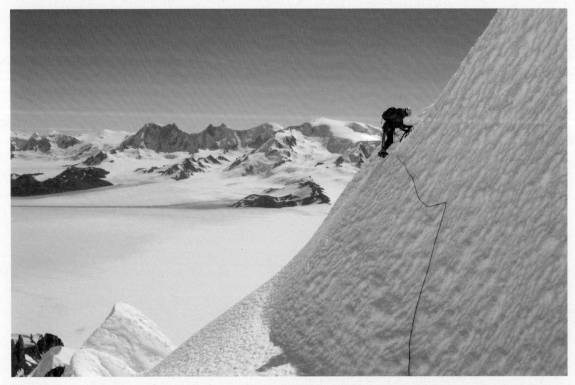

Colin Haley down climbing a short ice face connecting El Arca de los Vientos to the Ragni Route on the west face of Cerro Torre during the first ascent of the Torre Traverse, January 2008, Patagonia. *Photo: Rolando Garibotti*

to a crag, you'll want to do a bunch of pitches, if possible, to get in the necessary hours. Consider down climbing pitches, if possible, to build this skill, and to add more training time into each pitch. Concentrate on pace and efficiency. Do not rush or try to climb speedily. This only leads to mistakes and wasted energy. Efficiency is the hallmark of an alpinist.

If you have only eight weeks to execute a Base Period before getting on your goal climbs, you should complete only the Max Strength sessions plus the volume we've discussed above. Your muscular endurance will come on your climbing trip.

Muscular Endurance Plus Volume

From this point until you head out on your big expedition of the year you'll be ready to shift to a new emphasis that includes two different types of climbing days: muscular endurance climbing days and volume climbing days. This is the final part of the Base Period, which can last up to sixteen to twenty weeks. In the climb-to-train scenario, there is no need to execute a Conversion Period.

Climb for Difficulty: Muscular Endurance

This is the fun stuff that everyone wants to do and most climbers do a lot of, but normally they do it without the periodized approach: Go climbing and try as hard as you can! Twice a week you'll climb full pitches, concentrating on difficulty. You've already completed eight weeks of Max Strength bouldering and cragging workouts. These new sessions focus on Muscular Endurance. This means that you can start climbing to failure at the crag.

These days will look like a typical sport climber's day and will be spent at a crag or in a climbing gym. Do one or two easier pitches to warm up and then get on routes that are hard for you—that you can fall on. Try to plan your hardest routes as the third to fifth pitches of the day when your strength will be at its peak. This is the time to redpoint your sport climbing projects. As the day progresses, do slightly easier and easier routes that will be still difficult to complete due to building fatigue. This session is easily accomplished in a good climbing gym.

Personal Records on Long Routes

For one to a maximum of two days of the week (that aren't rest days) you'll climb long routes. It's OK to push the pace a bit, as long as you don't sacrifice efficiency. The other three to four days will be easy and recovery days only so that you can go hard on these workouts. If you feel heavy while doing these climbs, which is likely, it's OK to push

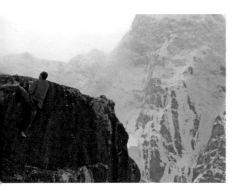

Marko Prezelj does a Max Strength maintenance workout (aka: boulders), in K7 base camp, the north face of K6 West (23,300', 7,100m) looms behind. *Photo: Steve House*

through that as long as you take enough rest days. Race to the base of your climbing objective with a full pack at top speed to create a Muscular Endurance workout for your lower body. This is like what we prescribed to do artificially with the water-carry workouts.

With speedy approaches and speedy climbing these will be hard days and will build up to hard weeks. The big weeks will be really hard physically and psychologically; all you will be able to do is eat, rest, and climb. Adequate recovery needs to be a priority during this period, so take days off and do easy recovery workouts like relaxed runs so that the hard days can be truly hard.

Organize Your Climbing to be Progressive

Let's lay out your entire Base Period, which will be at least eight weeks, and preferably closer to twenty weeks. Start writing down climbs you'd like to do. Group these climbs into easy, medium, and hard—or even better, categorize them in multiple ways: by technical difficulty, aerobic difficulty, and general alpine skills such as climbs requiring bivouacs, or containing loose rock, or requiring you to move fast on moderate terrain.

As you progress through the Base Period weeks of climbing you can refer back to these lists, even adding new climbs. The lists are helpful to identify when you could benefit from a certain route.

Principles to Remember:

- Continuity—Don't break the cycle of building by taking extended breaks.

- Gradualness—Each week should be a little harder than the last, but not much. Remember the rule of thumb not to increase your volume more than 5 to 10 percent per week.

- Modulation—Take a rest when you feel fatigued and head out climbing when you start to feel your strength returning. At the least you should drop the volume and intensity by 50 percent every three to four weeks to let your body absorb the load you have been heaping onto it.

Now, call your climbing partner, crack open a (light) beer, and get to work mapping out your season's climbing.

TAKE A ROAD TRIP

When you are climbing to train, and you're nearing the end of a long Base Period, a road trip is a good way to dial up your climbing-specific fitness before tackling a big project. For a full-time alpinist planning an expedition to the Karakoram, a spring Canadian Rockies trip would be perfect before leaving and is a progression Steve has followed many times. Ideally the structure of the climbing on your road trip should mimic the balance between long days and Muscular Endurance days, as in the final eight weeks of the Base Period discussed above.

If the weather during any period of your road trip is especially bad, you will have an excessively easy week. Here are some tips for an alpine climbing road trip:

- If you have a hard week of climbing, or do any one climb that requires more hours of actual climb and descent time than your biggest training week, fifteen to twenty hours for most, then make sure you take the next three to five days off and do only recovery-type workouts. Three days is the absolute minimum amount of rest you will need after this much effort. If the weather is good, you might not choose that, but know that if you keep hammering, your body will slow down and you will not be getting stronger. If you want to get stronger after doing a climb, you must rest after each major, demanding route.

- We all like to party on vacation. But this is a training camp, not a vacation. Don't disrupt your sleep patterns by staying up late and sleeping in. When you're alpine climbing you go to bed when it gets dark and you wake up before it gets light; get used to it.

- It is possible for fit climbers to stack less demanding climbs for a bigger training effect. This is the time-honored *link-up*. This is common practice in a training camp scenario when the full recovery is delayed till the end of the camp. If in Canmore, Alberta, an example would be Brewer's Buttress, followed the next day by the north face of Mount Stanley, followed by the Kain Route on Mount Louis, followed by the regular route on Ha Ling Peak, for four consecutive long days of easy-to-moderate climbing. This would give most parties a total of forty-plus hours of climbing in addition to the approach time. Then take between three and five recovery days.

- If you have a long period of bad weather, use the time constructively. Create whiteout navigation plans for routes you have in mind. Read guidebooks. Study maps. Do the approach to the base of a route. Scout descents. Go to a climbing gym or head out bouldering. Strength maintenance is good to do up to twice a week during this phase, not more. Bad weather is a good time to do some Max Strength maintenance (discussed in chapter 8). No gym is required; these will not be overly taxing if you have done a good strength progression to this point. If not climbing, you need to do an aerobic maintenance workout at least once a week. We recommend easy jogging or a long hike.

Lots of different sports use a training camp as a way to prepare for the competitive season. The idea is to get the team together in a great location, with other teams, and play and/or train to convert that base fitness to sport-specific fitness. (Think of baseball's spring training.) If you can't get away on a road trip, you may be able to have a training camp near your home.

CLIMB!

Now you're ready to attempt your biggest alpine climb of the year. For many alpine climbers, the year's big goal will be an expedition or an extended trip to a distant mountain range. Two weeks or a month of climbing in the Alps, Alaska, or the Himalaya or Karakoram ranges are the usual goals.

Below are some suggestions we, and many others, have learned the hard way:

- If you've been climbing to train, consider the one to two weeks of packing and travel to be your taper.

- Have multiple objectives, some that are doable in difficult conditions if the weather does not cooperate.

- Once you arrive at your destination, build up with easier weeks in the beginning, climbing harder, more intensely through the expedition. The intention is to peak on your route.

- Remember, it's easy to maintain your fitness now that you have it.

- Pacing yourself in the beginning can make the difference between success and failure at the end. Remember the tortoise and the hare. If you have followed a structured training plan for a year and stayed healthy, you are going to be stronger than you've ever been in your life! The big temptation is to go out of the starting blocks hard. Don't do it if you don't have to. The result is that you will fade, or get sick, toward the end of the trip right when you need to be your fittest to climb the highest peak or the most difficult route. If you are going to be on an expedition for a month or two, keep the big picture in mind.

RECUPERATE AND REGENERATE

After every big climbing trip or expedition, we strongly recommend taking time off from climbing. Spend time with your family. Eat pizza. Go to the beach. Anything but climbing. Rest—both the body and mind. It will pay off in terms of years and longevity.

A Word of Caution

Alex Lowe was one famous climber who enjoyed training and who frequented the weight room. He even experimented with creatine when the craze hit in the 1990s. (It works, but it makes you heavier.) He once told Steve that he felt he needed to be out all the time, to be pushing on risky routes and climbing in the mountains as much as possible. He reasoned that this kept him sharp. This was how he stayed in tune with the environment. Tragically, he was killed by a huge, naturally triggered avalanche in the Himalaya.

Charlie Fowler, who was Scott's frequent partner throughout the 1970s, told him that he had averaged over 300 days of climbing a year for several years. On his first trip to Chamonix around 1980, he was there for forty days and did thirty routes including several high-stakes solo ascents. He loved to be out in the environment and relished being on the edge of control. Sadly, he was also killed in the mountains.

Mark Twight once advised Steve that as a climber, "You can't live there all the time." The "there" is the dangerous and unforgiving alpine environment. Mark needed an occasional break from the mountains, and the authors believe that we all do.

In your twenties and early thirties, ambition often burns hot. If executed well, the training programs presented in this book will get you to a level of fitness you probably never imagined you could have. Strength fuels ambition. Climbing to train is fun, and powerful. Be prepared. Be smart. Be careful.

Les Droites

By Barry Blanchard

The spring-green leaf buds glowed in the rising sun as my climbing partner Kevin Doyle and I walked to the foreman's office to quit our jobs. It was June 1980 when we flew to Chamonix, France, intent on climbing the Alps until our money ran out. We were each twenty-one years old and dreamed of climbing the routes of our heroes: Harrer, Bonatti, Rébuffat, Terray, Lachenal, Messner.

John Lauchlan was another hero of mine. John was also from Calgary, but older than us. John was the first Canadian to have pushed his climbing to a world-class level. That summer he lived in the woods outside of Chamonix.

By the end of August, Kevin and I had tallied eleven alpine routes between us. The golden granite of Bonatti's Pillar had passed through my hands, as did the blue, blue ice of Couturier Couloir. My spikes had locked with the cement-gray ice of Mont Blanc du Tacul's East Face. Climbs that had felt the touch of our heroes. Kevin and I convinced ourselves that we were ready for the north face of Les Droites. This was a hard route, a grande-course, and the weight of it settled onto my psyche like a blanket of chainmail. I was overwhelmed. How in the hell was a guy who three years ago knew more about steer riding than about climbing, going to get up a route as big and as hard as the north face of Les Droites?

Warm air surged onto my face as I stepped into Chamonix's Alpenrose Bar. It was raining outside, and humidity and cigarette smoke condensed on the low ceiling. We heard the muffled clink of glasses, the murmuring of French, and laughter.

I spotted John at a crowded table behind regiments of empty beer glasses, a steak sandwich the size of my forearm in front of him. I waved and he rose and threaded his way through the crowd. An aura of electricity enveloped us and for ten minutes he raved to me about his recent ascent of the MacIntyre-Colton Route on the north face of the Grandes Jorasses. John and his partner had made the third ascent of the route in record time.

"What are you and Kevin's plans?" John asked.

He was a classy guy; he always asked about my plans. I didn't want to say, "Les Droites," because saying it would have it exist in the world beyond Kevin and me. I crammed my balled-up hands deeper into the pockets of my khaki painter's pants and looked down to my yellow Nikes. When I looked up, John's gaze was unwavering. No getting out of this one.

"Well . . . we're kinda thinking about the north face of Les Droites."

John locked his buzzing blue eyes onto me. "Do it—it is perfect for you guys."

I let go of the breath I'd been holding. "Oh man, I don't know if we're up to it yet. I don't know if Kev and I are there."

"No. No way. You guys can do it. I climbed it in July; I know it, it is right for you." He dropped his eyes to his hands, the sun had baked them to chocolate leather, his palms swept up to a peak. "The lower face is just like doing the north face of Mount Athabasca, and you guys have done that. Then you do Takakkaw Falls, you've done that too," his hands mimed the swinging and planting of ice tools, "then you top it off with Cascade Falls." His palms opened to the ceiling in a "so what?" gesture. "It's just three pieces of Canada on loan to France! All you have to do is put it all together in one day; you can do it, lad!"

The route unfolded as John had predicted it would. Kevin and I climbed a grande-course alpine route thanks to John breaking it down into terms that a steer rider could understand.

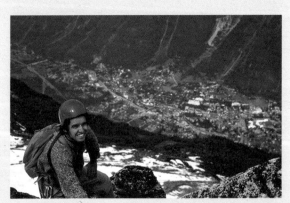

Barry Blanchard in 1980. *Photo: Kevin Doyle*

An IFMGA-certified mountain guide living in Canmore, Alberta, Barry Blanchard has put up first ascents around the globe, but is perhaps best known for his groundbreaking ascents and intimate knowledge of the Canadian Rockies.

Opposite: Twenty years after his ascent of the north face of Les Droites, Barry Blanchard attempts a new route on the south face of Nuptse East (25,603', 7,804m). *Photo: Marko Prezelj*

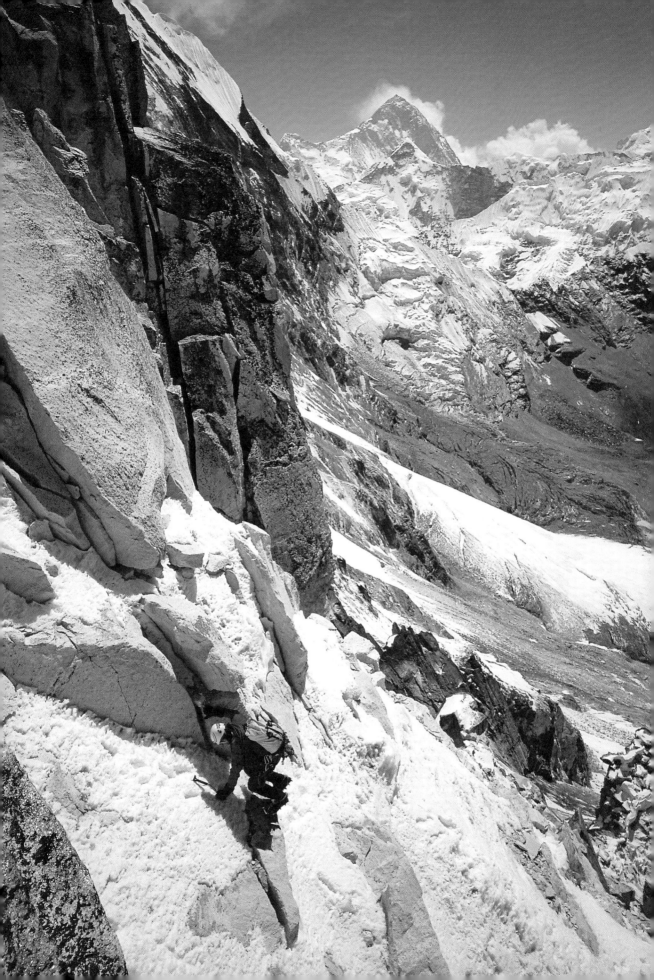

Two Attempts on the Southeast Face of Kyzyl-Asker

By Ines Papert

When I saw the 3,900-foot (1,200-meter) southeast face of Kyzyl-Asker in an old photo for the first time, I knew I wanted to climb it. I felt a great desire to try its difficult ice and mixed climbing along the steep line that topped out directly on the summit. The foundation of realizing success on a challenging objective is a bottomless enthusiasm for the route. That is a prerequisite if you want to succeed.

Many teams had already tried and failed on this wall, which only served to further inspire me. However, first I had to figure out why other teams had managed to complete only a third of the wall. The reason was clear: the aspect and the timing. The wall faces the sun nearly all day and this causes the ice to melt early causing deadly rock and ice fall. So I decided to go there in late autumn, when the nights are significantly colder and the sun is lower.

I know from experience that you cannot start too early with training for an objective, and I started right away in my home region of Berchtesgadener Land, Bavaria. To get mentally accustomed to the very low temperatures and expected bivouacs, I ran the local trails in the coldest and worst conditions. During the summer months I carried my climbing pack plus a paraglider up the west face of Hoher Göll Mountain. This benefitted me in two ways: First, I got used to the heavy load on my back, and my endurance increased rapidly. Second, I saved my knees from countless miles running downhill with a nice flight down to the valley.

The southeast face of Kyzyl-Asker deserves clean and committed climbing, so I planned to climb it in alpine style, without any bolts. Because of this I needed to plan my lead-up climbing trips very carefully. I chose Scotland since there were many trad climbing routes with long approaches there—and lots of bad weather. After a two-week trip to Scotland and numerous routes climbed, I felt ready for my big objective.

I trained and prepared for this climb for a year. I train and climb intuitively. When I am climbing, I give 100 percent. And as my dear, departed friend and climbing partner Hari Berger used to say, "The training stimulus only starts when it starts hurting." If after two days my body tells me to take a break, and I want to stop, I try to climb a few more routes. In these situations I often think of what Hari said, and this helps me make the extra effort.

I attempted Kyzyl-Asker twice with different partners. On our first attempt in 2010 we climbed to 650 feet (200 meters) below the summit in one day. Despite repeating all of the preparation, training, and planning, we were not successful on the second expedition. Unfortunately I had not been able to team up with the same extremely motivated people again. Shortly after arriving in base camp on the second attempt it became obvious that my partners weren't able to deal with the mental and physical difficulties of the expedition.

What did I learn? To listen to myself and decide whether I am ready for the objective, and if it inspires me. To weigh the realistic chances. To consider the objective hazards. To choose my partner(s) very carefully, and check beforehand if their levels of motivation are the same as mine. Preparing and training together is of the utmost importance. I learned that team discussions are really important. And to train mentally, as well as physically, for the objective.

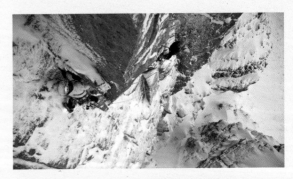

Ines Papert leading Blood, Sweat, and Frozen Tears on Ben Eighe in the Northern Highlands, Scotland. *Photo: Hans Hornberger*

Professional climber and multiple-time world champion in competition ice and mixed climbing, Ines Papert now focuses her climbing and training towards big rock, ice, and mixed routes throughout the world. Her most recent accomplishments have included 4,600-foot (1,400-meter) high mixed routes on Baffin Island and multi-pitch rock climbs up to 5.13c (8a+). Her self-taught climb-to-train progression is exactly what we prescribe in this chapter.

Opposite: Kyzyl-Asker (19,100 feet, 5,820m), Kyrgyzstan. *Photo: Thomas Senf*

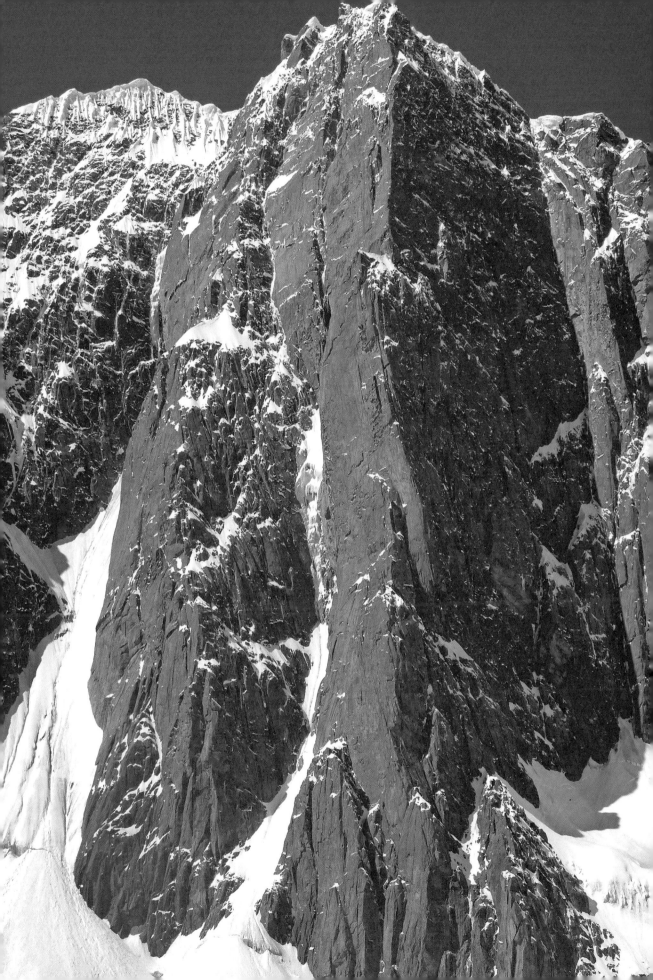

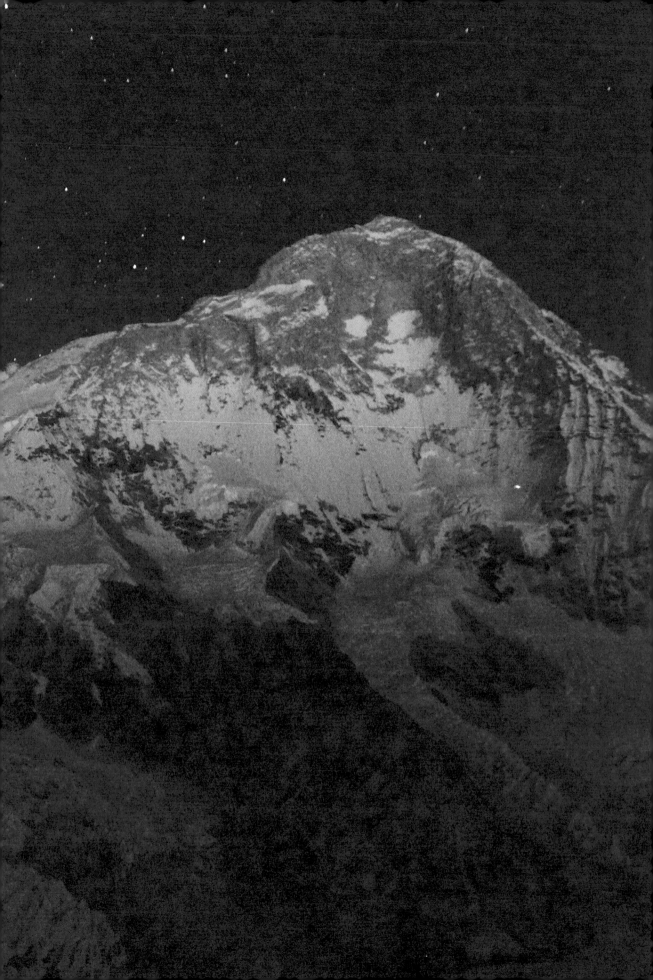

Chapter 15

The Art of Self-Knowledge

"Climbing is a sport, but climbing in the mountains, like ocean racing or crossing a desert, takes place in rather different conditions from those of the common run of sports. A runner, a boxer, or a rugby player, however serious he is, can always retire from the field if he is overcome by an excess of fatigue, having pushed himself too far or started off too fast, or if there is a sudden downpour. If necessary, he can push himself to the limit, drop exhausted in his tracks, and be carried off to rest immediately. But a climb is not a sort of game, which can be stopped at any time. Even if you are at the limits of endurance, if your feet feel like lead, if your head is swimming with exhaustion; even if nothing but an extreme effort of will keeps you going, even if lightning is flashing across the sky, you cannot sit down and say: "I've had enough, I'm giving up." And even when you do get to the top, the route is not finished, as we saw on Annapurna and elsewhere. This is undoubtedly the hardest of rules to accept, but it is nevertheless an attraction: on every ascent the climber must risk his whole self."

— GASTON RÉBUFFAT, French alpinist, writing in
The Mont Blanc Massif: The Hundred Finest Routes

Opposite: The huge central expanse of the west face of Makalu (27,825′, 8,481m) has seen numerous alpine-style and lightweight attempts since the early 1980s. The light visible is Steve's during a 2008 solo attempt on the wall that ended at 21,650 feet (6,600m). *Photo: Marko Prezelj*

Since men first began ascending mountains, climbing has been defined and revised by those who were best prepared. Mountains are dangerous and unpredictable. As Rébuffat points out, on every climb you must risk your whole self. With so much at stake, it is no wonder that diligent preparations are undertaken—and rewarded.

Hermann Buhl, the great Austrian climber, pedaled his bike from his home near Innsbruck south across the Italian border to the Dolomites, where he would climb new routes on those soaring rock pinnacles and then pedal home. He carried snowballs in his bare hands in the winter to build his resistance to frostbite. He became the first climber to ascend an 8,000-meter peak without supplemental oxygen in 1953, shortly after Hillary and Norgay stood atop Everest.

When Reinhold Messner was a student, he and his brother Günther would traverse back and forth across the walls of his university's campus in order to build their finger strength. In 1968, climbing in the Dolomites and with Günther belaying, Reinhold led a pitch of 5.11d in stiff leather mountaineering boots far up the sheer wall of the Pilastro di Mezzo after a cramped bivouac. He was twenty-four years old at the time and that is regarded as the first pitch of that difficulty ever free climbed.

The next year Reinhold walked to the 4,000-foot (1,219-meter) north face of Les Droites, a sweeping ice-covered granite face that, despite being just a couple of hours from Chamonix, had seen only three prior ascents. Messner climbed a new route, solo, onsight, in a single afternoon. Later that year the brothers established the now-classic Messner Route on the Dolomites' proudest big wall, the south face of the Marmolada.

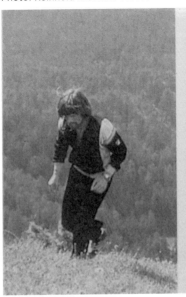 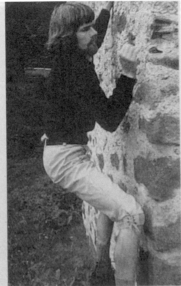

The young Reinhold Messner training.
Photo: Reinhold Messner collection

One year on, in 1970, Reinhold and Günther stood on the 26,660-foot (8,126-meter) high summit of Nanga Parbat. They had just climbed the Rupal Face, the biggest mountain wall in the world. On the descent Günther was tragically lost, and Reinhold suffered severe frostbite, losing all of his toes and parts of a finger. With the bone-end close under the skin on that damaged digit, he knew he would never be able to rock climb well again. He turned to high-altitude climbing.

In training for Himalayan summits, Messner would run uphill, eventually achieving the ability to ascend 1,000 meters (3,281 feet) in thirty minutes. In 1975 he and Peter Habeler walked two weeks to Gasherbrum I and after acclimating they climbed the peak in three days. This was the first alpine-style ascent of an 8,000er. In 1978 the two partners became the first to climb to the summit of Everest without using supplemental oxygen. In 1984, Messner and Hans Kammerlander became the first to enchain two 8,000-meter peaks in alpine style. By the time he was forty-two years old he'd ascended all fourteen 8,000-meter peaks without using supplemental oxygen. He has established 700 new routes in the Dolomites and been to the summits of 8,000-meter peaks eighteen times.

Hans Kammerlander, as part of his training, climbed the 4,600-foot (1,400-meter) high north face of the Ortler in Italy then immediately mounted his bike and rode 154 miles to the trailhead at the Tre Cime di Lavaredo and soloed the 1,800-foot (550-meter) high Cima Grande within 24 hours. Another time he climbed the Matterhorn four times by four different routes in one marathon day.

These accomplishments are overwhelming; how can such things be humanly possible? They must all be supermen! But they're not. They are dedicated alpinists who prepared well, as if their lives depended on it.

In 2002, when Steve started training with his first coach, he didn't know any alpinists training in a specific, structured way for alpine climbing or using a coach. Now this training is becoming more and more common among European alpinists, both professional and amateur. (Perhaps this is due to the popularity of Ueli Steck and his story of reporting to the Swiss Institute of Sport for physical testing and being told he was unfit. As Ueli told Steve, at first he was disappointed. Then he became inspired by what he might accomplish if he was truly fit, so he hired a coach and engaged in a serious training plan. Two years later he raced up the north face of the Eiger in two hours and forty-seven minutes.)

Consider for a moment that each year more than 600,000 people in the United States train for and run a marathon. Most of them run for fun and/or for fitness. Their methods of preparation are many. Of all those marathoners, only a tiny handful have run a near-record time of less than two hours and ten minutes in a marathon. In conventional sports it is clear that the more people involved in serious training, the more the sport will advance. In rock climbing in recent years we have seen this phenomenon manifest in the vast number of people climbing

5.13 and above. The popularity of climbing gyms and structured rock climbing training has expanded the base of good climbers, and natural human competition has driven standards even higher. The more people who climb 5.14, the more will climb 5.15. The larger the base of people training for alpine climbing, the better the top alpinists will be.

Today, if you train for alpine climbing, you may cast yourself outside of your climbing partners and friends. It's lonely work without training partners who share your goals. Those who do, we hope, will become recognized as leaders. In time, others will join these pioneers.

You can speed the process by becoming a recruiter. Get your partners to the weight room. Show them how much you've improved after six months of training. As we write these words, maybe a few dozen people train for alpine climbing. What will happen to alpinism when 1,000 people are training daily? Or 20,000?

In Steve's own career he's climbed the Slovak Direct on Denali in sixty hours, the Infinite Spur on Mount Foraker in twenty-five hours, K7 up and down in forty-four hours, and the Rupal Face to a 26,660-foot (8,126-meter) summit via a new route in six days. We don't offer these records as a boast, we are well aware that alpine climbing is still in its infancy and that these benchmarks are destined to be beaten. Steve is convinced that the Slovak can be climbed in less than eighteen hours, and that the Rupal Face could be climbed, by a fit, acclimated team, in a single forty-eight-hour push. When Steve, Mark Twight, and Scott Backes climbed the Slovak Direct, Steve was working as a mountain guide and doing a few pull-ups now and again, not really training at all. He climbed the Rupal Face after he'd been training, with help from Scott, for a mere three years. His partner on that climb, Vince Anderson, engaged in no organized training at all. Alpinism is in its infancy when it comes to discovering what is humanly possible.

Each generation has to mark out its own limits, exceed its own impossible. We believe that this both hampers us and drives us forward. People have a need to break new ground for themselves. The previous generations were full of talented, ambitious, strong climbers who have set the bar high. Future generations are not going to raise that bar using a helter-skelter method.

Steve's most recent alpine project has been to climb the west face of Makalu in alpine style. He has been to that peak three times now, spent five months at the base camp. Yet his highpoint is still 1,500 feet (457 meters) below the highpoint established by Voytek Kurtyka and Alex MacIntyre in 1982. Voytek and Alex climbed without harnesses to save weight. One helmet was carried, for the belayer. Their bivouacs were sitting affairs on small ledges chopped in the ice.

By contrast Steve and Marko Prezelj started up the face carrying a small tent, food for a week, fuel for eight days. They belayed where Kurtyka and MacIntyre dared to climb unroped. Perhaps their fitness was not sufficient; perhaps their approach was too heavy. The formula for success on this great problem lay beyond their reach. The problem did not get harder between 1982 and 2011, but their personal readiness, their ability, their imaginations were not up to the task. What was impossible in 1982 seems even more distant in 2011. Steve and Marko were not up to par with the great climbers who went before them. We can each only express what we, ourselves, today, are capable of.

We believe that the self-improvement ethic, the tilting-at-windmills romanticism, the drive of climbers, runs deep. And progress, like everything in this age, seems to compress. Steve made five expeditions to the Himalaya before standing on one, insignificant, summit. In 2012, twenty-two-year-old Hayden Kennedy, together with Kyle Dempster and Urban Novak, climbed new routes on 22,749-foot (6,934-meter) high K7 and Kyle and Hayden climbed 23,901-foot (7,285-meter) high Ogre 1 later that same summer. Climbers like these can chart the direction of the new alpinism if they so choose.

Each one of you with the dedication to take to the gym, to lace up running shoes, to drip sweat onto dusty trails while hauling gallons of water up steep mountainsides, you will push the boundaries in your lives. But it won't be because of the records you set or the summits you conquer. Training for climbing big mountains trains the mind as the body takes shape. It is here, in the mind, where your personal advancements are made. The performances of any climber on any given day are a reflection of that individual, or team's, evolution. In this way the beginner shares kinship with the elite.

Our ultimate goal in writing this book is to offer a road map for you to transform your personal climbing. We know there will be value for many people who follow a basic training plan. You will dramatically boost your fitness, increase your enjoyment of climbing, and discover something of yourself. You will be faster and safer in the hills. Not everyone can set a new standard. But for those who dare to try, this book can take you as far as you have the will to go.

As you train, reflect upon the stories you've read of Yaniro, Habeler, Kurtyka, Messner, Troillet, Steck, and Papert. Study those who broke the barriers of their time. Consider the why and the how of it. Training gives your body greater capabilities, no doubt. But most importantly, it disciplines your mind. It is a practice that takes self-control, planning, vision, a belief in yourself and in your ability to improve and evolve. Remember that it is your mind that holds the words *possible* and *impossible*. It is your imagination that sees limitations, just as it is your imagination that figures out how to prepare yourself for a new level. The climbs you will succeed on will simply be physical expressions of what you already knew you could do. First in your mind, then in your body. This is the art of self-knowledge.

Some of you completing this book now will write the next chapters in the history of climbing. We look forward to meeting the climbers who train full time for a full decade, or two. These will be the climbers who will redefine what is possible, who will boggle our minds with the next great ascents. Some of you will become the source of our future inspiration. Your great ascents begin now, as you set down this book. Imagine a goal, write a training plan, lace your boots, do a workout. It begins with you. It begins today.

Glossary

1RM: See One Rep Max.

Adenosine Triphosphate: ATP is a molecule that acts as an energy-transfer medium within each cell. It is one of the end products of cellular metabolism. These same processes for which ATP supplies the energy in turn break the molecule down to its precursors of ADP (Adenosine Diphosphate) and AMP (Adenosine Monophosphate) so that the cycle of re-synthesis of ATP can begin again. The rate at which ATP can be re-synthesized determines the rate of work of which the human organism is capable.

Aerobic Metabolism: In our usage we are referring to the cellular respiration process that takes place within the mitochondrion whereby fuels in the forms of fat, carbohydrate, and protein are broken down and combusted in the Krebs cycle to produce ATP. It is the primary energy production pathway for endurance events lasting more than about two minutes. The by-products are CO_2 and ATP.

Aerobic Threshold: A measure of the intensity of exercise where the production of ATP begins to involve significant contribution from glycolysis. At this point blood lactate begins to rise above the resting level. The convention is to choose a blood lactate concentration of 2mmol/L (millimole per liter) as indicative of the increased glycolysis. Another handy marker of the aerobic threshold is the depth and pace of ventilation. When your breathing becomes too strong to maintain through your nose, you are at the aerobic threshold (AeT). This is a very important physiological marker of intensity for endurance athletes, as it marks the upper level of the most important training zone to use in developing aerobic capacity, the cornerstone to all endurance activities lasting over two minutes. The marker is very trainable and will move higher as measured by both speed of movement and heart rate. Top endurance athletes can have an AeT that is within 10 percent of their anaerobic threshold.

Anabolic: The metabolic process of combining smaller molecules into larger ones. The synthesis of protein that results in new structures within the body is an example of anabolism. Hormones that stimulate the metabolism of protein synthesis are known as anabolic steroids. Training has its effect due to the anabolic process stimulated by the training bouts themselves.

Anaerobic Metabolism: Strictly, this means a chemical reaction that takes place without oxygen as one of the reactants. In terms of exercise, it refers to the cellular respiration process that takes place outside the mitochondrion but within the muscle cell, whereby energy is produced to fuel muscle contractions without the use of oxygen. Two types of anaerobic metabolism occur. For very short (ten seconds or less) bouts of very high-intensity exercise, high-energy phosphate fuels stored in the muscle cell as ATP and creatine phosphate (CP) can be used to produce energy for muscle contraction. For longer duration, high-intensity exercise glycolysis provides the energy needs. When the requirement for power is great enough that not all of it can be met through aerobic glycolysis, the shortfall will be made by anaerobic glycolysis. Lactate is produced during glycolysis and can be used as a marker of intensity of exercise since it rises in a nonlinear relationship with the rate of glycolysis.

Anaerobic Threshold: The maximum steady state intensity of exercise that can be sustained for no more than about thirty minutes. The limit to this intensity of exercise is the blood's increasing acidity, which inhibits energy production. The acidity is a product of glycolysis, which fuels high-intensity exercise. Blood lactate concentrations also rise with the acidity and can act as a good marker for this level of exertion. Lactate is a metabolic substrate that is consumed in aerobic metabolism. The anaerobic threshold is the highest intensity where lactate production equals the metabolism of lactate. Because of this, several other common names exist for this point: lactate balance point, maximum lactate steady state, onset of blood lactate accumulation. The actual existence of such a distinct physiological point and how to measure it are debated among exercise scientists, but every endurance athlete and coach knows that there exists an intensity above which he goes only on borrowed time.

Biogenesis: The production of new organisms from existing ones. Mitochondria undergo biogenesis as the means of increasing both their size and number within the cells.

Body Weight: The resistance to movement is provided only by your own body weight (such as a pull-up or a push-up).

Breakaway Breathing: The stage of ventilation when both the rate and depth of breathing increase to the point where you can only speak in short phrases.

Carbohydrate: An organic compound made up only of carbon, hydrogen, and oxygen. In terms of dietary makeup, the carbohydrate group comprises mainly grains and of starches. In general, the more highly processed the food, the higher the carbohydrate content.

Cardiac Output: The amount of blood being pumped by the heart in one minute. It is the product of the stroke volume as measured in liters per beat and the heart rate as measured in beats per minute.

Capillary: The smallest of the body's blood vessels. The cross section of capillaries is on the order of the size of a red blood cell. They transport the blood along with the nutrients and oxygen that it carries into intimate contact with the organs and muscles.

Catabolic: The metabolic process of breaking larger molecules into smaller ones for the release of energy. Extensive catabolism of the body's protein structure can have a debilitating effect.

Catalyst: A substance that increases the rate of a chemical reaction by lowering the activation energy required for the reaction to take place. The catalyst is not consumed in the reaction.

Circuit: A strength workout where one completes one set each of several exercises in quick succession before returning to the first exercise and repeating the circuit. Can be repeated multiple times with various rest periods as needed for different training effects.

Core: Vernacular for the musculature of the torso. The core is referred to as the critical link between the shoulder girdle and the pelvis. All athletic movements involve the core in either a static stabilizing role or in a dynamic role of transmitting motion.

Core Strength: Strengthening of the core musculature in both its static and dynamic roles is critical for all athletes. Many exercises exist for core strengthening by either isolating the core or by directing forces generated in the limbs through the core to an opposing limb or resistance from gravity.

Creatine Phosphate: Also known as phosphocreatine, abbreviated PCr or CP, this is a readily available source of high-energy phosphate in skeletal muscle and the brain. The CP reserve is small, lasting only five to eight seconds of an intense effort. The CP can anaerobically donate a phosphate group to ADP to form ATP for muscular contraction. During periods of low-intensity exercise, excess ATP can be used to re-synthesize CP by giving up a phosphate group to the creatine to form CP by a process known as phosphorylation. This continual give-and-take mechanism allows CP to replenish and be available for repeated bouts of high-intensity work.

Diuresis: A change in cellular fluid balance that results in an increase in urine production.

Duration: The length of time of an exercise bout or training session.

Emotional Intelligence: The ability to identify, assess, and control one's own emotions, and to identify and asses the emotions in others.

Endurance: The ability to resist fatigue during exercise. For high-intensity exercise, endurance is measured in minutes, whereas in low-intensity exercise endurance is measured in hours or even days. Duration is inversely proportional to intensity. Proper endurance training helps one increase the time to fatigue at a given intensity.

Enzyme (aerobic and anaerobic): Biological catalysts responsible for the myriad chemical reactions that sustain life. As with other catalysts, they speed up the chemical reaction by lowering the activation energy of the reactants and are not consumed during the reaction. In some cases they speed up the reaction by over a million times.

Fast Twitch Fiber: A type of muscle fiber that is on the higher power end of the fiber spectrum. These fibers contract more rapidly and with greater force than their slow twitch relatives. They are larger in cross section, have lower mitochondrial density and lower-density capillary beds suffusing them, and rely more heavily on glycolytic metabolism for ATP production. They have less endurance than the slow twitch fibers but can be trained for more endurance.

Fat (dietary): A diverse group of chemical compounds that are insoluble in water. Fats can be categorized into saturated, unsaturated, and trans fats. The chemical bonds in fat allow it to store almost twice the chemical energy per unit of mass than carbohydrates and protein. Because of this, fats provide a large reservoir of energy for low- to moderate-intensity exercise.

Frequency: The number of times each week that an exercise routine is completed.

Functional Adaptation: Changes to the human organism as a result of the recurrent systematic stress of training. The adaptations to training fall into two general categories: functional, those that relate to the function of the various body systems, and structural, those that relate to the body's structures.

Glycolysis: The metabolic process that converts glucose (a form of sugar derived from carbohydrates) into pyruvate and ATP. In aerobic glycolysis the pyruvate becomes acetyl CoA and enters the Krebs cycle. Glycolysis is the primary energy supply for ATP synthesis in high-intensity exercise because glycolysis proceeds at a faster rate than the production of ATP via the Krebs cycle.

Hemoglobin: Abbreviated Hb or Hgb, this is the oxygen-carrying molecule in the red blood cell.

Hypertrophy: In strength training, this is the method that induces the fastest rate of muscle growth. The increase in muscle volume can be caused by increased sarcoplasmic volume or an increase in the contractile proteins.

Innervate: To supply with nerves.

Insulin: A hormone central to regulating carbohydrate and fat metabolism in the body. Insulin causes cells in the liver, skeletal muscles, and fat tissue to absorb glucose from the blood. In the liver and skeletal muscles, glucose is stored as glycogen, and in fat cells it is stored as triglycerides.

Intensity: A measure of the power developed by the human body in exercise. Intensity is a measure of the rate of energy consumed by the body. Intensity determines the preferential fuel the muscles use. It also determines the kind of adaptations that will be caused by the training. Common measures of intensity include heart rate, perceived exertion, blood lactate levels, and percentage of VO_2 max.

Krebs Cycle: Also known as the citric acid cycle, it is a multistep metabolic process that takes place within a cell's mitochondria and results in the production of ATP.

Lactate Balance Point: The point where lactate production is equal to lactate re-metabolism. This is considered the point of maximal intensity that can be maintained for a long duration of many minutes without a subsequent rise in blood lactate level. Also known as the anaerobic threshold (AnT), maximal lactate steady state (MLSS), and onset of blood lactate accumulation (OBLA). This metabolic point has a direct relation to the time to exhaustion at VO_2 max intensity and, as such, bears strongly on the endurance of an athlete. It depends largely on the ability of the active muscles to oxidize lactate. Hence, the aerobic capacity of the slow twitch muscle fibers, along with the lactate shuttle process, is largely responsible for endurance at high-intensity levels of exercise.

Lactate Threshold: See Lactate Balance Point.

Lactic Acid: A chemical product of glycolytic metabolism in muscle cells. It is almost immediately dissociated into lactate and a hydrogen ion (H+). Lactate then has two main pathways available to it whereby it can be used as a fuel: (1) It can be converted to pyruvate, which can then enter the Krebs cycle of aerobic metabolism; (2) it can be converted to glucose in the liver by the process of gluconeogenesis. The release of the hydrogen ions can have the effect of lowering the blood's pH (or increasing its acidity). If this continues without adequate buffering, it results in a burning sensation in the muscles and a forced slowing of the pace.

Lipolysis: The metabolic process of breaking down long chain lipids or fatty acids into segments that can enter the Krebs cycle.

Load (weight): The amount of resistance used. For the transition period, use a load 50–75 percent of your one rep maximum. For the max strength period, use a load 85-90 percent of your one rep maximum, or enough to allow only five reps.

Local Muscular Endurance: The concept of training relatively small muscle groups for endurance without imposing a large load on the cardiovascular system. This effect is accomplished by making the muscular load high through added resistance. This causes the aerobic capabilities of the high-power muscle fibers, which are responsible for the movement, to be the limit on exercise, not the cardiovascular system's ability to supply oxygen to those muscles. The fatigue from this sort of training will be localized to the small group of muscles alone.

Macrocycle: From conventional sports. A period representing one complete cycle of training resulting in the preparation for a major event. In climbing, this period will usually coincide with an annual cycle of training, hard climbing, and the regeneration/recovery necessary before embarking on another annual cycle. It is possible to have two macrocycles in one year.

Maximum Lactate Steady State: See Lactate Balance Point.

Mesocycle: The intermediate-length periods that make up a macrocycle. In this book, and in the climbing context, we limit ourselves to the following mesocycles: Transition (back into training), Base (basic conditioning), Specific (climbing oriented), Taper (before a major objective), and Recovery (rest and recuperation). Each mesocycle has a unique purpose as a preparation for the next phase of training.

Metabolism: In general this refers to all chemical reactions that occur within an organism. In our case we are mainly interested in the energy production necessary to yield ATP molecules and produce muscular work.

Microcycle: Usually a week of training that includes several different training stimuli.

Mitochondria: The tiny (0.5–1 micrometer) organelles within all animal cells responsible for the majority of ATP production. Due to their crucial role in cellular energy production, they are often called the powerhouse of the cell. In exercise we are mostly interested in the mitochondria in the muscle cells, which undergo adaptation due to training.

Motor Unit: A group of muscle fibers and the motor nerve that innervates them.

Muscular Endurance: The ability to do repeated muscular contractions of the same kind against a resistance. In many cases (such as the number of consecutive pull-ups or push-ups you can do) the muscular endurance is not limited by cardiovascular endurance. However, in many athletic undertakings (such as front-pointing up a steep ice face quickly or running the 800-meter track race) the limitations of the two systems of cardiovascular and muscular endurance are closely linked and interdependent.

Muscle Fiber: Also known as myocyte or muscle cell, this is an elongated multi-nucleus cell in human skeletal muscle tissue.

Muscle Fiber Conversion: Muscle fibers respond directly to the training stimuli imposed upon them. Chronic training of a particular type over many months has the effect of changing the muscle's characteristics and in some cases seems to convert it to either slower or faster twitch. Multi-year studies indicate that prolonged endurance training will result in improved endurance of the faster twitch fibers within an endurance-trained muscle.

Negative Energy Balance: Also called calorie deficit. A common condition among endurance athletes when the volume of work performed is greater than calorie input. This situation is very common on an extended alpine route. It is why alpinists, along with ultra-endurance athletes, need to have such a well-developed fat metabolism. The body's fat stores are the only energy resource that can sustain this sort of extended exertion. The better trained these energy pathways are the higher power output (faster rates of climbing) they will allow.

One Rep Max: The maximum load you can lift with one repetition of an exercise movement.

Onsight: The ability to climb a route the first time it is viewed. Not using any rehearsal of a route or having prior knowledge of the climb. Adds significant difficulty to many climbs where prior knowledge or rehearsal can save precious energy.

Periodize: A structured organization of training used in all modern sports to allow the athlete to focus time and energy on one or a few desired training adaptations.

pH: The measure of the acidity or alkalinity of a substance. Used in chemistry and biology to indicate the relative acidity of a compound.

Power: Equals work divided by the time to complete the work; the rate at which work is done. Often confused with energy or work. The crucial differentiating element of power from work or energy is the measure of time in the denominator.

Recovery Time: This is a rest interval between sets of the same exercise or between different exercises when using a circuit.

Redpoint: The successful climbing of a route without weighting any of the pieces of protection after rehearsal of part or all of the route.

Repetition or Rep: One complete exercise movement cycle. One pull-up movement would be one rep.

Set: A group of repetitions. One set can contain from one rep to many, many reps in the case of muscular endurance training.

Slow Twitch Fiber: A class of muscle fibers that have greater endurance then their fast twitch neighbors. The slow twitch fibers are endowed with more mitochondria, denser capillarization, and higher levels of aerobic enzymes. They are smaller in cross section and contract with less force than the fast twitch fibers.

Strength Reserve: The difference between your maximum strength and the normal level of strength needed to do the movements of an activity. A higher strength reserve will generally imply greater muscular endurance, but not in extreme cases.

Strength Training: Any one of several methods of training directed at improving the contractile qualities of the muscles.

Stroke Volume: The volume of blood ejected from the heart with each contraction of the cardiac muscle. This is a highly trainable quality. Endurance training leads to an increase in stroke volume up to a point that is probably largely determined by one's genetics.

Structural Adaptation: The changes to the body's structures brought about by chronic training.

Supercompensation: That post-training period during which the parameter that was trained rises to a new performance capacity than it did before the training occurred.

Taper: To reduce the training load significantly after a training buildup to allow the body to reach a higher level of performance.

Triglycerides: A type of fat within the blood that facilitates the transfer of energy either to or from the adipose fat stores of the body.

Ventilatory Threshold: A notable shift in breathing depth and rate that indicates a change in cellular respiration, and hence metabolism. Useful as a real-time indication of the intensity of exercise.

VO$_2$ Max: The measure of the maximal aerobic power an animal can develop. Measured by comparing the rate of inspired and expired oxygen during a multistep exercise test to voluntary exhaustion.

Work: From physics. Work equals force times distance over which the force is applied. An example would be that a 50-pound weight lifted 10 feet has had 500-foot pounds of work done to it.

Appendix

Helpful Nutrition Tables

Calories per 100 Grams of Select Common Climbing Foods

Breakfast

	Calories per 100 grams
Granola	365
Cream cheese	357
Instant oatmeal	352
Bagel	100
Bananas	90
Eggs	51

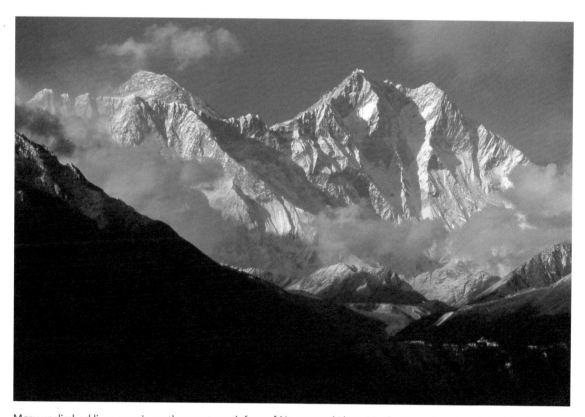

Many unclimbed lines remain on the great south face of Nuptse and Lhotse in the Everest region of the Himalaya.
Photo: Marko Prezelj

Midday

	Calories per 100 grams
Almonds	600
Cashews	552
Peanuts	584
Nutella	540
Peanut butter	530
Peanut M&M's	500
Dark chocolate	465
Sardines in water	430
Sausage	388
Gummi bears	358
Dried mango	350
Triscuits	333
Raisins	302
Beef jerky	300
Pita bread (1 piece)	165
Chapatti	300
Tortilla, whole wheat (1 piece)	110
Whole wheat bread	275
Salmon	247
Strawberry jelly	210
Tuna	115
Cheddar cheese	84
Cream cheese, lowfat, 1 Tbs	30
Swiss cheese (1 oz)	106

Dinner

	Calories per 100 grams unless otherwise noted
Olive oil	857
Instant mashed potatoes	590
Ramen noodles	447 (1 packet contains 385 calories)
Instant refried beans (before rehydrating)	441
Annie's mac & cheese	385
Butter	365
Quinoa (weight before cooking)	360
Instant black bean soup	352
Instant miso soup	125
Pasta (1 cup cooked)	200
Rice, white (1 cup cooked)	242
Couscous (1 cup cooked)	176

Energy Gel Products

Gel	Calories/package	Weight (grams)	Grams of carbohydrate	Kcals/gram of gel
GU Roctane	100	33	25	3.3
GU Energy Gel	100	33	25	3.3
Honey Stinger Energy Gel	120	40	29	3.0
Clif Shot Energy Gel	100	34	22	2.9
Powerbar PowerGel	110	42	27	2.6
Hammer Gel	90	38	21	2.4

Popular Energy Food

	Calories per 100 grams
PowerBar Triple Threat Energy Bar	418
Hammer Perpetuem	391
Spiz	382
Hammer Sustained Energy	376
Clif Bar	352
Clif Shot Bloks	333
GU Chomps	300

Candy Bars

	Calories per 100 grams
Skor Toffee Bar	512
Peanut M&M's	500
M&M's	492
Snickers Bar	475
Nature Valley Granola Bar	452
3 Musketeers Bar	433

Protein, Fat, and Carbohydrate Content of Select Common Climbing Foods

Food	Protein (g)	Fat (g)	Carb (g)	Energy (kcal)
Almonds, dry roasted, 1/4 cup	8	18	7	206
Beans, 1/2 cup cooked	8	0.5	24	129
Beef (3 oz, lean)	30	8	0	199
Bread, whole wheat, 1 slice (1.5 oz)	2.5–3	2.5	21.5	119
Cheese, cheddar, 1 oz	7	9	0	114
Cheese, Swiss, 1 oz	8	8	2	106
Chicken, dark meat, roasted, 3 oz	23	8	0	174
Chicken, white meat, roasted, 3 oz	26	3	0	140
Cream cheese, small package, 3 oz	5	29	3	291
Cream cheese, low-fat, small package, 3 oz	6	12	6	168
Couscous, 1 cup, cooked	6	0	36	176
Egg, 1 large	6	5	1	77
Fish (non-oily such as cod, halibut), 3 oz	19	.5	0	89
Fish (oily such as salmon), 3 oz	20	4	0	118
Hamburger, regular, 3 oz	20	18	0	246
Hamburger, extra lean, 3 oz	24	13	0	225
Lentils, 1/2 cup cooked	9	Trace	20	115
Milk, whole, 8 oz	8	8	11	146
Milk, 2%, 8 oz	8	5	11	122
Milk, nonfat, 8 oz	8	Trace	12	83
Low-fat chocolate milk, 1% fat, 8 oz	8	2.5	9	158
Pasta (spaghetti) cooked, 1 cup /4.9 oz	8	1	43	220
Peanuts, oil roasted, 1/4 cup	10	19	7	221
Peanut butter, 2 Tbs	8	16	6	188
Pita bread, whole wheat, 1 large piece (2.3 oz)	6	2	35	170
Potato, baked, 1 large (7 oz)	5	Trace	43	188
Ramen, 1 package	8	15	56	385
Rice, white, regular, cooked, 1 cup (5.6 oz)	4	0	45	205
Tortilla, 1 piece 7-8" diameter	4	4	24	144
Turkey, dark meat, roasted, 3 oz	24	6	0	159
Turkey, white meat, roasted, 3 oz	25.5	0.5	0	167
Tuna, water packed or fresh, 3 oz	23	0.5	0	106
Tuna, oil packed, drained, 3 oz	25	7	0	168

Various Protein-Rich Supplements by Calories and Protein/Fat/Carbohydrate Ratios.

All nutrition information was obtained from the nutrition facts labels.

Protein supplement	Amount	Source of protein	Energy (kcal)	Protein (g)	Fat (g)	Carbohydrate (g)
Twinlab 100% Whey Fuel	1 scoop, 33 g, in 6 oz water	Whey protein concentrate and isolate (from milk)	130	25	2	4
Myoplex Original (Ready-to-Drink)	17 fluid oz	Milk protein concentrate, calcium caseinate, whey protein isolate	300	42	7	20
Heavyweight Gainer 900	4 scoops, 154 g	Beef protein, whey protein concentrate and hydrolysate, egg albumen	630	35	9.5	101
Met-Rx Protein Plus bar	1 bar, 85 g	Milk protein concentrate, whey protein isolate and concentrate, calcium caseinate, egg white, L-glutamine	310	32	9	32

Recommended Reading

9 Out of 10 Climbers Make the Same Mistakes; Dave MacLeod, Rare Breed Productions, 2009.

Above the Clouds: Diaries of a High-Altitude Mountaineer; Anatoli Boukreev, St. Martins Press, 2001.

Advances in Functional Training: Training Techniques for Coaches, Personal Trainers and Athletes; Michael Boyle, On Target Communications, 2010.

The Altitude Experience: Successful Trekking and Climbing Above 8,000 Feet; Mike Farris, Globe Pequot Press, 2008.

Annapurna: The First Conquest of an 8000-meter Peak; Maurice Herzog, Lyons Press, 2010.

Better Training for Distance Runners, 2nd Edition; Peter Coe and David Martin, Human Kinetics, 1997.

Beyond the Mountain; Steve House, Patagonia Books, 2009.

The Block Training System in Endurance Running; Yuri Verkhoshansky, Self-published e-book, 2008.

Conquistadors of the Useless: From the Alps to Annapurna; Lionel Terray, The Mountaineers, 2008.

Everest: The West Ridge; Thomas Hornbein, The Mountaineers, 1998.

Extreme Alpinism: Climbing Light, Fast, and High; Mark Twight, The Mountaineers, 1999.

The Feed Zone Cookbook: Fast and Flavorful Food for Athletes; Biju Thomas and Allen Lim, Velo Press, 2011.

Feed Zone Portables: A Cookbook of On-the-Go Food for Athletes; Biju Thomas and Allen Lim, Velo Press, 2013.

Going Higher: Oxygen, Man, and the Mountains, 5th Edition; Charles Houston, MD, The Mountaineers, 2005.

Lore of Running, 4th Edition; Timothy Noakes, MD, Oxford University Press, 2001.

The Mont Blanc Massif: The Hundred Finest Routes, Revised Edition; Gason Rébuffat, Baton Wicks Publications, 2005.

Mountaineering: The Freedom of the Hills, 8th Edition; The Mountaineers, 2010.

Nancy Clark's Sports Nutrition Guidebook, 5th Edition; Nancy Clark, Human Kinetics, 2013.

Nanga Parbat Pilgrimage: The Lonely Challenge; Hermann Buhl, The Mountaineers, 1998.

Periodization: Theory and Methodology of Training, 5th Edition; Tudor O. Bompa and G. Gregory Haff, Human Kinetics, 2009.

Periodization Training for Sports, 2nd Edition; Tudor O. Bompa and Michael C. Carrera, Human Kinetics, 2005.

Savage Arena; Joe Tasker, St. Martin's Press, 1983.

Science of Sports Training: How to Plan and Control Training for Peak Performance, 2nd Edition; Thomas Kurz, Stadion Publishing Co., 2001.

The Science of Winning: Planning, Periodizing, and Optimizing Swim Training; Jan Olbrecht, Self-published, 2000.

The Seventh Grade: Most Extreme Climbing; Reinhold Messner, Oxford University Press, 1974.

Solo Faces; James Salter, North Point Press, 1988.

Special Strength Training: Manual for Coaches; Yuri Verkhoshansky and Natalia Verkhoshansky, Self-published, 2011.

Starlight and Storm: The Ascent of Six Great North Faces of the Alps; Gaston Rébuffat, Random House, 1999.

Training for Climbing, 2nd Edition; Eric Hörst, Globe Pequot Press, 2008.

The White Spider; Heinrich Harrer, Penguin Putnam Inc., 1998.

Winning Running: Successful 800m and 1500m Racing and Training; Peter Coe, The Crowood Press Ltd., 1996.

Zen Mind, Beginner's Mind; Shunryu Suzuki, Shambhala Publications, 2010.

References

"Altitude Acclimatization and Illness Management." September 2010. *US Army Technical Bulletin, Medical #505.* Washington, DC: Headquarters, Department of the Army.

Amann, Markus, Lee M. Romer, Andrew W. Subudhi, David F. Pegelow, and Jerome A. Dempsey. 2007. "Severity of Arterial Hypoxaemia Affects the Relative Contributions of Peripheral Muscle Fatigue to Exercise Performance in Healthy Humans." *Journal of Physiology* 581: 389–403.

Anand, I. S., Y. Chandrasekhar, S. K. Rao, R. M. Malhotra, R. Ferrari, J. Chandana, B. Ramesh, K. J. Shetty, and M. S. Boparai. 1993. "Body Fluid Compartments, Renal Blood Flow, and Hormones at 6,000 Meters in Normal Subjects." *Journal of Applied Physiology* 74: 1234–39.

Armstrong, L. 2002. "Caffeine, Body Fluid-Electrolyte Balance, and Exercise Performance." *International Journal of Sports Nutrition and Exercise Metabolism* 12 (2): 189–206.

Armstrong, L., A. C. Pumerantz, M. W. Roti, D. A. Judelson, G. Watson, J. C. Dias, B. Sokemon, D. J. Casa, C. M. Maresh, H. Lieberman, and M. Kellogg. 2005. "Fluid, Electrolyte, and Renal Indices of Hydration During 11 Days of Controlled Caffeine Consumption." *International Journal of Sports Nutrition and Exercise Metabolism* 15 (3): 252–65.

Ashenden, M. J., C. J. Gore, D. T. Martin, G. P. Dobson, and A. G. Hahn. 1999. "Effects of a 12-Day 'Live High, Train Low' Camp on Reticulocyte Production and Hemoglobin Mass in Elite Female Road Cyclists." *European Journal of Applied Physiology* 80: 472–78.

Ashenden, M. J., C. J. Gore, G. P. Dobson, and A. G. Hahn. 1999. "Live High, Train Low Does Not Change the Total Hemoglobin Mass of Male Endurance Athletes Sleeping at a Simulated Altitude of 3000 Meters for 23 Nights." *European Journal of Applied Physiology* 80: 479–84.

Ashenden, M. J., C. J. Gore, G. P. Dobson, T. T. Boston, R. Parisotto, K. R. Emslie, G. J. Trout, and A. G. Hahn. 2000. "Simulated Moderate Altitude Elevates Serum Erythropoietin but Does Not Increase Reticulocyte Production in Well-Trained Runners." *European Journal of Applied Physiology* 81: 428–35.

Auerbach, Paul, 2012. *Wilderness Medicine,* 6th ed. Philadelphia: Elsevier Publishing.

Bärtsch, Peter, and Simon R. Gibbs. 2007. "Effect of Altitude on the Heart and Lungs." *Contemporary Reviews in Cardiovascular Medicine* 116: 2191–202.

Billat, Veronique, P. M. Lepretre, A. M. Heugas, M. H. Laurence, D. Salim, J. P. Koralsztein. 2003. "Training and Bio-Energetic Characteristics in Elite Male and Female Kenyan Runners." *Medicine and Science in Sports and Exercise* 35 (2): 297–304.

Bompa, Tudor and G. Gregory Haff. (1983) 2009. *Periodization: Theory and Methodology of Training,* 5th ed. Champaign, Illinois: Human Kinetics.

Bramble, Dennis and Daniel Lieberman. November 2004. "Endurance Running and the Evolution of *Homo.*" *Nature* 432: 345–53.

Brooks, George A. 1986. "The Lactate Shuttle During Exercise and Recovery." *Medicine and Science in Sports and Exercise* 18 (3): 360–68.

Burke, L. M., D. J. Angus, G. R. Cox, K. M. Gawthorn, J. A. Hawley, M. A. Febbraio, and M. Hargreaves. 1999. "Fat Adaptation with Carbohydrate Recovery Promotes Metabolic Adaptation During Prolonged Cycling." *Medicine and Science in Sports and Exercise* 31.

Brurok, B., J. Helgerud, T. Karlsen, G. Leivseth, and J. Hoff. 2011. "Effect of Aerobic High Intensity Hybrid Training on Stroke Volume and Peak Oxygen Consumption in Men with Spinal Cord Injuries." *American Journal of Physical Medicine & Rehabilitation* 90: 407–14.

Calbet, J. A., R. Boushel, G. Radegran, H. Sondergaard, P. D. Wagner, and B. Saltin. 2003. "Why is VO2 Max After Altitude Acclimatization Still Reduced Despite Normalization of Arterial O2 Content?" *American Journal of Regulatory, Integrative, and Comparative Physiology* 284 (2): 304–16.

Chapman, R. F., J. Stray-Gundersen, and B. D. Levine. 1998. "Individual Variation in Response to Altitude Training." *Journal of Applied Physiology* 85 (4): 1448–56.

Chen, G. H., R. L. Ge, X. Z. Wang, H. X. Chen, T. Y. Wu, T. Kobayashi, and K. Yoshimura. 1997. "Exercise Performance of Tibetan and Han Adolescents at Altitudes of 3,417 and 4,300 Meters." *Journal of Applied Physiology* 83 (2): 661–67.

Cibella, G., G. Cuttitta, S. Romano, B. Grassi, G. Bonsignore, and J. Milic-Emili. 1999. "Respiratory Energetics During Exercise at High Altitude." *Journal of Applied Physiology* 86 (6): 1785–92.

Clark, Nancy. 2013. *Nancy Clark's Sports Nutrition Guidebook,* 5th ed. Champaign, Illinois: Human Kinetics.

Coleman, Ellen. 2003. *Eating for Endurance*, 4th ed. Boulder, Colorado: Bull Publishing Co.

Costill, David and S. W. Trappe. 2002. *Running: The Athlete Within*. Traverse City, Michigan: Cooper Publishing Group.

Coyle, Edward, 1995. "Fat Metabolism During Exercise: New Concepts." *Sports Science Exchange, Gatorade Sports Science Institute* 8 (6).

Coyle, Edward, A. E. Jeukendrup, A. J. Wagenmakers, and W. H. Saris. 1997. "Fatty Acid Oxidation is Directly Regulated by Carbohydrate Metabolism During Exercise." *American Journal of Physiology* 273 (2): 268–75.

Csikszentmihalyi, Mihaly. 1990. *Flow: The Psychology of Optimal Experience*. New York: Harper and Row.

Daniels, Jack, 2005. *Daniel's Running Formula*, 2nd ed. Champaign, Illinois: Human Kinetics.

Davies, Kelvin J., Lester Packer, and George Brooks. 1981. "Biochemical Adaptations of Mitochondria, Muscle, and Whole Animal Respiration to Endurance Training." *Archives of Biochemistry and Biophysics* 209 (2): 539–54.

Dunford, Marie and Andrew Doyle. 2012. *Nutrition for Sport and Exercise*, 2nd ed. Belmont, California: Wadsworth Cengage Learning.

Faoro, Vitalaie, S. Huez, S. Giltaire, A. Pavelescu, A. van Osta, J. J. Moraine, H. Guenard, J. B. Martinot, R. Naeije. 2007. "Effects of Acetazolamide on Aerobic Exercise Capacity and Pulmonary Hemodynamics at High Altitudes." *Journal of Applied Physiology* 103 (4): 1161–65.

Farris, Mike. 2008. *The Altitude Experience: Successful Trekking and Climbing Above 8,000 Feet*. Guilford, Connecticut: Globe Pequot Press.

Fink, Heather H., Lisa A. Burgoon, and Alan E. Mikesky, 2006. *Practical Applications in Sports Nutrition*. Boston, Massachusetts: Jones and Bartlett Publishers.

Goddard, D. and U. Neumann. 1993. *Performance Rock Climbing*. Mechanicsburg, Pennsylvania: Stackpole Books.

Gollnick, P. D. 1985. "Metabolism of Substrates: Energy Substrate Metabolism During Exercise and as Modified by Training." *Federal Proceedings* 44 (2): 353–57.

Gomez-Cabrera, M. C., E. Domenech, M. Romagnoli, A. Arduini, C. Borras, F. V. Pallardo, J. Sastre, and J. Viña. 2008. "Oral Administration of Vitamin C Decreases Muscle Mitochondrial Biogenesis and Hampers Training-Induced Adaptations in Endurance Performance." *American Journal of Clinical Nutrition* 87 (1): 142–49.

Hackett, P. H. 2010. "Caffeine at High Altitude: Java at Base Camp." *High Altitude Medicine & Biology* 11 (1): 13–17.

Hargereaves, Mark. 2006. *Exercise Metabolism*, 2nd ed. Champaign, Illinois: Human Kinetics.

Harms, S. J. and Robert C. Hickson. 1983. "Skeletal Muscle Mitochondria and Myoglobin, Endurance, and Intensity of Training." *Journal of Applied Physiology* 54 (3): 798–802.

Hickson, Robert C. 1981. "Skeletal Muscle Cytochrome C and Myoglobin, Endurance and Frequency of Training." *Journal of Applied Physiology*. 51 (3): 746–49.

Ingjer, F. and K. Myhre. 1992. "Physiological Effects of Altitude Training on Elite Male Cross-Country Skiers." *Journal of Sport Sciences* 10 (1): 37–47.

Jacobs, Robert, R. Boushel, C. Wright-Paradis, J. S. Calbet, P. Robach, E. Gnaiger, and C. Lundby. 2013. "Mitochondrial Function in Human Skeletal Muscle Following High-Altitude Exposure." *Journal of Experimental Physiology* 98 (1): 245–55.

Jeukendrum, A. and M. Gleeson. 2010. *Sport Nutrition: An Introduction to Energy Production and Performance*, 2nd ed. Champaign, Illinois: Human Kinetics.

Jones, Graham. June 2008. "How the Best of the Best Get Better and Better." *Harvard Business Review*.

Kenney, W. Larry, Jack Wilmore, and David Costill. 2012. *Physiology of Sports and Exercise*, 5th ed. Champaign, Illinois: Human Kinetics.

Kurz, Thomas. 2001. *Science of Sports Training: How to Plan and Control Training for Peak Performance*. Island Pond, Vermont: Stadion Publishing Co.

Liebenberg, Louis. 2008. "The Relevance of Persistence Hunting to Human Evolution." *Journal of Human Evolution* 55 (6): 1156–59.

Lin, Jiandie, H. Wu, P. T. Tarr, C. Y. Zhang, Z. Wu, O. Boss, L. F. Michael, et al. Aug. 15, 2002. "Transcriptional Co-Activator PGC-1 Alpha Drives the Formation of Slow Twitch Muscle Fibers." *Nature* 418: 797–801.

Mainwood, G. W. and J. M. Renaud. 1985. "The Effect of Acid Base Balance on Fatigue of Skeletal Muscle." *Canadian Journal of Physiology and Pharmacology* 63 (5): 403–16.

Martin, Daniel, D. Z. Levett, M. P. Grocott, and H. E. Montgomery. 2010. "Variation in Human Performance in the Hypoxic Mountain Environment." *Journal of Experimental Physiology* 95 (3): 463–70.

Martin, W. H. III, G. P. Daisky, B. F. Hurley, D. E. Mathews, D. M. Bier, J. M. Hagberg, M. A. Rogers, et al. November 1993. "Effect of Endurance Training on Plasma Free Fatty Acid Turnover and Oxidation During Exercise." *American Journal of Physiology* 265 (5 Pt1): E708–14.

Mujika, Iñigo. 2012. *Endurance Training: Science and Practice.* Self-published. Basque Country, Spain.

Muza, S. R., C. S. Fulco, and A. Cymberman. 2004. "Altitude Acclimatization Guide." *US Army Technical Bulletin, TN04-05.* Washington, DC: Headquarters, Department of the Army.

Noakes, Timothy. February 2009. "Evidence That Reduced Skeletal Muscle Recruitment Explains the Lactate Paradox During Exercise at Altitude." *Journal of Applied Physiology* 106: 737–38.

Noakes, Timothy. 2012. *Waterlogged: The Serious Problem of Overhydration in Endurance Sports.* Champaign Illinois: Human Kinetics.

Noakes, Timothy, Juha E. Peltonen, and Heikki K. Rusko. September 2001. "Evidence That a Central Governor Regulates Exercise Performance During Acute Hypoxia and Hyperoxia." *Journal of Experimental Biology* 204: 3225–34.

Nordsborg, Nikolai, C. Siebenmann, R. A. Jacobs, P. Rasmussen, V. Diaz, P. Robach, and C. Lundby. June 2012. "Four Weeks of Normobaric 'Live High-Train Low' Do Not Alter Muscular or Systemic Capacity for Maintaining pH and K+ Homeostasis During Intense Exercise." *Journal of Applied Physiology* 112: 2027–36.

Pette, Dirk and Gerta Vrbova. June 1999. "What Does Chronic Electrical Stimulation Teach Us About Muscle Plasticity?" *Muscle Nerve* 22: 666–77.

Phillips, Stuart. December 2006. "Dietary Protein for Athletes: From Requirements to Metabolic Advantage." *Applied Physiology Nutrition and Metabolism* 31: 647–54.

Reeves, J. T., B. M. Groves, J. R. Sutton, P. D. Wagner, A. Cymerman, M. K. Malconian, P. B. Rock, P. M. Young, and C. S. Houston. August 1987. "Operation Everest II: Preservation of Cardiac Function at Extreme Altitude." *Journal of Applied Physiology* 63: 531–39.

Romijn, J. A., E. F. Coyle, L. S. Sidossis, A. Gastaldelli, J. F. Horowitz, E. Endwert, and R. R. Wolfe. September 1993. "Regulation of Endogenous Fat and Carbohydrate Metabolism in Relation to Exercise Intensity and Duration." *American Journal of Physiology* 265: 380–91.

Rusko, H. K. September 1992. "Development of Aerobic Power in Relation to Age and Training in Cross-Country Skiers." *Medicine and Science in Sports and Exercise* 24: 1040–47.

Ryan, M. 2012. *Sports Nutrition for Endurance Athletes*, 3rd ed. Boulder, Colorado: VeloPress.

Scott, Gardiner A., J. C. Martin, D. T. Martin, M. Barras, and D. G Jenkins. October 2007. "Maximal Torque- and Power-Pedaling Rate for Elite Sprint Cyclists in Laboratory and Field Tests." *European Journal of Applied Physiology* 101: 287–92.

Sidossis, Labros S., R. R. Wolfe, and A. R. Coggan. March 1998. "Regulation of Fatty Acid Oxidation in Untrained vs. Trained Men During Exercise." *American Journal of Physiology* 274: 510-15.

Spriet, L. L., K. Sonderlund, M. Bergstrom, and E. Hultman. February 1987. "Skeletal Muscle Glycogenolysis, Glycolysis, and pH During Electrical Stimulation in Men." *Journal of Applied Physiology* 62: 616–21.

Staron, R. S., R. S. Hikida, F. C. Hagerman, G. A. Dudley, and T. F. Murray. 1984. "Human Skeletal Muscle Fiber Type Adaptability to Various Workloads." *Journal of Histochemistry and Cytochemistry* 32 (2): 146–52.

van Patot, M. C., L .E. Keyes, G. Leadbetter III, and P. H. Hackett. Spring 2009. "Ginkgo Biloba for Prevention of Acute Mountain Sickness: Does It Work?" *High Altitude Medical Biology* 10: 33–43.

Wang Xiaomei, C. L. Zhang, R. T. Yu, H. K. Cho, M. C. Nelson, Corinne Bayuga-Ocampo, J. Ham, H. Kang, R. Evans. March 2004. "Regulation of Muscle Fiber Type and Running Endurance to PPAR Sigma." *PLOS Biology* 2: e294.

West, J. B., J. S. Milledge, A. Luks, and R. B. Schoene. 2013. *High Altitude Medicine and Physiology*, 5th ed. Boca Raton, Florida: Taylor & Francis.

Widrick J. J., S. W. Trappe, David Costill, and R. H. Fitts. August 1996. "Force-Velocity and Force-Power Properties of Single Muscle Fibers from Elite Master Runners and Sedentary Men." *American Journal of Physiology* 271: C676–83.

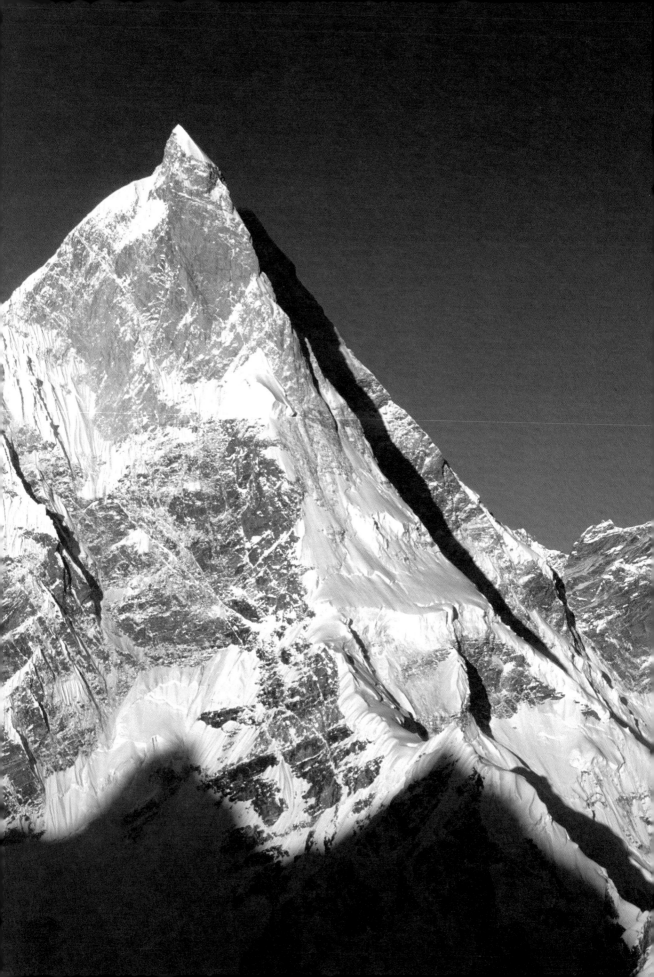

Index

Page numbers in italics indicate photographs.

Opposite: Masherbrum (25,659', 7,821m), also known as K1, was first ascended by Americans in 1960, and that expedition became the basis for the highly successful 1963 American Everest Expedition. The original route is unsafe now due to changes in the glaciers; one other route has been established on its west side. The northwest pillar and north faces, seen here, represent ultimate challenges for the future generations of alpinists. The upper headwall of the north face overhangs for several thousand feet. *Photo: Marko Prezelj*